Organizationally Minded Nursing
LEADERSHIP

Catherine Gilliss
PhD, RN, FAAN

Dean and Styles Professor of Nursing
Associate Vice Chancellor for Nursing Affairs
University of California, San Francisco, School of Nursing

Bobbie Berkowitz
PhD, RN, NEA-BC, FAAN

Dean Emerita, Columbia University, School of Nursing

Jean Johnson
PhD, RN, ACC, FAAN

Emerita Dean and Professor School of Nursing
George Washington University

Paula Milone-Nuzzo
PhD, RN, FHHC, FAAN

President and John Hilton Knowles Professor
MGH Institute of Health Professions

Patricia Reid Ponte
RN, DNSc, FAAN, NEA-BC

Associate Professor of the Practice
Boston College William F. Connell School of Nursing
Affiliate Associate Clinical Professor
University of Washington School of Nursing

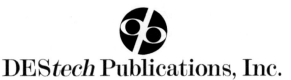

DEStech Publications, Inc.

Organizationally Minded Nursing Leadership

DEStech Publications, Inc.
439 North Duke Street
Lancaster, Pennsylvania 17602 U.S.A.

Printed in the United States of America
10 9 8 7 6 5 4 3 2 1

Main entry under title:
    Organizationally Minded Nursing Leadership

A DEStech Publications book
Bibliography: p.
Includes index p. 349

Library of Congress Control Number: 2022949318
ISBN No. 978-1-60595-668-8

HOW TO ORDER THIS BOOK

BY PHONE: 877-500-4337 or 717-290-1660, 9AM–5PM Eastern Time

BY FAX: 717-509-6100

BY MAIL: Order Department
DEStech Publications, Inc.
439 North Duke Street
Lancaster, PA 17602, U.S.A.

BY CREDIT CARD: American Express, VISA, MasterCard, Discover, PayPal

BY WWW SITE: http://www.destechpub.com

Table of Contents

Section II—Understanding the Elements of Organizational Life

Foreword

An Academic Perspective

Reading this book, I remembered a graduate student who once took a course of mine. She came to class annoyed at her boss who was not helping her be successful in her clinical position. After she described her situation, I asked her, "What do you think your boss needs from you?" It was clear from her response that she thought it was an inappropriate question and even believed that meeting the expectations of her manager constituted toadying behavior. I disagreed with her and said, "Even if you don't personally like your boss, it's being savvy to understand whether your work meets her expectations and those of the organization. Every leader counts on others to do certain things at their level so they can deliver outcomes at another level." One week later, this student sought me out again to let me know that the approach worked, and their relationship had improved. She had started to ask regularly, "What does my boss/organization need from me?" more than, "What do I need from my boss/organization?"

What this student really needed to exert leadership in her clinical role was the content of this book because it focuses on nurses' learning to think organizationally. But she would not be alone in thinking her leadership would be empowered only if her manager understood her professional needs rather than her also needing to understand the building blocks of organizational life—e.g., mission, vision, values, teams, communication, governance, policies, resources, planning, and change.

Nurses largely function within complex organizations—hospitals, universities, military, health departments, government, industry, and the like—so why didn't she understand? Historically, the emphasis in the literature has been on *leadership as personal* (the attributes a good leader should possess) rather than on *leadership as achieving organizational mission* (what leaders need to know to establish an organizational culture of performance excellence). In healthcare and academia, there also has been an underlying predisposition to think that the provider-patient relationship or the student-teacher relationship is infinitely more important than how the establishments in which we function operate, and only those who self designate as being on the administrative track need to bother with figuring out the context in which their employment is embedded. In short, we equate organizational savvy with mind numbing bureaucratic thinking, and that is a mistake.

Well, the world has changed. All registered nurses (RNs) and advanced practice registered nurses (APRNs) have to operate increasingly in circumstances in which leadership can be exerted only if one understands systems thinking no matter the job title. Those who report to you need to be clear about what they are expected to do so you can meet your role expectations, and you need to understand how what you do fits into the mission and values of the overall organization. And this book is an excellent means of developing these sensibilities.

Most chapters begin with vignettes from clinical and academic leadership, so the reader can think about some of the dilemmas faced by nurse leaders. And most chapters end with questions that encourage the reader to reflect further on the vignettes. Since each chapter begins with both a clinical case study and an academic case study, I found this approach to be particularly effective in healing the historic divide between practice and education. For example, if you are a faculty member, the academic vignette will force you to think about your work setting and the clinical vignette will encourage you to think about what you need to do to prepare your students for those kinds of settings.

One of the major strengths of this book is the five authors. Collectively they represent a broad range of leadership experiences. All made their reputations in clinical areas that encourage big-picture, systems thinking: Gilliss (family care), Berkowitz (community health and policy), Johnson (patient safety), Reid Ponte (oncology), and Milone-Nuzzo (home care). They have led in both public and private institutions, and in unionized and non-unionized settings. Gilliss, Berkowitz, Johnson, and Milone-Nuzzo have all served as deans; Reid Ponte has held executive positions at the Dana-Farber Cancer Institute, Brigham and Women's Hospital, and the American Nurses Credentialing Center. All have had extensive experience heading professional organizations and serving on national boards. Milone-Nuzzo is now president of an inter-professional organization.

Dr. Darrell Kirch, former president and chief executive officer of the Association of American Medical Colleges, spoke at Milone-Nuzzo's installation as the sixth president of the Massachusetts General Hospital Institute of Health Professions. In his remarks, he called her a "multiplier," which he described as someone who brings people together to make positive changes in an organization. That is exactly what this book is about; it aims to help nurses learn to think of themselves as having a multiplier effect on their organizations.

ANGELA BARRON MCBRIDE, PhD, RN, FAAN
Distinguished Professor and University Dean Emerita
Indiana University School of Nursing

A Clinical Perspective

Ever wish you had a practical "go to" resource for navigating your entire nursing career leadership journey regardless of whether you were a novice or expert leader in a service setting? Have you ever been struck by the observation that your ability to lead and drive change were intertwined with the organizational culture, mission, vision, values, and decision-making structure? Have you ever felt alone as an organizational leader? I have.

Fortunately, this timely book has been written just for you. No matter where you are along the continuum of leadership, this book will help you become even more effective in leading and managing change in your organization.

We live in an interconnected world of speed, connectivity, instant communication, and complexity. Change is constant. Knowledge, adaptation, imagination, and leadership are essential, especially when responding to the unexpected and uncertain future as we so vividly highlight our incredible experience with the COVID-19 pandemic. Leaders and the workforce have had to run twice as fast to stay in the same place!

The World Health Organization (WHO) designated 2020 as the Year of the Nurse and Midwife. Little did we anticipate that the pandemic would feature the heroic nature of nursing's work while challenging our organizations (clinical and academic) like never before.

Imagine the incredible pace of change needed for healthcare service organizations to adapt to the rapidly evolving pandemic. How does one lead when traditional strategic responses are not in the communication plan or procedure manuals as information is constantly evolving? How does a leader flexibly steer the organization in a socially just manner in the midst of enormous challenges while providing the necessary support to the workforce? How does the leader care for the staff while also caring for self?

As I reflect on my career and leadership journey, I am struck by the insight that each successive position—starting in academia, then professional associations, and finally in service settings—built on the learnings and challenges of leading in these different types of organizations. Each role enhanced my awareness, learning, and understanding of leadership within the organizational context. This book would have been invaluable as a resource guide to better understand the linkages between my role as a leader and the organization's success.

It has been a joy to have had the opportunities to work with each author in various situations over our careers. They individually and collectively bring a wealth of diverse leadership experiences across the academic-service continuum. Together they have written this book targeted for novice to expert nurses who aspire to be and/or who are already in formal leadership positions.

The structure of the book is unique. The format embeds key literature combined with clinical and academic vignettes and key questions to ask oneself, as well as invaluable personal reflections, case studies, and questions. *This book makes you think.* I found myself reflecting on my own past service leadership situations and wondered: how else might I have handled that situation? What else could have been done?

This book will be invaluable across your career journey, whether you are just starting out or are an experienced nursing leader. It is rare to have a team of talented, accomplished nursing leaders share their personal stories and leadership lessons with such openness and honesty.

This book provides hope through theory + practical + real life experiences. It is a foundation and inspiration for nursing leaders everywhere as we take on the enormous challenges of steering our organizations toward health and health equity for all people in a globally interconnected world that is changing at warp speed.

Now let's get reading and reflecting in hopes of making the world a better place for all!

MARILYN P. CHOW, PhD, RN, FAAN
Vice President, National Patient Care Services and
Innovation, Kaiser Permanente, Retired
Professor, *University of California, School of Nursing*

Preface

Who should read this book?

This book is designed for nurses who want to lead more effectively in health delivery and academic organizations. Our goal is to help nurses who are working in the health sector and in colleges and universities become more effective leaders for the organizations they lead, ultimately advancing the individuals within the respective workforces and the products produced by the organizations, whether academic or health service. This book is designed to have meaning and to be useful for both novice and expert nurse leaders who are already in formal leadership positions or aspire to be, as well as those learners who are preparing for a future in leadership.

If any of these questions are ones that you ask yourself periodically, this book is for you:

- How do I know if my organization values what I value?
- How can I tell where my organization is headed?
- How can I best use my talents to influence my colleagues and the organization from whichever role I hold?
- How can I understand and act effectively when I see behavior or a decision that seems unjust or unfair?

Why did We Write this Book?

Unlike many texts on leadership, this book focuses on the relationship of the leader and the organization. Despite the fact that most nurses carry out their work within organizations, most texts on leadership are *not contextual*, that is, they ignore the fact that leadership occurs in the social context of an organization. We believe that leadership is a relational activity and we assume the stance that socially just leadership is synergistic, dynamic and ever-evolving as are the individuals within the organization. We recognize that organizations grow and develop, and guiding that development is one of the essential responsibilities of the leader. Our goal in this text is to guide nurses toward leadership that is effective, credible, inclusive, just and organizationally minded.

For many reasons, leadership positions are often lonely positions. Such is the case for nurse leaders whether in academic or clinical settings. Although the development of a professional network for sharing experiences and information is one important resource for you, as a leader, we believe that this book also serves as a resource. For that reason we wrote this book to include a balance of theoretical explanations, practical experience and personal anecdotes.

Given the advanced stage of our careers, we saw this collaborative project as an opportunity for the five of us to reflect on our careers and pass along knowledge about our successes and failures, our "lessons learned" (including those we are still learning), the challenges and joys of working in organizations, and the wisdom and pain we have all experienced. The ultimate aim of our effort is to offer perspectives on successful organizational leadership to other nurses who aspire to lead well.

What is the Focus of this Book?

As indicated, our treatment focuses on the organization and how leaders can effectively understand and intervene to lead organizations. The content focuses on what we see as the most important characteristics or properties of the organization, the work of the leader in relation to the organization and how to understand the organization to effectively manage change. We share principles, frameworks, approaches and perspectives about organizations, as well as some practical advice. A unique aspect of our work is our willingness to share personal experiences from our long and largely successful careers. And we have included anecdotes which are not all pretty!

The characteristics of the leader are secondary to the main purpose of our focus. We view the leader as an agent whose goal is to shepherd the organization to some productive, just end.

How is the Book Organized?

The book is developed in three sections. In Section I we introduce the reader to thinking organizationally. In Section II, we discuss some key concepts, including organizational attributes and common organizational work required to understand before leading. In Section III, we address leadership development, growth, and offer some lessons learned. Each chapter begins with a vignette from an academic and a clinical setting. At the conclusion of the chapter we invite the reader to return to the vignette and consider how the chapter content can inform the leadership challenges and possible interventions. Throughout most chapters, we ask the reader to reflect on their own experiences in relation to the subject at hand.

Prologue

We started thinking about this book together in 2017. The final days of writing and editing are taking place in late 2022.

We wouldn't have imagined the need to reflect on a very specific limitation of the book in a decisive and transparent way back when we started imagining such a book. And this is it: we are five white women who grew up in the United States. We also all identify as nurses, white, cis-gender, married/widowed and middle age, from middle class upbringings. We were educated in and have worked in organizations in the United States, primarily.

We are now beginning to understand that our socialization as well as our identities and experiences limit our capacity to see things without racial prejudices (Irving, 2014, Waking up White and Finding Myself in the Story of Race). We realize that no one is free of prejudice, it's impossible to be (Diangelo, 2018, White Fragility). However, we are now realizing, as we had not before, that as leaders in healthcare and academic organizations we have been complicit with policies and structures that have been created to oppress minority groups, particularly people of color but also other groups. We are now beginning to understand structural/systemic racism (Kendi, 2019, How to Be an Antiracist) and (Kendi, 2017, Stamped from the Beginning), and to appreciate how we have contributed to its continuation. As individuals and as leaders, we are committed to eliminating structural racism knowing the work may well outlast us.

We are each on a journey of coming to terms with our own prejudices, our white privilege, and finding ways to become more effective members and leaders of communities and organizations. We are trying to find ways to initiate major change specifically related to structural racisms in organizations we work and lead in and we integrate content related to this critically important work within each chapter. Our experience tells us that there are common themes to address, but that effective solutions must be tailored to the organizational cultures and practices. As you read this text, we hope you will think with us about how to approach the work in an effective way.

Pathways to Leadership

Gilliss: Pathway to Leadership

Depending on who you ask, there are any number of people who would have said I was headed to a career in leadership. My younger brothers will tell you I was always bossing them around. My seventh- grade classmates helped me post flyers when I ran a successful campaign for class secretary. My high school classmates worked with me, as Pep Club president, to paint and hang butcher-block posters in the halls before game day. In college I served as president of my junior class. Professionally, however, I did not set out with plans to hold a leadership position. The process was "organic."

My call to leadership roles was borne of a call to serve, to organize people to get things done. My insights of the fundamental commitment to make positive change came a bit later, as I had some experience and enjoyed the opportunity to reflect on my satisfaction with the work. My commitment to serve and make things better is enduring. Two phases come to mind, phrases repeated by two people close to me: "Leave it better than you found it," words first spoken by my soon-to-be husband who was a former Boy Scout on one of our early camping trips. The second, excerpted from a Robert Browning poem, was often repeated by my father throughout my childhood: "*A man's reach should exceed his grasp, Or what's a heaven for?*" To me these sentiments suggested that a person should aspire to make things better.

My first significant professional leadership responsibility grew out of a call from my departmental peers who recruited me as a candidate for department chair. An extended search had not produced a good fit between the needs of the department and the qualities and accomplishments of our candidates. My colleagues urged me to submit my name, suggesting that I was as qualified as any of our external candidates. I knew that was not true, but I did begin to wonder whether I could be successful in the position. I certainly understood the internal issues we faced and I had a beginning reputation beyond the school.

After a successful term as chair, I was curious for a larger challenge and moved into a deanship, where I learned some hard lessons. I declined an offer to lead at a school viewed to be among the nation's best, in favor of one where the offer of leadership involved effecting change. Although I learned that I loved the work of the academic leader, I did not fully understand some critical lessons about organizational culture, change management, and role clarity. The lessons were painful. After more than six years, I moved into a second deanship, one in which the lessons I had learned were put to good use. As opposed to the well-developed and deeply traditioned environment where I had first served as dean, the next organization was young, innovative, and for a number of logical reasons, under-developed. It was also my undergraduate alma mater. The culture of reform and innovation was well-matched to my philosophy of leadership and my leadership style. The university leadership was extraordinarily supportive of our school and me as a leader. We were able to build a close and supportive school community that worked tirelessly to achieve our goals. We developed stronger ties throughout the campus and a reputation for excellence in our field. Without question, we exceeded everyone's expectations.

Most recently I accepted my "encore deanship." Some colleagues have exclaimed, "You must be crazy! Who would do this again?" I would. I am now serving my doctoral alma mater at the institution where my career began. I anticipate that the lessons learned from my previous deanships will inform this assignment, which calls for a combination of skills sharpened in the first two positions.

Once again, it is the call to serve combined with the opportunity to improve that attracts me. And in the meanwhile, I have come to think of leading large organizations as my clinical practice. I once told my university president that I was an organizational interventionist. He, an English professor, looked at me in a manner suggesting that this term was not in his lexicon.

I am motivated to share lessons on leadership in hopes that others will be more successful than I was. My work in leadership has been influenced by the writings of and personal mentorship of a number of great leaders.

- Watching Ingeborg Mauksch and Loretta Ford in the late 1970's and beyond, taught me to be bold and to stay the course.
- Barbara Durand, who was tirelessly committed to patients, students, faculty colleagues and friends demonstrated humanity as a teacher and administrator. She was pretty funny too.
- Angela McBride and Rhetaugh Dumas helped me to understand what an organization expected from its leader and guided me in demonstrating my commitment to those organizations and fulfilling the expectations of the person to whom I reported.
- Mary Champagne showed me how a former dean could continue to lead supportively from elsewhere in the organization.
- Marilyn Chow has whispered new ideas in my ear at exactly the right time, as evidence of her superb skills as a peer and mentor.
- Nancy Woods, who has never uttered an unkind work in her life, has demonstrated the balance and equanimity to which I will always aspire (and likely never achieve) and the importance of continuing a life including music!

- Martha Hill guided me to a method of faculty engagement at exactly the right moment, and it made all the difference.
- Doreen Harper has been a constant in my life since 1972, when we began graduate school together. Her Myers-Briggs profile differs from and complements my own, reminding me to attend to what I might otherwise overlook.

To them, and to those who have contributed to the scholarship of leadership and written of their leadership experiences, I offer my thanks.

Berkowitz: Pathway to Leadership

As a child growing up in a rural community during the 50's and 60's, I had limited exposure to experiences that might fuel a young girl's desire for adventure. Nevertheless, I was a child with big ambitions but was shy and introverted. A long illness and hospitalization while in grade school exposed me to an experience that was difficult and frightening but an inspiration for my future profession. From my child's perception, nurses were the most powerful people in my hospital environment and through them I gained a sense of confidence and competence in my ability to persevere, what we think of as resilience. If I could learn from my experience with illness, I may be able to manage other complex challenges. Those feelings remained with me as I grew older and struggled with the dissonance of ambition and shyness. I was unsure how to change the dynamic. I decided to enroll in acting lessons and successfully auditioned for and performed in every school play in junior high and high school. In the broader context of risk taking, this may seem mild; but for me, it launched a change in the way I perceived myself. This confirmed my choice of nursing as a career and enabled my pathway to leadership. This early experience created a new narrative for myself as a young woman who could take risks and manage and learn from a challenge. That has remained my way forward over these many years in leadership.

Early understanding and critical self-appraisal as a child launched a "reboot" of my personality but other choices have framed and guided my leadership style and leadership values. Early in my career as a nurse I chose to practice in public health. It was closest to my values, enabled a personal connection to the individuals, families and communities I wanted to serve, and provided significant independence in decision making. It also provided variety in my practice on a day to day basis and served up an endless opportunity to improvise, innovate, problem solve, empathize, communicate, and take risks. I worked in a rural public health department with skilled mentors; the chief medical officer and the chief nursing officer. They were generous in providing opportunities for growth and learning and often pointed out strengths and weaknesses that I overlooked. They taught me something new every day and encouraged me to pursue advanced education and rewarded me with leadership opportunities. I became a supervisor then director of nursing under their watch and they supported me when I decided to pursue a PhD. Much of what I learned about leadership I learned from them: a sense of humor is essential, service to the community is an expectation, empathy is at the core of caring, listening is virtuous, criticism is valuable, teach something and learn something every day, intellectual development is not optional; and. my favorite: opportunities are for the taking.

I took my mentor's many lessons along with opportunities in larger and more complex positions in public health, policy, government, and academia. I have had many incredible role models during my career, but the lessons I learned in that rural public health department created the foundation and core of my leadership.

Johnson: Pathway to Leadership

There are as many roads to leadership as there are leaders, I never saw myself as a leader nor did I aspire to lead anything. I now recognize that in many ways I was an informal leader who could convince others – such as my older sister, to engage in stunts that were definitely not approved by our parents. I was late coming to nursing. My first degree was in economics with a focus on developing economies. I discovered that I am an experiential learner so I have a history of fully engaging in whatever it is that my passion at the time draws me to. With my degree in economics I set out by myself to see the world and traveled extensively experiencing many cultures and ways of being. I settled for a while on a Greek island, fell in love, got very sick and while reflecting on my life I determined that if I survived I was going to do something meaningful. I realized that some of the most meaningful experiences in my life was as a volunteer at Condell Memorial Hospital in my hometown of Libertyville Illinois. As a result of that work, I worked as a nursing assistant during summers and college vacations and loved that. I decided that I would return to the US, enroll in nursing school and set off on a path that has been incredibly rewarding.

So how does this relate to becoming a leader? I believe we build on all of our experiences. The building blocks from my youth and early adulthood of being curious, taking risks, and challenging the way things are coupled with my love of nursing contributed to not only getting a BSN, but then an MSN as a geriatric nurse practitioner when it was a new role for nurses, and eventually my PhD in health policy. I am a great believer in need, opportunity and timing as major contributors to leadership as well as passion to create change and innovation. The need and the timing are usually beyond our control but being open to opportunity is within our control and I would say that I have been a world-class opportunist. My challenge is that everything seems like an opportunity and I must prioritize. My formal leadership experience began when I was a newly minted NP who came to Washington DC. Being a newly minted geriatric NP, I found an opportunity with George Washington University to work on a geriatric curriculum for medical students and be part of a geriatric care team. I also connected with a newly established NP program and soon became the director. I had never taught a course, been in academics nor officially led anything. I accepted and have continued to embrace opportunities to do work that I highly value. Since then, I have had the opportunity to lead interprofessional education, be the founding dean of a school of nursing, provide leadership to professional organizations, work internationally and many other very satisfying projects--and to promote the best nursing care possible.

Milone-Nuzzo: Pathway to Leadership

My pathway to leadership was probably more unexpected than that of my co-authors. I was the youngest of 4 children born to parents who were not college educated. They wanted more for their children than they had, and we all had a strong focus on education growing up. As the youngest, I was given a lot of latitude and for most of my K-12 educational experience, I was a mediocre or below student. I often felt the only purpose for school was to have the opportunity to have a good time with friends. During my junior and senior year in high school, my parents began talking to me about college. I let them know I preferred not to attend college but wanted to go to work instead. They reminded me that the rule was everyone in the family went to college and I would be no different from my brother and sisters. My mother said "I think you would be a good nurse." By some miracle I was accepted to nursing school and by the end of the first week, I was hooked. I loved everything about nursing school. I loved the science courses, I loved learning how the body worked and how disease affected normal physiology. I loved taking care of patients and I loved the way I felt in my student nurse uniform. I felt taller, thinner and smarter than I ever felt before. I loved making people feel better at the worst times in their lives. Therein began my love affair with our profession.

After a very short stint as an in-patient hospital nurse, I had the opportunity to teach in an LPN program. My love of teaching drove me to continue my education so that I could have a career in academia, at this point not considering leadership as an option. In my first academic position, I had the opportunity to see academic leadership, and sometimes the lack thereof, in action. I saw the impact a great leader can have on an organization and its members. I witnessed the importance of personal and professional integrity in the role and I saw the negative effects when it was not there. I saw how a leader can shape the future of an organization. It was during this first academic position that I aspired to a career in academic leadership.

I used my doctoral program very intentionally to fill in the gaps I felt were missing in my knowledge base. By the time I entered doctoral education, I knew I wanted to be a Dean so I entered a program in higher education administration with minors in economics and finance and adult learning. My dissertation was on managing interpersonal conflict among faculty in schools of nursing. All of this study provided me with the foundational theoretical knowledge that I thought would be necessary for an academic leader. That preparation served me well, but I needed to gain experience and credibility. It was at that point I made one of the most risky decisions of my career. By the time I finished my doctorate, I was tenured in a state college in CT. I was only 35 and could have stayed there for the rest of my career. At the same time, a three year soft money position was being advertised at Yale University School of Nursing for someone to help them launch the first curriculum for advanced practice nursing in home care. They were very clear that it was for 3 years and no more. I applied, was offered the position and left my tenured position to engage in that important work.

Three years turned into fourteen and I had multiple leadership roles during those great years culminating in appointment as Associate Dean for Academic Affairs. I learned so many leadership lessons during my time at Yale . . . the importance of being credible in your work and the role of experience in establishing credibility, that there are no small problems for the people you are leading and probably the most important lesson taught to me by my mentor at Yale, Catherine Gilliss, that as a leader, there is never a casual comment. People will listen, interpret, analyze and often act on what you might have said as an off the cuff comment. The other important thing I learned was that when you get into the role of the Dean, your primary role is to help others be successful in their role. By encouraging others and helping them get in the place to be successful, a leader magnifies their impact. Your true success as a leader is seen in the success of others. When I left Yale to become a Dean, I had learned so much about myself as a person and a leader .

I had never had a real mentor in my career until I met Catherine Gilliss at Yale. Since we met in 1998, she has served in that role for me, first as my dean and then as a most trusted friend and colleague. Although I had heard all the presentations and read the articles on the importance of having a mentor, it was not until I had a mentor that I realized how important it really was.

For my entire career, I have been influenced by what I have seen other leaders do in their careers. I have always been in awe of the giants in nursing and since I was a young nurse, I aspired to be like them. I still get excited when I get to be in the company of our nursing legends. I have learned as much about leadership from great leaders as I have learned from those who I felt fell short of that mark. I have always worked hard to do more than what was expected of me. I have tried to lead with integrity of spirit and action and authenticity of voice. I have loved the leadership roles I have had.

Reid-Ponte: Pathway to Leadership

Many nurses influenced my career trajectory and my leadership practice including my mother who was a nurse. I worked during high-school and college at MGH, Boston, MA where my mother worked. I think of this hospital and the nurses and others who worked there as helping shape me from a formative standpoint. For instance, my first job there was in the kitchens of the Phillips House which was a building for "private patients." I met and worked with two Black women, Rose and Marianne who took me under their wings.

Several faculty from my undergraduate program inspired me to want to learn and integrate their values with my own. During that time I also learned so much from two close friends who were nursing students in the same program and we roomed together over two years. They influenced me in such a profound and positive way as a nurse and person and they continue do so today

My first nurse manager was thoughtful, focused and very helpful to me in my growth and development. Further along, when I became a nurse manager it was notable that the professional development offered to novice nurse leaders provided by that hospital nursing service also was formative and piqued my interest in human behavior in organizations. I remain close to one of those leaders till this day.

Later, several wise and effective nurse leaders helped me understand systems, standards, structures and processes and how they contribute to excellence in care delivery, shared decision making as well as clinical workforce and organizational outcomes. I also learned from several physicians, social workers, pharmacists and administrative colleagues what true partnership and collaboration means.

Even later, the importance of healthy work environments, effective labor relations, quality improvement, cultures of safety, interdisciplinary collaboration and patient and family centered care were promulgated and advanced by nurses and others who were instrumental in my career and life. I learned how to listen carefully to people as a Nurse Executive Team Member then later a Chief Nursing Officer both in unionized organizations. I learned about the power and politics that all organizations have—both good and bad.

My graduate and doctoral programs were completed while I worked, so although the faculty and the learning activities influenced my thinking and practice, they were not as prominent in my development and career trajectory as the practice environment nurse leaders were. One particular nurse leader actually supported me taking doctoral courses during the workday. She was ahead of her time. A doctoral class mate, this nurse leader (now retired) and I meet on zoom monthly to discuss and debate important societal and political issues.

My dissertation focused on the nurse patient/family relationship, patient distress and nurse empathy which was an extension of my own values and beliefs as is commonly the case in dissertation research projects and served to bolster my own commitment to these principles which formed the basis of my leadership practice, education and scholarship throughout my career.

Currently, I am inspired by colleagues, friends and community members, many of whom are clinical and administrative nurses, deans, associate deans, chief nursing officers, faculty members, students, nurse practitioners and nurse anesthetists, business owners, association leaders and volunteers, and board members.

My husband has been a constant source of joy, reflection and learning for my entire post college life and I have learned great humility and how love is the basis of everything from him and our sons, one who is a nurse practitioner and the other who serves in the U.S. Army and each of their wives who are in the same roles/careers as their husbands are. My father died when I was 5 years old, my three siblings have been instrumental in the person who I have become as well as of course, my mother; and her sister and brother in law who were prominent forces in our lives from childhood to adulthood.

I have learned to trust myself and have learned the importance of mindfulness in life and leadership with social justice as the backbone of everything. I am clearer than ever that what I value drives who I am and I want to spend time with people who have similar values or if not, who are open to dialogue, discourse, reflection and personal growth with the intention of making the world a better place.

I have never had a formal mentor although many individuals have helped me greatly. An executive coach who I worked closely with for 15 years was central to my self-development and leadership effectiveness and is now a very good friend. She helped me understand my own strengths and use them wisely, she helped me see my gaps in leadership and living and helped me to be more equanimous and to better face power politics and social injustice.

I was not advised by any one person on how to direct my career or specifically how to sculpt my leadership practice. Early in my career, I learned about leadership theories and approaches, for effective problem solving, decision making accountability, process improvement and outcome management through my own reading, taking courses, experience at work, from healthcare consultants and of course through my masters and doctoral programs. I now integrate these experiences and content into the courses I design and teach.

I was very fortunate to be a fellow in the Robert Wood Johnson Nurse Executive Program mid-career, which positioned me to have extraordinary personal and professional connections and colleagues around the nation and to have top notch competency based professional leadership development. I have learned a great deal from and care a great deal for several fellows in this program and one particularly who is a dean, continues to serve as an inspiration to me.

Not long ago, I completed a 14 year relationship with the ANA most recently as President of the American Nurses Credentialing Center (ANCC). That experience positioned me to have global influence related to organizational nursing excellence and professional development. I am so grateful for those nurse leaders, two of whom were RWJ Nurse Executive Fellows, who paved the way for my leadership in those organizations.

I am now a faculty member at Boston College with a joint appointment at the Connell School of Nursing and Woods College of Advancing Studies Masters of Health Administration Program and I teach part time at Simmons University. I am a member of the Lahey Hospital Medical Center board of trustees and in the capacity serve on the Beth Israel Lahey Health system-wide quality assessment committee.

Although I very much enjoyed leading change and assuring extraordinary clinical, workforce and organizational outcomes in my past roles in health service, I love the work of preparing others to take the lead.

My inherent interest in continuous learning, self-improvement and self-care positioned me to seek and attain leadership positions in healthcare organizations in which I used my talents, knowledge and skills to influence others. I really love organizational life. I am now realizing that I was socialized to think that white privilege was the norm and that the organizations I worked in were (and still are) structurally racist as most organizations at least in the United States are today.

I am beginning to consider how I will lead when not employed by an organization has begun to surface. The idea that I need to lead in the community as a nurse to assure no individuals or groups are oppressed is at the basis of my thinking. I am working hard to increase my knowledge through reading lay and scientific literature and participating in discussions and forums to better understand our history, society and politics.

I am prioritizing learning and growing differently now that I am clearly aware of my prejudices, privileges and racist tendencies. I am clear about the great opportunities that I have had because I am a white woman. I am working on not holding back, not being afraid to make mistakes, to take a stand particularly related to not being complicit with current norms of oppression. I am fiercely committed to assuring that all individuals and groups are equally treated with dignity and respect.

My major efforts are focused on helping nurses and advanced practice nurses use their expertise and voices within their families, communities and organizations to identify, reduce and ultimately eliminate inequities and oppression of individuals and groups through population health with an emphasis on our roles in improving the social determinants of health for all.

This is the work of the nurse for decades to come and although we might say that this has always been our work, we have not come near to meeting this objective. Now, during this time of collective awakening, we have an opportunity to be central to improving the lives and health of all people

To do this effectively, nurses in organizations need to practice and to lead with great skill and conviction—at the bedside, in the community, in their own families, in boardrooms, in churches, in businesses and wherever else we are. I see this book as a small but mighty component of the toolkit necessary to help nurses to do this crucially important work.

The Framework for Understanding the Leadership of Organizations

CHAPTER 1

Overview of Organizations and the Role of Leadership

INTRODUCTION

Each of us has spent a significant part of our professional lives in organizations. Organizations, guided by their mission, vision, and values (MVV), provide enabling structures, resources, and guidelines to allow people to work efficiently and effectively. Some organizations meet their missions and continuously improve the quality of work and the outcomes they produce, whereas others seem to impede productivity and work quality. How do they differ? Importantly, what does leadership have to do with organizational functioning? Based on our leadership experience and our reading of scientific literature, we believe that the most effective organizations are led by leaders who understand the complexity and intricacies of organizations in addition to the specific work to be done.

An organization is a living entity, often composed of hundreds, and even thousands, of people. The organizationally minded leader's challenge is to guide the collective of individuals in the organization to be as effective and constructively impactful as possible. Effective leaders understand the unique characteristics and dynamics of the organizations they lead and routinely take these qualities into consideration as they frame their leadership work. Yet much of the leadership literature addresses the personal skills and talents of the leader rather than the work of leadership within the context of the organization. The focus of this text is organizational leadership—the role of leaders in organizations and the description of best practices based on the authors' collective experience of working in organizations since the 1960s. Our intent is to share lessons learned, strategies and tactics that can serve to guide both novice and more experienced leaders as they navigate the diverse types of organizations in which nurses lead.

3

CHARACTERISTICS OF HEALTHCARE ORGANIZATIONS

Organizations share similar characteristics, and all have unique aspects. Among the similarities are the need to have a financially sustainable plan and to consistently address efficiency, the quality of the product or service, and the environmental changes that may impact the organization. There are several important characteristics of healthcare organizations that are unique compared to other organizations. These differences greatly influence the work of leaders within them. Several of these differences are described below:

- Healthcare organizations are social institutions in which deeply personal relationships exist between the "customers" and those employed to provide services. Although most organizations work to build relationships with their customers and suppliers, healthcare organizations are structured to build relationships with their customers as a primary objective. In healthcare, relationships with staff, providers, and the people served by the organization are often very personal and intimate. Healthcare providers, clinicians, and staff touch patients; inquire into the most intimate details of one's life; and act to extend and save lives, as well as counsel and educate individuals, families, and communities.
- Healthcare organizations reflect society as a whole. In the United States (US), healthcare organizations have not provided equal access to high quality, safe healthcare as a result of structural racism and the dominance of leaders who do not reflect the diversity of our population. Change will require policies that revamp access to care, care delivery redesign, and building of trust among communities of people of color.
- A paradox of needs and supply drives healthcare delivery services. Although in most markets demand drives supply, in healthcare supply drives demand. This paradox has been demonstrated repeatedly by those looking at practice patterns across the US. For example, when there are more magnetic resonance imaging (MRI) machines, we see higher volumes of MRIs. This results in a complex relationship between the healthcare organization and its customers.
- The products of organizations that deliver healthcare are more difficult to measure than companies that manufacture goods. Although one can count the number of patients cared for and know the overall cost of a care episode, the "care product" is more difficult to define. There are numerous and variable inputs into care of a patient, including physical assessment, care planning treatments, monitoring, education, and more. There has been significant movement toward examining patient experience and outcomes of care, and this movement will continue.
- Healthcare is a multiproduct business and includes a wide array of services, including preventative care, chronic and acute care, and extended or conva-

lescent care. Services are directed toward people who are healthy and those who are ill. Services include nursing care, medical care, social services, occupational and physical therapies, and others. Within each of the services there are other services, for instance, phlebotomy, radiology, and nutrition therapy.

- Although all organizations face uncertainty, healthcare organizations face high uncertainty in at least three levels: national regulatory, state regulatory, and organizational. National and state regulators have shifted their focus to value, which has forced organizations to change the way they obtain reimbursement and measure outcomes. As we write this book, the COVID-19 pandemic has resulted in enormous uncertainty in both academic and clinical organizations and has placed significant stress on individual workers, as well as the organizations in which they work.

- Healthcare organizations are highly complex and include both high tech and high touch elements. High touch services demand a high level of patient-provider interaction. Unlike services that can be automated, healthcare requires personal relationships and is carefully tailored to address individual differences in illness and the patient/situation. Some high-tech organizations can produce lines that are highly automated such as pharmaceutics, soft drink manufacturers, car companies, and many others. Healthcare incorporates technology more broadly with electronic health records, monitoring equipment, sophisticated equipment for treatments, and automated processes such as requesting and receiving supplies. Patients want the best technical care and also want providers who demonstrate compassion in the delivery of care. The work of leaders includes preparation of systems and providers that can do both.

- Social injustice, structural racism, and other forms of discrimination must be identified and eliminated within healthcare organizations. The COVID-19 pandemic has brought health inequities into stark relief. The social determinants of health have contributed to rates of infection and death that have disproportionately affected persons of color, the poor and those living in crowded housing, and the elderly. Health is a human right and the delivery of healthcare must include equitable access to care that is relevant and culturally appropriate for the consumer.

Recognizing the properties associated with the social unit of the organization will inform the leader's choices about when and how to lead. Within nursing we prepare clinicians with skills to address the social systems significant to the structures, processes, and outcomes of care. For instance, we assume that the outcomes of a child's care are related to the influences of the family, such as the ability of caregivers to recognize the child's needs and respond appropriately to those needs. Likewise, we assume that the functional health of a family has a relationship to the surrounding social system of the community—its environmental factors and the availability of healthy food, transportation, and policies that promote recreation, safety, and meaningful exchange. However, even as we recognize the mutual influences of these nested social systems in our clinical understanding, we seldom extend the leader's relationship to the organization to focus on the organization's interconnected social systems and think about actions as interventions in those social systems. We often fail to fully take into account that the organization influences the individual and the individual influences the organization.

We believe that the individual, as leader, designs leadership interventions based on an understanding of the organization, its development and characteristics, and its relationship to the individuals who are part of the organization. In doing so, there is a dynamic interplay of leaders and social systems within the organization. This fundamental belief will guide our presentation of ideas to help the nurse leader, regardless of the setting, to more effectively consider when and how to lead. Leadership, then, is the work of intervening in an organization to effect intentional positive change aimed at meeting the mission and strategic priorities of the organization.

As nurses, most of us began our career in a healthcare delivery system of some kind: hospital, home care, long-term care facility, community clinics, schools, or retail. Our first role may have been focused on patient care where the primary responsibility was the delivery of safe care to several patients. Later, we may have assumed a supervisory or management position, where we had responsibility for several individuals and accountability for certain outcomes, and our role remained focused on accomplishment of a set of operational tasks. Eventually assuming leadership responsibility within the organization, nurses change their focus from a singular or set of discrete tasks to a concern for a larger group, including multiple subgroups or the entire organization. What is involved in in making the transition from interventions that are individually focused to those that are organizationally focused? How does the leader impact the evolution of and capabilities of the entire organization? How does decision-making in one unit of an organization impact the work of another unit? The organizationally minded leader comes to see the emergent properties of the organization and intentionally assesses, plans, intervenes, and evaluates at the level of the organization.

DEFINITION AND ASSUMPTIONS OF ORGANIZATIONAL LEADERSHIP

We believe that organizational leaders need to bring their emotional and relational understanding of people and the culture of the organization as well as the technical analytical abilities based on knowledge and experience to leading within organizations. We define organizationally minded leadership as:

Leadership that intervenes based on an understanding of the organization, its development and characteristics, and its relationship to the individuals who are part of the organization. Organizationally minded leadership recognizes and values the organizational context and intentionally acts to influence the social system of the organization.

In addition to the definition of organizationally minded leadership, there are several assumptions of organizational leadership that are important to understanding this framework of leadership. The assumptions are:

- Organizations are made up of people wanting to contribute positively and meaningfully who have a unique set of identities, talents, expertise, needs, fears, and life challenges that can enhance or create barriers to working effectively.
- Leading an organization effectively requires technical, interpersonal, adaptive, and emotional understanding of self and others to effectively connect individuals and groups to organizational priorities and goals.
- Individuals and groups are parts of social systems within organizations. Effective leaders care about social groups as well as individuals. They care about the multiple identities that individuals and groups value.
- The overall impact of the organization is greater than the sum of its parts.

We believe that understanding leadership within the organizational context is critical to improve our healthcare systems—moving them from fragmented organizations that leave providers burned out to ones that are person-centered and meet the needs of those who work in the organization and those who are served by it. Organizations today are facing large and complex challenges. Healthcare organizations face changes in public funding; declining financial support from third party payers; workforce shortages; increasing clinical, administrative and technical complexity; and considerable uncertainty. Universities are challenged by the public's growing concern of the high cost and relative value of higher education, the job-readiness of its graduates, and keeping up with technology and facilities that attract the best students.

Leaders who understand how to assess their organization and how to work effectively within their particular system will be the most effective in their role regardless of the formal leadership position held. The link between assessment and intervention is decision-making. Every assessment leads to a decision to act or not act, and if the decision is to act, the assessment determines what the action or intervention should be.

The nature of formal and informal leadership is similar in that both are needed to be effective. The scope of influence may vary, as will the degree of accountability, based on the actual position. Leadership success will depend on the ability of the leader to consider the elements we set forth in this chapter and the more detailed explanation that follows in the remainder of this text. Our examples will move between the academic and service sectors because we believe that the process of leadership and the best practices of successful leaders have commonalities across settings and roles.

Each chapter is organized in a way to allow the reader to relate the important content to an academic and clinical case study that begins each chapter. Critical elements of organizationally minded leadership are then explored from both a theoretical and experiential perspective weaving in real life examples of leadership from the authors. Over the course of each chapter, you will also be asked to reflect on your own leadership experience related to the chapter content. At the end of each chapter, there are critical thinking questions that ask the reader to use the content in the chapter to explore the case study in depth. The vignettes presented, critical thinking questions, and reader's reflection on their leadership experiences allow for application of essential content and will contribute to the leader's growth.

GETTING TO KNOW YOUR ORGANIZATION: WHAT TO LOOK FOR

The following section provides a brief overview of topics that are covered in greater depth in Chapters 3–15 and is designed to provide a framework to orient you to the substantive content of this text.

Organizational Culture

Organizational culture is defined as the underlying beliefs, assumptions, values, and ways of interacting that contribute to the unique social and psychological environment of an organization (Cancianlosi, 2017). Culture is set by the vision and values of an organization, but it is carried forward and manifested in the organization through customs, norms, and beliefs of the people working in the organization. For instance, an organization's values statement indicates a commitment to recruit exceptional people who will excel. To live that vision, the organization should commit to a meaningful onboarding program for new employees on the basic resources and customs of the organization. As is often said, "You can ignore what people say but watch what they do!"

Leaders play an integral role in setting workplace culture, and they need to understand that the organizational culture provides the context for how work gets done and how people feel about being a member of the organization. Does the organization have a culture of quality? Does it foster organizational learning and investment in the employees? Or is the culture focused on maintaining the status quo or maximizing success rather than employee growth or customers satisfaction? Culture may been implied in the behaviors of leaders, for instance, do the leaders attend and offer appreciation during the Nurses' Week Awards Ceremonies? Does the Department Chair or Dean or Associate Dean provide remarks of appreciation at the retirement of a senior faculty member? Do leaders conduct or make provision for exit interviews, showing an appreciation for learning the criticisms of their organization as well as enjoying the kudos?

Leaders must understand their role in the sustainability of an organization's culture. Culture provides a roadmap for the acceptability of behavior within an organization. The rules of conformity set by culture help people achieve their goals which, in turn, also increases job satisfaction (Tsai, 2011). Building teamwork into the organizational culture always improves the job satisfaction of employees. Organizational culture and job satisfaction are linked, and the leader has a role in setting a positive course through culture establishing norms.

One area where organizational culture is displayed is in how an organization recognizes and rewards employees. Although some organizations are better at this than others, most organizations engage in some form of recognition and reward for employees who contribute collectively and individually to the mission. Organizations have different approaches to recognition and rewards, including cash bonuses, merit raises, public recognitions, titles, and promotions. The goal of rewards is to recognize positive behaviors and to increase the likelihood that those behaviors will be repeated by the employee as well as others in the organization. For a full discussion of organizational culture, see Chapter 3.

Consider: **How would you describe the culture of the organization in which you currently work or learn? Is it a culture that supports, recognizes, and rewards people for work well done? What would you change about the culture?**

Mission, Vision, and Values

Organizational leaders need to be clear about the consistency of their values and beliefs with the organization's MVV. Alignment is critical. If there is no alignment (unless a leader is brought in to change the MVV), the fit will ultimately not work well, and the leader will be frustrated in their role. Examples of MVV for both an academic as well as a clinical organization are below. These descriptions provide clear information on the purpose of the organization, what it hopes to accomplish, and its core values. An academic organization might represent its MVVs as listed in Table 1.1 and the MVVs of a clinical entity appear in Table 1.2.

Not only is it necessary to have alignment of the leader's and organization's MVV statements, but also it offers direction to why the organization exists, its goals and aspirations, and the values it lives. These core statements serve as touchstones for decision-making by all members of the organization, including its leaders. An in-depth discussion of organizational MVVs will be presented in Chapter 4.

Table 1.1. Mission, Vision, and Values of an Academic Organization.

Mission: The Harris University School of Nursing is a diverse community of scholars and clinicians, committed to educating the next generation of transformational leaders in nursing. We advance nursing science in issues of global importance and foster the scholarly practice of nursing.

The **mission** of the **Harris University School of Nursing** is to create a center of excellence for the advancement of nursing science, the promotion of clinical scholarship, and the education of clinical leaders, advanced practitioners, and researchers. Through nursing research, education, and practice, students and faculty seek to enhance the quality of life for people of all cultures, economic levels, and geographic locations.

Vision Statement: Together transforming the future of nursing, to advance health with individuals, families, and communities.

Core Values:
- Excellence
- Integrity
- Collaboration
- Respect
- Innovation
- Diversity and Inclusiveness

Table 1.2. Mission, Vision, and Values of a Clinical Organization.

The MVVs of the **Colfax Medical Center and Children's Hospital** convey the reasons we exist as an organization, what we aspire to as an organization, and the way we will work to get there. They are unifying forces that link all of us together.

Mission: Our mission—the reason we exist—is Caring, Healing, Teaching, and Discovering.
Vision: Our vision—what we want to be—is to be the best provider of healthcare services, the best place to work, and the best environment for teaching and research.
Values: Our values statement—our guide to the individual and organizational behavior we expect—is embodied in the acronym PRIDE:

P for Professionalism, how we conduct ourselves and our business
R for Respect for our patients, families, ourselves, and each other
I for Integrity, always doing the honest, right thing
D for Diversity, understanding and embracing the diverse beliefs, needs, and expectations of our patients, community, and employees
E for Excellence, what we strive for in everything we do

Consider: What are your most important values that drive how you lead? Are those values consistent with your organization's MVVs? How do the organization's MVVs influence your leadership philosophy?

Strategic Planning

Strategic planning is one of those administrative activities that many people find burdensome, but it is essential to the success of an organization. A strategic plan gives the leader a roadmap for decision-making, financial planning, and determining the strategies that they want to pursue, especially in the face of competing priorities. Strategic planning provides direction and goals, aligns resources with those goals, creates a plan of action, and provides the information about success through rigorous evaluation. The strategic planning process of an organization should inspire its members to think about aspirational goals and objectives, those areas where the organization can distinguish itself from its competitors.

Leaders recognize the critical role that members of the organization play in the development and implementation of the strategic plan. Engagement of members of the organization serves several purposes. It allows the leader to hear a broad perspective of ideas from different parts of the organization and from individuals with different perspectives about the organization's mission. Engagement also supports buy-in from the members. If people know that they have a voice in determining the path forward of an organization, they will be much more inclined to work toward that goal. Strategies for developing and implementing a strategic plan include using data to analyze the current status, conducting a SWOT (strengths, weaknesses, opportunities, and threats) analysis, and managing the pace of change.

The final step of the strategic planning process involves both examination of the plan itself and the metrics that define the outcomes of the plan. Defining how to measure the critical strategic initiatives gives the leader a picture of how effective the implementation process has been. Too often, a strategic plan is developed and then put on a shelf, not to be opened again until it is time to do the next strategic plan. A functional strategic plan that is developed as a community effort, uses data to evaluate its current state and plan for the future, and has a tactical plan that includes metrics for evaluation is an important organizational asset. The strategic planning process is detailed in Chapter 5.

Consider: What has been your experience in developing the strategic plan in your organization? Since it was developed, how has the leader used it to define the work of the organization or as the basis for decision made? In what ways could you see using the strategic plan in your current organization.

Organizational Governance: Structure, Roles, and Accountability

Whether large or small, all organizations have a form of structural order. Structure should support the function and goals of the organization and clearly reflect who is accountable to whom and for what. Depending on the purpose of the organization, the form might focus on clinical "service lines," or clusters of service providers by discipline or function. An academic organization might be organized into subgroups by academic departments or degree programs. The organizational chart displays the ways in which an organization is ordered. The level and degrees of detail within an organizational chart vary from organization to organization, but the display will generally reflect the functional units and the reporting structure or chain of command and lines of authority. Traditionally, clinical entities are structured in a hierarchical format, wherein there is a clear, formal chain of authority and clear reporting relationship. These structures are often described as "vertical" and contrast with the less formal and more "horizontal" structures in academic organizations. These differences can be tied to the work of the organization. For instance, in academic settings in which creative collaborations are encouraged and the qualifications of faculty are often homogeneous, shared decision-making is often encouraged at the "ground level." This contrasts with the clinical environment, in which hierarchical structures are most often present to ensure established clinical standards are followed as the stakes (life/death) are high. The need for accountability is high in both sectors, but the outcomes are obviously quite different.

Consider: Does the structure of your organization adequately support the functions? What does your organizational chart tell you that you didn't know? Who is accountable for what? In what ways is knowing the organizational chart useful in your work?

The governance function of organizations sets out the orderly process for how work is actually accomplished. Regardless of the overall structure, organizations distribute roles and responsibilities to those who are employed or are contracted to serve in them. Roles and responsibilities must be identified for the participants to understand their jobs. Clinical nurses are expected to deliver high quality, safe patient care according to an established set of standards. The unit leaders are expected to staff each shift with an adequate number of qualified staff. The chief nursing officer is expected to provide each unit leader with the resources necessary to staff the unit safely and focus on operational excellence. The chief nurse executive is generally charged with collaborating with other executive level leaders to develop the plan for strategic advancement. In the educational setting, the chief academic officer, usually the dean, accepts overall responsibility for implementation of quality educational programs that are appropriately staffed, resourced, and accredited. Likewise, within the academic setting, the dean may delegate portfolios of organizational work to others, including associate deans, but the expression "the buck stops here" reflects the dean's ultimate responsibility for outcomes. Department chairs may be responsible for hiring and faculty development; chief finance officers design budgets and monitor revenues and expenses.

Within complex organizations, people may have a variety of roles and responsibilities. Not only is the staff nurse responsible for taking care of a certain number of patients, but also is expected to participate in quality improvement activities, committee work relevant to a specific unit or the overall organization such as the risk management committee, and perhaps teach nursing students or orient new nurses to organization. Faculty and staff within an academic organization also have several "hats," including teacher, researcher, committee member of the school of nursing or the university, and many more. All employees in effective organizations know their roles and what is expected of them and are empowered to think about better ways of attaining the organizational goals. The importance of sorting out who does what and who is accountable for decisions will be discussed in detail in Chapter 6.

Consider: **What are your roles and responsibilities in your organization? Is the set of responsibilities noted in your job description reflective of what you do? Who makes what decisions in your organization? What is the decision-making structure and process in your organizational unit? Where do you currently fit in the organizational structure?**

Organizational Ways of Operating: Policies, Procedures, Guidelines, and Committees

In addition to specifying how responsibilities are distributed, organizations have preferences for getting work accomplished. Academic organizations are renowned for the shared governance approach to decision-making, in which administrative leaders and elected faculty work together to establish policies and processes. Decision-making that sets policy is often done by committee, creating lengthy timelines that are painfully slow compared with most industries. In addition to committees, academic institutions also have faculty and staff organized by educational program or degree, or whether they are primarily researchers, teachers, or clinicians.

Policies, processes, and systems are ways of accomplishing work. Having all staff understand these is essential to effective functioning. Some systems and processes are unique to an organization and others are more commonly "tried and true." In most organizations, the important systems and processes are written down and transmitted to individuals new to the organization in their orientation. Individuals new to organizations want and need to be clear about the MVVs of the organization, expectations of them, how work gets done, and the standards for success. Even though there are written guides for negotiating the systems and processes of an organization, people rely on colleagues for information. Organizational culture is reflected in the policies and processes guide, but culture is often experienced. It is a way of being in the organization, with some organizations having people supportive of each other and others having a competitive environment.

Organizations that rely primarily on word of mouth to transmit the important ways of accomplishing the work of the organization are often less effective. The word-of-mouth message may differ from the organization's stated policies. The establishment of defined processes helps achieve defined outcomes and provides a sense of security and reliability to those doing the work. When systems and processes are not clear and information is transferred by word of mouth, greater variation in outcome results. In a clinical setting where reliability is needed to ensure outcomes, patients are at risk from misinformation.

Because organizational policies, procedures, and systems can vary from organization to organization, policies and procedures are important to share with new members of the organization. When a nurse is new, someone in the organization should be dedicated to reviewing the policies and procedures, and these should be readily available both in hard copy and online. In an academic setting, the faculty handbook or student handbook serves as the repository of such policies. In the clinical delivery setting, policy and procedure books are used to guide practice decisions. Based on rapidly changing evidence, institutional policies are now kept current by use of an intranet. Whatever the format, these institutional policies and standards to which clinicians, faculty, staff, and students are held regarding delivery of care serve to guide the conduct of the organization's membership. A more detailed discussion of policy and guidelines follows in Chapter 7.

Consider: How do you find a policy or procedure related to a specific question in your organization? Remember when you first joined your organization, how were the policies and procedures introduced to you? What is the process and how often are your policies and procedures changed and updated?

Resources

All organizations have a defined set of resources and the ability to accomplish a set of activities. Five commonly discussed resources include money, time, human capital, reputation, and space. Money, as represented in the budget, is a critical resource and an important indicator of the organization's values. Being true to the mission and vision of the organization will help to set the course for the scope and priority of the activities to undertake, both core operational and strategic activities. The leader should have a good understanding of the financial picture of the organization and how the money is generated and spent, which is reflected in the organization's budget. A budget shows the sources of income, costs, and investments. Funding is often a source of competition between units within an organization with each unit vying for the funds necessary. Nursing personnel is the largest budget item for hospitals and long-term care organizations. When an organization needs to cut costs, often the nursing personnel budget is a place for possible cuts. Knowing the overall financial picture of an organization is essential in having adequate funding for nursing care, faculty positions, and other organizational strategic priorities. Currently, nursing education is seen as an important source of revenue for academic institutions and the challenge to leaders is to ensure that at least a certain portion of tuition and other income stays in the school to fund faculty and invest in new program development.

The leader must be able to clearly articulate the work of the organization and how time is spent in service to the organization's mission and vision. Organizations whose activities are too broad are at risk of not accomplishing their core activities. People in the organization may appear to be busy, but they are not accomplishing their goals and may be squandering resources. How much of the organization's time is spent in meetings? Are the meetings efficient? "Death by meeting" is said to characterize many academic organizations.

Reputation can be viewed as an organizational resource. Reputations are slow to change and can serve to bolster pride in an organization in difficult times and even steer talent and new resources toward the organization. Just as reputation can rise, reputations can fall precipitously. Part of the leader's responsibility is to evaluate the gap between the *reputation* and the *reality* of an organization. The leader must assess how good a job the organization can do given the strengths and skill gaps of employees. Being willing and able to provide constructive feedback to individuals who are not working up to expectations is a critical characteristic of effective leaders. Similarly, under-performing units with significant gaps between the reputation and reality may need to have the highest-level leaders enlisted to get their help to secure additional resources, make staff changes, and do whatever is necessary to close the gap.

For leaders in healthcare, a reputation of providing high quality care is critical. Rankings, and therefore business, depend on reputation and quality of service. Although reputation has many definitions, a useful conceptualization is that "reputation consists of familiarity with the organization, beliefs about what to expect from the organization in the future, and impressions about the organization's favorability" (Lange, Lee, and Dai, 2011). There are many sources of information about organizations, for example, The *U.S. News & World Report*, *Consumer Reports*, blogs, health websites such as the compare websites, social media groups, and more. Finding information about an organization is easy using one of the search engines. Google not only is the name of a company, but also is a verb. Use of technology-based information is going to increase, and organizational leaders will need to know how to use technology to best advance the organization. A survey by *Binary Fountain* (2020) found that 41% of respondents use online ratings and reviews when selecting a physician provider. More people are using social media and internet-based sources to make decisions. Health education and service organizations will be responding with changing goals and priorities depending on information and ratings from consumers.

Space is often seen as a symbol of power. The corner office or the windowed office holds high status. The dean's office is larger than the office of the staff assistant. Location also conveys status; for instance, to be located in a new hospital building or on a new campus may be viewed as superior to being in the basement of a building with seismic flaws. And we have begun to understand that the structure of our workspaces will influence efficiency of work in terms of how we move through and use the space, as well as how we feel in terms of comfort of the space. For instance, do we have wide halls with soft seating where people can congregate for informal meetings and furnishings, such as a fireplace or a piano to invite members of the organization to sit, relax, and interact.

Because an organization's resources are often limited, it is imperative that leaders be clear on how they are spending scarce resources to further the organization's missions and vision. Organizations can be resource-rich or resource-poor, and resources can vary across time, depending on the local or national economy or even the availability of safe, affordable housing. A full description of financial leadership is developed in Chapter 8.

Consider: **Review your organization's budget. What does it tell you about the financial health and priorities of the organization? How much time do you spend in meetings? Could this time be used more productively? How does your organization support professional development activities? How is your organization ranked by a variety of sources such as *The Blue Ridge Report* or *U.S. News & World Report*? Is the space you work in inviting and supportive of working efficiently?**

Human Capital Resources

Resources can also take the form of employee talent or human capital. Organizations will have unique characteristics that distinguish them from other organizations. However, organizations are collections of individuals, and each person must meet the needs of the organization by learning how to perform their work within the organization. The development of talent and talent management is a critical skill for the leader to develop.

It is often said that the most important resource in an organization are its people. The people in an organization have the responsibility for implementing the mission, producing the outcomes, and representing the organization to the community. Having the right people in the organization doing the right work with the skills to be able to adjust as the organization evolves is critical for success. The importance of the leader investing in the support, development, and satisfaction of the people of the organization cannot be overstated.

The human resource (HR) office of 10 years ago is very different from the contemporary HR office of today. In some cases, it is not even called human resources. Alternative names sometimes seen are human capital office, people operations, employee experience office, or partner resources. HR professionals spend less time on issues of employee oversight and discipline and more time on creating a workplace that supports the mission of the organization, enhances its culture and is inclusive and welcoming for all members of the organization. Common areas of involvement are talent acquisition, developing equity advocates, and making sure that federal and state regulations related to hiring and retention are followed. Acquiring and retaining human capital resources is discussed in Chapter 9.

Consider: **How have you interacted with your HR office in your organization? What is perception among your peers about the role of the HR office? Is it developmental and supportive or punitive? How do you think the HR office in your organization can be more responsive to the employees?**

Organizational Decision-Making

Decision-making within organizations is designed to select a course of action to achieve specific goals. Decisions are based on an analysis of the cost and benefits of an action. The costs and benefits can be based on financial impact, reputation, social mission, and other considerations. It is how people in the organization engage, and the type and level of engagement will vary according to assigned roles, culture, personal style, and preference for valued outcomes. For instance, organizations may decentralize decision-making to the "grass roots" or "front line" as a general philosophy and structure. Other organizations make decisions based on data that support a particular outcome (e.g., financial results) or without data, based on intuition or hunch. Recently, organizations have come to examine their decision-making process more precisely, using criteria related to specific goals and then evaluating the results against the criteria.

Without a careful and thoughtful structure and process, poor decisions can compromise patient care and the educational experience of students and faculty. Decision-making can be compromised because of a lack of information and expertise, implicit bias, and not having key stakeholders as part of the process. Importantly, as decisions are made, all relevant parties need to know and understand the decision! The failure to acknowledge that a decision has been made can result in confusion and requests to re-examine the decision, a process that can become cyclical and delay progress. The ways in which we frame decisions and use data will be the focus of Chapter 10.

Consider: **What decision-making groups are you part of and how are decisions made with each group? Do decisions within your organization include data and important stakeholders? How are decisions disseminated?**

Quality and Safety in Organizations

High quality care and patient safety as well as high quality of educational programs is the aim of clinical and academic leaders. Although quality improvement efforts have been based in a practical approach, more rigorous and scientific approaches are expanding. Quality improvement methods have been pioneered through efforts in manufacturing resulting in Toyota Production System, Lean, Six-Sigma, and others. These methods share common steps, including the definition of the problem, design and planning of the improvement effort, implementation and evaluation of the intervention, and finally sustaining and spreading the improvement. Important nationally accepted aims for clinical quality include STEEEP (safe, timely, equitable, efficient, effective, & patient centered) (*see* Figure 1.1).

In addition, the quadruple aim provides a broad brush set of goals, including affordability and patient satisfaction with care, with a focus on population health and a healthy workplace. Frameworks for quality education programs are program standards through organizations such as the Commission on Collegiate Nursing Education and the National League for Nursing Accrediting Commission. Successful completion of pre-licensure as well as advanced practice registered nurse programs leads to the quality control of licensure and certification.

Measures are the backbone of quality. The development of clinical measures requires rigorous research to ensure the validity, reliability, and usefulness of the measures. The rigor has become more critical as measure results have been linked to clinical payment. The ranking of nursing education pro-

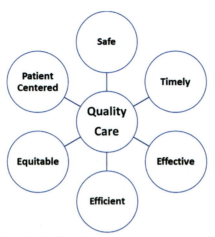

FIGURE 1.1 IOM Aims for Quality (Source: National Academy of Medicine, 2001, 5–6).

grams is based on the submission of data related to all aspects of educational programs including student experience, available resources, and research. We also need to ensure that the measures give us information that is actionable. A framework for measures developed by Donabedian in the 1960's remains useful in both clinical and academic organizations and includes measures of structure, process, and outcome. More in depth information about quality and safety is in Chapter 11.

Consider: **Is quality central to the mission and vision of the organization you work in? How is the importance of measuring quality communicated throughout your organization?**

Organizational Communication Styles

Whether written or spoken, all organizations have styles of communicating, including who speaks to whom and when and about what. Networks of communication can include both internal and external channels through which formal and informal communications are transmitted. *External formal* networks might include groups of individuals who help you accomplish the work in your organization, such as the role of the Oncology Nurses Association for nurses who work within the specialty of oncology care. Whether in education or care delivery, this large professional organization of nurses sets standards, shares information, raises funds to support scholarships and awards for its members, and provides support for career advancement.

External informal networks are also the source of important information and may be more difficult to access, because they are often unknown to others outside the network. For instance, a group of eight nurses who work in the same organization or are in different organizations may share interests in a common area and hold a private Zoom meeting every month to support one another and share information that is not yet public but will help them do a better job.

Internal networks, formal and informal, may provide many similar functions and are also important to an organization and its members. Internal networking helps people make the connections and learn ways of accomplishing their work. The stronger the interoffice relationships are, the more success there will be with collaboration and communication between employees. Some networks will provide information about career opportunities; others will share the "gossip" before it becomes public. As a leader of an organization, participating in educational programs or events may introduce you to others who share common interests and challenges. Volunteering for a leadership role will provide the opportunity to meet other leaders in your organization. Volunteering in this capacity not only introduces you to people outside your usual circle of colleagues, but also it is a great way to show your leadership skills. Some organizations have regular newsletters or video clips, whereas others organize after hours happy hours. In all cases, it is useful to know how information is shared internally, both formally and informally.

Important, but often overlooked, is the role of rumor in organizations. If you want to understand where information goes and who carries messages, you can seed an informational message of your own and watch where it travels. This can be an informative way to assess the informal movement of messages.

Although communication is part of our everyday lives, approaches to communication must be intentional and tailored to the circumstances of the situation. Engaging in difficult conversations, communicating with your boss, or communicating in a crisis requires thoughtfulness and leadership skills to be effective. Dimensions of effective communication are explored in Chapter 12, which also provides in-depth information about communication skills, strategies and tactics.

Consider: **How do you get information within your organization? Primarily, with whom do you communicate? Who communicates with you? With which external organizations does your organization communicate? Which electronic platforms does your organization use?**

The Importance of Teams

The value of teams in healthcare continues to be demonstrated in both patient and provider satisfaction and in the quality of patient and student outcomes.

Teams are two or more people who work together toward a shared goal/s and the accomplishment of the mission of the organization. Teams can be defined as several nurses working together or a nurse, physician, physical therapist, and social worker collaborating on a patient situation. An example of an academic team could be two faculty members who are teaching a course in healthcare in prisons. One faculty member from the School of Nursing is an expert on the health of prisoners and the other faculty member from the School of Liberal Arts is an expert in the state correction system. The importance of interdisciplinary teams or interprofessional teams is that each member of the team brings a unique skill set and perspective that allows for a better clinical or academic outcome. Having a team in which members have different skills, experiences, and knowledge provides a wider array of ideas that can be brought to bear on a decision.

Many clinical care delivery organizations use teams composed of people with different expertise or points of view to make policy or to deliver care. Effective teamwork has multiple benefits, including exchange of ideas that promotes problem solving, adding capacity and complementary styles, learning from other members of the team, and fostering the sense of belonging that is critical to job satisfaction. In academia, team teaching is a frequently used model to allow students to learn from experts in two areas. Regardless of the team setting, the goal of all teams is to be high-performing. High-performing teams are able to work effectively together to achieve their objective and contribute to the mission of the organization.

Effective leaders know how to develop collaborative teams able to achieve expected goals. Working in a team allows employees to experience the rich diversity seen in many organizations and benefit from the diversity of thought that makes problem solving more effective. Composing teams and fostering team development will be discussed in greater detail in Chapter 13.

> *Consider*: **What teams have you been part of in your organization? How effective have they been? What role do you usually play when you are part of a team? Do you often rise to the position of leader? If so, why do you think that happens? What challenges have you seen play out in dysfunctional teams? Would you prefer to work in a team or independently? Why?**

Change and Innovation

Although organizational leaders need to be clear about the roles and responsibilities of everyone in their sphere of responsibilities, it is also important to empower people to think about ways of providing better care or employing more effective and creative teaching methods. It is important for the leader to create a balance to empower creativity while maintaining known standards reflected in guides to systems and processes. An example is the recognition of the demographic shift that is occurring in higher education represented by a decrease in the number of high school graduates and the shrinking applicant pool. If an admissions office were to continue to follow a traditional system of recruitment and admission that was successful 10 years ago and not include some new ways of thinking about an applicant's qualifications, the system would not change. Likely, the ability of the organization to recruit a diverse and more representative group of students would be limited. Disruptions in organizations can be caused by external trends that may come on slowly and predictably, or by extreme and unpredicted changes, such as the COVID-19 pandemic. Regardless of the type of disruption, change can be difficult for people and for organizations. Some organizational forces push toward change while countervailing forces maintain the status quo.

Innovating in health care delivery and nursing education is essential to advancing the discipline of nursing and improving the product delivered to patients or students. The work of the leader in times of change, including assessing organizational forces, managing change, and innovating will be discussed more fully in Chapter 14.

Consider: How has change occurred in your organization? Have the affected employees been involved in the change process? Has the change process been seen as positive with those who are most affected? How would you describe your organization's receptivity to change? What are the biggest barriers to change in your organization?

ORGANIZATIONS DEVELOP AS DO THE PEOPLE WITHIN THEM

Social systems evolve or devolve over time. Most nurses study human development and assume that people will grow and change over time. Various classic developmental theorists address these changes; some focus on concepts of developing cognition such as the work of Piaget (1964) or Kohlberg's (1984) moral development, whereas others such as Erikson (1950) focus on human interaction across the life cycle. One dimension of the work of nursing is observing patterns across time, some of which involve growth and development of individuals.

The social system of the family is similarly thought to develop over time (e.g., Duvall, 1962) through a set of epigenetic stages that are set/reset according to the age of the oldest child. Interventions with the family should be stage appropriate. Similarly, the social system of the group may also be viewed as having stages such as Tuckman's (1965) "forming, norming, storming, performing, adjourning." Understanding the stage of group development and the challenges faced by the group at any given stage is a significant consideration for a group leader planning interventions.

Understanding organizational development is important to the organizationally minded leader. Most theorists discuss the development of organizations as an aspect of change. In other words, the framework for organizational development addresses how organizations are behaving at baseline, how they behave as change begins and, finally, how to support organizations in establishing a fixed pattern after change. Although change theories such as those proposed by Kotter (2012) or Lewin (1951) can be useful for understanding organizational change, leaders often use these theories in combination with theories about other concepts. For instance, understanding Benner's Skill Acquisition Framework for Nursing (1984) will guide a nurse manager to think about the best way to support and develop an individual nurse. Understanding theories of group development (Tuckman, 1965) will guide the dean who is working toward a cooperative agreement between several department chairs.

In addition, organizations have past histories and current cultures, and these can represent barriers (or facilitators) to change. For instance, organizational pride and contentment can blind the organization's members, who focus on the historical greatness and accomplishments of the past, overlooking the fact that the current environment is vastly different from the past. The belief that "we have never done that before" can be so strong as to deter those who might propose that "we can do it now, and we must."

Importantly, in beginning leadership work, the individual members of the organization are often the focus of the leader's attention. Understanding communication theory, and human behavior and development, is a plus, but the point of organizationally minded leadership is to consider how to view the individuals as part of the organization and how to view the emergent properties of the organization.

Work of the Organizationally Minded Leader

Given the overview of the qualities of the organization described in this chapter and the promise to provide additional depth on these qualities in subsequent chapters, it should not be a surprise to the reader that these qualities have something to do with organizationally minded leadership. Organizations, as social systems, display *emergent* properties. Emergent properties are those that result from the interaction of other smaller parts of the system that do not display those properties by themselves. For instance, the 45 nurses working in a medical surgical unit may provide far more support to one another than the 45 individual nurses who work on the cardiology unit. The quality of group supportiveness may also be displayed in the academic department of family health care but may not be apparent in the department of continuing education. These emergent properties can be changed by intentional leadership interventions; however, intervention begins with a conscious awareness, or assessment, of the properties featured by each unit or microsystem within an organization.

As with other clinical interventions, assessment serves as the basis for designing interventions. Interventions are implemented with an outcome in mind; those outcomes need to be evaluated and additional interventions considered if needed.

Guidance for the Organizationally Minded Leader

The leadership literature offers considerable guidance to the would-be leader. That guidance often includes directives on individual behavior, for instance, to develop a set of core characteristics, including trustworthiness, character, compassion, competence, selflessness, and integrity. Additional characteristics have been recommended to these core and classic attributes, and these are believed to address the complexity of effective leadership in today's organizations. Organizationally minded leaders should do the following:

Be Credible and Develop Trust with those They Lead

Leadership is about relationships. Credibility is the cornerstone of effective leadership (Kouzes & Posner, 2017, Covey, 2006). To accomplish this, leaders must have integrity, others must resonate with their intentions, they must be capable and viewed as such by others, and they must produce results consistently that resonate with the organization and those who they lead. These qualities and relationships occur over time and leaders must constantly be aware of the trust level experienced by those they serve.

Embrace Change and Envision the Future

New approaches to organizational structure are possible because of advances in technology and new views on centralized authority. In many organizations, it is not necessary for every member of an organization to be present for each day of work. For example, a faculty member may work from home, attending meetings by video conference and providing online office hours for students. Trips to campus would be infrequent and mainly for teaching classes or attending meetings where a videoconference connection is impossible. In the clinical setting, this structural flexibility might not be possible, but embracing innovations in the use of technology in all settings has the potential to improve the efficiency and effectiveness of organizations.

Leaders should also be open to the possibility that hierarchical authority paradigms may not be the best way to organize a system. Allowing members to have the authority for the work they are closest to might, in fact, be a much more efficient way to organize. Distributing authority provides for more fluid boundaries and efficiencies that cannot be produced in a stiff hierarchical structure.

Use and Share Data for Making Decisions

The ability to look past the horizon and see the opportunities and challenges that are coming toward the organization is an important characteristic of an organizationally minded leader. To create a picture of the future, leaders should be adept at mining data and gathering perceptions from their team to identify issues and trends that are needed to anticipate the future. Much of this work takes time. Leaders may need to adjust information technology systems to answer an important question or may need to plan a retreat to discuss a critical issue. Although time is always in short supply, it will be necessary to invest in this work to be fully prepared for the changes as they arise. Leaders should also plan time for in depth thinking, analysis, and reflection for themselves. Most leaders spend their days going from meeting to meeting and task to task. There is little time left for the in-depth thinking and analysis that is necessary for creating a clear picture of the future. Planning for that time, just as one would plan for a meeting, is essential.

Be an Expert Communicator and Collaborator

One of the most important responsibilities within the organization is to communicate clearly, effectively, and efficiently. Communication is a key medium of effecting organizational change. In many organizations, the amount and type of communications within the organization is a source of discontent among the employees. Deciding how much to communicate and when is a challenge for leaders. Too much communication turns everything that is sent out to employees into white noise. No one pays attention to even the really important information. Too little communication allows people to wonder about what is happening in the organization and feeds the rumor mills that inevitably exist.

Being an expert communicator not only involves sharing information, but also requires the leader to be an effective and strategic listener. It is important to know when to convene the team to hear their perspective on an issue. Asking for input and listening actively allows team members to feel as though they are valued members of the organization.

Support Risk Taking and Resilience in Self and Others

Because both successes and failures happen every day in organizations, it is critical that leaders role model these behaviors. Leaders, like everyone, are fallible and letting those they work with know this creates a sense of psychological safety within organizations. Leaders should encourage curiosity, questions, disagreements, and respectful debates with the aim of ensuring transparency and trust. In many organizations, there is a culture that defines the amount of risk the organization will feel comfortable with. Organizationally minded leaders understand that risk tolerance and work in ways that are consistent with the culture of the organization. In today's organizational climate, the concept of risk is ubiquitous. As organizations innovate in products and services or embrace creative ideas that will distinguish them in the marketplace, some new initiatives will be successful and others will not. The ability to learn from the failure and put the organization on the right path is an important characteristic of an organizationally minded leader. The business literature often talks about the process of "failing fast." The goal is not to fail, but if one does fail, they learn quickly that the path they are going down is wrong. In response to that learning, one should tweak, reset, and then redo if necessary.

Create Governance Structures and a Culture in which Shared Decision-Making is Valued and in which the Voice of the Diverse Community, Consumers, and Those Who Work in the Organization is Consistently Present and Influential

Entrenched structural inequities that are subtle and complex exist in both academic and healthcare institutions. Racism is the most prominent oppressive inequity, although there are certainly more. Structural racism in healthcare delivery and education, including higher education, perpetuates the practices that result in inequities in health care delivery and outcomes.

Policies, procedure, norms, and practices of organizations often advantage white people and disadvantage people of color, and those who identify as LGBTQ. Because these differences are long-standing and the practices are assumed to work, the ways in which they work against some groups generally goes unnoticed. As a result, the leader must first recognize structural inequities and call the attention of others to the problem. The leader must render the problem visible.

As reported in 2018, based on the NCSBN National Nursing Workforce Survey, the diversity of the US population of registered nurses still lags the US population. The US population of minorities is 40% (US Census, 2021) and the population of registered nurses who identify as minorities is 30.9% (Zippia, 2021). Based on a developing literature, the ethnic, racial and gender diversification of the nursing profession is expected to better meet the needs of the population served and improve the educational and care delivery outcomes for the diverse US population.

Leaders must be ready and willing to change the policies and practices of the organization to create an environment that is more inclusive, respectful, equitable, and welcoming for all. The process of change begins with deeply listening to the members of the organization who are most directly affected by policies and practices that are racist. Often leaders get so used to the "way things are done" that they become oblivious to the pain and stress these policies and practices cause in the non-white and other oppressed members of the organization. Willingness to make change based on fully understanding the complexity of white privilege and racism as well as other forms of oppression is the first step. Examining the policies, practices, and power dynamics and beginning dialogues to co-create a new future is the second step, which can only happen when leaders fully appreciate the perceptions and lived experiences of all members of the organization. The goal is to create an inclusive, respectful, equitable, and socially just community for all people (Gilliss *et al.*, 2010).

Be comfortable making decisions and strengthen and encourage others to do so as well. Priority setting and the related decision-making is one of the most important roles of the organizationally minded leader. The organization and its members look to the leader to set the direction, give them information on the path forward, and help them to see how organizational challenges will be managed. All these expectations rely on a leader who can be an effective and efficient decision-maker. It will be important to recognize that not all decisions will be appreciated or welcomed by the members of the organization. Even if you seek input, weigh the options, and base your decision on data, there will be people in the organization who will not be pleased. By recognizing that "you can't please everyone" in advance of the decision-making process, the leader is better prepared to address any negative consequences of the decision.

Be positive, share a common purpose, and spread joy in the workplace. Many organizations today are experiencing periods of rapid, transformational change, which requires a transformational response. These responses are often labor intensive and can be physically and emotionally draining for the leader. Even in the face of significant organizational challenges, leaders should radiate positive energy and enthusiasm to the members of their respective organizations. Sharing a positive attitude and helping people be positive, not overwhelmed, in the face of difficult situations is an important role of the organizational leader.

To retain that positive energy and enthusiasm, leaders need to work on their physical and emotional well-being and find ways to help others do so as well. As healthcare leaders, we know the importance of maintaining health. Mindfulness, exercise, good nutrition, stress reduction, and work life balance are all essential components of health maintenance for the leaders. Leaders cannot manage the stress associated with most leadership roles and be effective role models for healthy behaviors if they do not practice these behaviors and support their staff members to do the same. The importance of and models for self-care for the leader are discussed in Chapter 15.

SUMMARY

This chapter provided the context for organizational leadership. A definition of organizational leadership was provided and the authors stated their belief that a focus on the organization is essential to creating change. Given the unique characteristics of the healthcare system in today's environment, leaders need to employ all the characteristics noted to create efficient and effective healthcare and academic organizations. The importance of working to create just and equitable systems of healthcare and education are integral to the work of the organizational leader. The importance of a social justice lens in all aspects of leadership is threaded throughout this chapter.

REFERENCES

Benner, Patricia (1984). *From novice to expert: Excellence and power in clinical nursing practice*. Menlo Park, CA: Addison-Wesley Pub.

Binary Fountain (2020). 2020 Healthcare Consumer Insight & Digital Engagement Survey. https://go.binaryfountain.com/2020-healthcare-consumer-survey-ebook.html

Cancialosi, C. (2017, July 17). *What is organizational culture?* Gotham Culture. https://gothamculture.com/what-is-organizational-culture-definition/.

Covey, S. R. (2006). *The speed of trust*. Simon & Schuster.

Duvall, E. M. (1962). *Family development* (2nd ed.). Lippincott.

Erikson, E. H. (1950). Childhood and society. W. W. Norton & Co.

Gilliss, C. L., Powell, D. L., and Carter, B. (2010), "Recruiting and retaining a diverse workforce in nursing: From evidence to best practices to policy." *Policy, Politics, & Nursing Practice* 11, no. 4: 294–301. https://doi.org/10.1177/1527154411398491.

Kohlberg, L. (1984). *The psychology of moral development: The nature and validity of moral stages*. Harper & Row.

Kotter, J. P. (2012). *Leading change*. Harvard Business Review Press.

Kouzes, J. M., & Posner, B. Z. (2017) *The leadership challenge: How to make extraordinary things happen in organizations*. Jossey-Bass.

Lange, D., Lee, P. M., Dai, Y. (2011). Organizational reputation: A Review. *Journal of Management, 37*(1), 153–184. https://doi.org/10.1177/0149206310390963

Lewin, K. (1951). *Field theory in social science: Selected theoretical papers*. D. Cartwright (ed.). Harper & Row.

National Academy of Medicine (2001). *Crossing the Quality Chasm: A New Health System for the 21st Century*. Washington DC: National Academy Press.

Piaget, J. (1964). Cognitive development in children: Development and learning. *Journal of Research in Science Teaching, 2*, 176–186. http://dx.doi.org/10.1002/tea.3660020306

Tsai, Y. (2011). Relationship between organizational culture, leadership behavior and job satisfaction. *BMC Health Serv Res, 11*, 98. https://doi.org/10.1186/1472-6963-11-98

Tuckman, B. W. (1965). Developmental sequence in small groups. *Psychological Bulletin, 63*(6), 384-399. https://doi.org/10.1037/h0022100

US Census Bureau (2021) http://census.gov/quickfacts/fact/table/US/PST045221

Zippia (2021) Registered Nurse Statistics by Race: https://www.zippia.com/registered-nurse-jobs/demographics/

CHAPTER 2

Thinking About Organizational Leadership Developmentally and Theoretically

INTRODUCTION

Thinking theoretically about leadership and organizations will guide you toward a systematic way of thinking about and understanding the current state of an organization and its composite features and matching leadership interventions to achieve a desired outcome. As noted in Chapter 1, the context for leading in healthcare organizations differs from leading in other industries. There are also differences between leading in the service sector of healthcare and leading in the academic sector within the broad community of healthcare.

Healthcare, which accounted for about 7% of Gross Domestic Product (GDP) in the late 1970s, has grown to represent nearly 18% of the GDP as of 2018 (CMS, 2020). Healthcare became the United States' (US) largest employer in 2017 (Thompson 2018), and the US Labor Department identified the US healthcare sector as a continued area for job growth over the next decade (US Bureau of Labor Statistics 2020). Recognizing today's vastness of the healthcare enterprise is a clarion call for effective leadership.

Healthcare organizations have continuously evolved since the establishment of the Pennsylvania Hospital of Philadelphia in 1752. Today, many different types of organizations comprise the health system, including provider organizations (hospitals, clinics, acute rehabilitation, schools, retail, long term care facilities, etc.), insurers, device and pharmaceutical manufacturers, and more. Healthcare systems are constantly changing with more provider groups merging or partnering with other types of organizations such as insurer groups, pharmaceutical groups, and major retail pharmacy chains merging with major health insurance organizations. Health systems include a variety of care segments including outpatient, acute care, home care, and other services. Each organization is complex, and the collective of interconnected organizational units into health systems produces an even more complicated organizational environment.

Academic environments that focus on preparing health care providers, scholars and researchers are also very complex given the unique relationships needed between the service sector and academic programs. The need for clinical placements, the recruitment of clinical research subjects and research collaborators require strong connections that have to be developed and nurtured. Academic programs that have overlapping content such as nurse practitioner and physician assistant education often have the additional challenge of internal negotiation for external resources such as clinical placements.

Our perspective on leadership varies somewhat from that of many other leaders, authors, and scholars. We believe that the point of leadership is to advance the work of the organization and that work is done by the people. As such, the work of an organization is both contextual and interactive. Our intention is to support the development of the reader's understanding of both the organization's features (as developed in Section II: Understanding the Elements of Organizational Life) and the interactive characteristics of an effective leader. We will examine strategies to guide the reader in how to interact or intervene within an organizational context in light of the organization's particular qualities or characteristics. We think of leadership as a set of organizational interventions that are informed by both empirical and non-empirical evidence, including theories and frameworks. This chapter defines organizational development and describes its historical evolution. The contemporary theories and frameworks that can be used to examine organizations are included.

In general, theories are thought to differ from frameworks in that proof exists for theories that supports their reliability and ability to predict and explain phenomena. Frameworks identify the salient features of a model but lack accumulated proof for their validity and reliability. The research literature on leadership is not well developed by scientific standards. Therefore, our purpose in this chapter is to promote a disciplined way of assessing, intervening, and evaluating leadership interventions.

What is Organizational Development?

Understanding organizational development is critical to being an effective leader in today's organizational context. The understanding of organizational efficiency and management of change has expanded greatly over the past several decades. Organizational development assumes that the organization develops over time, from a less developed form to a form that is more complex. Organizations can stall in their development, or even regress, depending upon the resources available to them and the challenges they face. Organizational development is system oriented in that it requires a focus on the whole of the organization as well as its component parts. Organizational development is also process-focused, requiring attention to the way events occur and whether they occur at all. This framework assumes that organizations are systems and that the behavior of individuals and groups are significant as a demonstration of an organizational phenomenon, and not just the random acts of those individuals or groups.

Within the framework of organizational development, leadership interventions are thought to take several forms, each aimed at changing the dynamics or functionality of the organization. Remembering that organizations are comprised of people and sub-groups, some interventions focus on changing human processes; for instance, changing an individual's communication, focusing on group dynamics, introducing a third party (consultant), or focusing on the development of a highly functional team. Other human process interventions might include confronting the group (or members of a group) by explicitly identifying a problem, disrupting intergroup relations, or intentionally disrupting the process of a large group.

Organizational dynamics can be also changed by technical or structural changes, such as the redesign of workflow or the restructuring of position responsibilities. An HR approach to intervention might include programs focused on diversity and wellness, or performance management and development (ex. through coaching). Strategic changes are influential by changing expectations, mission, and expected outcomes.

Although there are numerous definitions of organizational development theory, a working definition is the following:

> "Organizational Development is an effort planned, organization-wide, and managed from the top, to increase organization effectiveness and health through planned interventions in the organization's 'processes,' using behavioral-science knowledge." (Beckhard 1969)

This definition captures the key elements of organizational development that incorporates knowledge and reflects the role of science. It also makes individuals central as the source of change, and that change is the key to organizational effectiveness.

THE EVOLUTION OF ORGANIZATIONAL DEVELOPMENT

Early Phases of Organizational Development

A precursor to the development of organizational theory was the focus on the efficiency of manufacturing. Seminal work was done in the early 1900s by Frederick Winslow Taylor, a mechanical engineer, who was the first to bring a scientific approach to the work of an organization. Taylor promoted the idea of efficiency in the workplace and that the workers whose skills were best matched to the work to be done should be chosen for hire. He also suggested that training of workers will ensure competency and the importance of a working relationship between management and workers (Taylor, 1911). While Taylor's work laid the groundwork for organizational development, he considered workers an input, whose work could be precisely described and performed.

The 1940s saw the emergence of a more humanistic approach to workers. Kurt Lewin was a pioneer in the US who recognized the importance of understanding the motivations, needs, and values to produce a more effective workforce (Lewin, 1935). As a social psychologist, Lewin is sometimes referred to as the "grandfather of applied behavioral sciences" (Scherer, Alban, and Weisbord, 2016). Lewin consulted with the Harwood Manufacturing Company to understand why they were underperforming financially and losing workers at a high rate of turnover. The consultants interviewed managers and front-line workers and made observations. Their recommendation was to experiment with front-line workers to see how they would respond to change. This was an approach that was very unusual for the time.

The experiment was based on the assumption that individual behaviors were not only a function of personal factors but were influenced by the organizational context in which they occurred. In other words, context matters. Discussions among the workers and debriefing sessions revealed the value of "here and now" interactions (Scherer, Alban, and Weisbord, 2016) in creating changes in understanding about what was going on. As a result of this and other experiences, Lewin began the first "training groups" in the 1940s. Also known as the "T Group movement," launched at the National Training Laboratory (NTL) in Bethel, Maine, Lewin focused on the study of human relations, which led to the organizational development movement. These discussions came to be called "sensitivity training" sessions and were expanded by the NTL. "T-groups" focused on self-understanding and the development of self-awareness. The power of the small group emerged as a critical factor in influencing behavior and came to be understood as a basic unit of organizational change.

Lewin's work set the stage for modern day organizational development approaches through three areas of work: values, premises, and methods. The values encompassed a belief in democracy, the primacy of small groups, and the importance of science to inform social change. Lewin was an advocate for the importance of workers and managers forming a constructive relationship to improve the functioning of an organization, and that the workers were very important to change. Premises included field theory and the primacy of small groups. Field theory included all behavior, both internal and external forces, and the driving or restraining forces need to change. Driving forces push in the direction to cause change to happen, while restraining forces in an organization are those which are obstacles to change. Lewin suggested that interventions could be analyzed for ongoing consequences and could promote driving or restraining forces, based on the desired outcome of change. Small groups were viewed as the social unit within organizations that were the primary drivers of constructive change.

Lewin's methods included action research which were critical to understanding force field impact, and as an intervention undertaken to bring about positive social change that was necessary to organizational development (Lewin, 1946). Action research is seen as collaborative problem-solving, with members of a social system being involved in the investigations of their own field of forces and creating interventions to change the force field. This process was an iterative process similar to the quality improvement process used today of Plan, Do, Study, Act. Attention was on group dynamics exploring how groups form and function with change.

Another contribution in terms of his methods included the Three Step Model of change: unfreeze, movement (change), and refreeze. A pillar of Lewin's major work proposed a way of thinking about how social changes take place. The three phases, unfreezing, changing and refreezing, follow in sequence. Unfreezing involves moving to realize that a change is needed. Many circumstances can affect this phase, but creating urgency is a common approach to moving people along in their thinking. Budget cuts, imposed deadlines, and unexpected crises are all examples that can accelerate the process of unfreezing. Another strategy involves creating a more compelling vision for the future.

Changing involves exploring new behaviors or approaches and beginning to test these. In this phase, the need for change has been recognized and now the work shifts to finding acceptable new approaches to operating. The work of this phase is difficult. People do not accept change at the same rates so the early adopters may be ready to move while those resisting change lag behind. Keeping track of all parties is important to the work of leadership, so that those slow to change are still valued and respected.

Refreezing follows the period of change and involves institutionalizing the new changes or approaches. In refreezing, people may celebrate the successes associated with the change or may depart the organization in protest. Policies are rewritten, and more formalized rules are developed to support the new approaches.

Lewin generated a remarkable legacy in laying a framework for organizational development and in the 1960s and the 1970s, Lewin's work was expanded. The ideas that were prominent during this time frame included scientific positivism which suggests that the only authentic knowledge is scientific knowledge, and that such knowledge can only come from positive affirmation of theories through strict scientific method. Organizations were beginning to be seen as open systems that interact with their environment rather than mechanistic entities. Considerable attention was paid to team dynamics and team building. There was a positive view of people and their potential based on humanistic and existential psychology theories, such as those proposed by Carl Rogers (1951), Rollo May (1950), and Abraham Maslow (1943).

The 1980s and 1990s moved away from the world of objectivity and toward the world of social constructs and social sciences. Action research was expanded into action inquiry (a way of simultaneously conducting action and inquiry as a disciplined leadership practice that increases the wider effectiveness of actions [Steckler and Torbet, 2010]), and appreciative inquiry (a collaborative, group approach to making change in organizations) gained credibility. The focus on groups was extended to large groups and interventions that would be effective. Attention was given to the meaning of work and the language used within organizations recognizing that language was not just passively descriptive but was shaping reality. The idea of change moved from episodic in which there was a beginning, middle, and end, to realizing change as a chaotic, fluid, and organic experience. There began to be attention to broader social impacts, and a broader set of democratic ideals. Thought leaders, such as Edgar Schein (1984), proposed his organizational culture model, which was among the first to recognize that organizations had cultures that were based on assumptions, espoused values, and used artifacts and symbols to represent the organization.

Today, the field of organizational development is rich and varied, integrating more traditional ideas and newer views and mixing these in innovative ways. Blended approaches use many different areas of knowledge and inquiry to constantly work at understanding organizational development and change. Today's work is greatly influenced by what is considered the fourth industrial revolution, which includes the integration of technology-based supports into the workplace. The work in artificial intelligence, large data sets, machine to machine communication, robotics, sensors, self-monitoring devices, and many other technologies continue to challenge our understanding of organizational development and how people find meaning in their work.

Organizational Development Practitioner

Those employing organizational development as a guiding theory refer to themselves as "Organizational development (OD) practitioners" (Anderson, 2017). OD practitioners can, and often do, include consultants who are external to the organization; however, whether external to or internal to an organization, the work of the OD practitioner is to help the organization's members effect constructive change. When using the organizational development framework, the work of a leader is about assisting organizations to advance in their development. Some experts distinguish the role of the OD practitioner from the strategist, with the former focused on the internal resources and dynamics and the latter focused on the external environment (Cheung-Judge and Holbeche, 2015). That distinction seems to blur in the face of the rapid cycle changes seen in healthcare delivery and the educational systems that prepare healthcare providers. In this discussion, we assume that the leader has responsibility for both and will use the term OD practitioner to mean the leader.

Our Model of Organizationally-Minded Leadership

We have integrated a mixed model of theories and frameworks reflecting eclectic thinking about organizational development. Our model integrates our definition of organizational leadership as noted in Chapter 1.

The effective organizational leader recognizes and engages the interconnected components of an organization with relationship building being paramount to creating a culture of productivity, innovation, ethical decision-making, inclusivity, and compassion with organizations being greater than the sum of its parts. This definition requires one to be open to a variety of scientific traditions and thinking. To recognize the contributing theories and frameworks, as well as provide a way of thinking about leadership of organizations, we incorporate the theories of change, strategic management, systems, and humanism as shown in Figure 2.1. Throughout this book we have included select theories and frameworks as they relate to organizationally-minded leadership.

Humanistic Theories/Frameworks

Humanistic thinking related to organizations began in the 1930s with the work of Lewin who recognized the importance of developing the human capital of an organization. Psychologists such as Carl Rogers, who is considered the father of humanistic psychology, contributed to the thinking that considered a view that recognized the emotional needs of individuals (Rogers, 1961). Until the 1950s, psychology was dominated by the thinking that people had little control of themselves. From a psychoanalytic perspective, people were controlled by unconscious thoughts, and from a behaviorist perspective, biology dominated behavior. Rogers' model believed that people were motivated

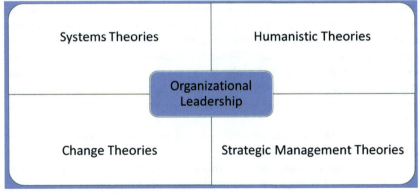

FIGURE 2.1 Organizational Development Leadership.

to achieve their full potential. He introduced thinking about the self in terms of self-worth, self-image, and ideal self. His model of person-centered therapy integrated unconditional positive regard, empathy, and congruence. In addition to Rogers, Abraham Maslow contributed to humanistic psychology with his paper *Theory of Human Motivation* (Maslow, 1943). This paper described a hierarchy of human needs that later was depicted as a pyramid beginning with the physiologic needs and rising to self actualization.

A major contributor to the movement toward humanism in the workplace was Mary Follett, who had a social service background and was one of the first, if not the first, woman consultant in organizational management. She noted that workers are most productive when they participate in decision-making and are part of any conflict resolution efforts between management and workers. Her work was remarkable, given she was a woman who challenged the hierarchical practices of the early 1900s. The work of Follett and the psychological humanism work of Rogers, Maslow, and others overlapped with the work of Elton Mayo in his Hawthorne experiments at Western Electric Company (Mayo, 1946). Mayo found that group dynamics were important in productivity and workers wanted to have meaning in what they do. Communication and cooperation between workers and management resulted in greater efficiency (Follett, 1927). The work of Argyris and Schein continued to explore humanism within organizations. Argyris noted that important aspects of the life of a worker include motivation, empowerment, and accountability (Argyris, 1964). Schein (2010) contributed to recognition of organizational culture having a powerful effect on productivity.

Today, there is a great deal of attention to the human factors in the workplace. There is the recognition of the importance of meaning in work, group dynamics, and human self-actualization. There is also the recognition of the role of a leader's emotional intelligence as very important to effective leadership and productive organizations. Emotional Intelligence is defined as the capability of individuals to recognize their own emotions and those of others, discern between different feelings and label them appropriately, use emotional information to guide thinking and behavior, and adjust emotions to adapt to environments (Colman, 2008). The seminal work of Goleman and others have strongly noted that emotional self-awareness and management, as well as social awareness and management, play a very major role in organizational effectiveness (Goleman, 1995). The emotional capability of a leader clearly helps to understand the humanistic needs of followers and supports the ability to act humanistically.

More recently, the Institute of Healthcare Improvement has promulgated the idea and related strategies of "Joy in the Workplace." The premise of a recent white paper is that finding purpose and meaning in work results in an increased level of engagement and improved overall organizational outcomes (Perlo *et al.,* 2017).

There is another major phenomenon in healthcare organizations and academia today related to dismantling structural racism. Racism and inequalities in social determinants of health set the stage for this unequal access to high quality care and racial disparities. Student admission practices, hiring of faculty and employee promotion are areas where structural racism is evident is in academia. There are several key steps organizations are taking today to eliminate structural racism, including improved data collection related to race and ethnicity, documenting the health impact of racism, assessing eliminating racist policies and practices at the individual and organizational levels (Baily, Felman, and Bassett, 2020).

Systems Theories/Frameworks

Systems theory is an approach to organizations that recognizes the interdependence of the parts that have defined functions as well as the interrelated responsibilities. The organization influences and is influenced by the external and internal environments. If one part of the organization is affected by an external force the entire organization is affected, which likens the enterprise to an organism with interdependent parts, each with its own specific function and interrelated responsibilities. Von Bertalanffy (1956), a biologist, provided an early framework for understanding that when elements are in interaction, they influence one another providing positive and negative feedback that impact future interactions. Inputs, processes, and outputs all have the power to influence how the system operates and therefore, influencing one will influence the others. Peter Senge (1990), in his acclaimed book on system thinking, defined system thinking as a holistic approach to analysis that focuses on the way that a system's constituent parts interrelate, and how systems work overtime and within the context of larger systems.

Strategic Management Theories/Frameworks

Strategic management frames an organization's ability to attain its goals. A practical definition of strategic management is:

> An organization's process of continuous planning, executing, monitoring, analyzing, and assessing all that is necessary for an organization to meet its goals and objectives in pursuit of a future direction (LBL Strategies Team 2020).

Models of strategic management are numerous. We have found Thompson and Strickland's 7 Forces Model (Thompson & Strickland 2001) especially useful. This model considers:

1. Industry's dominant economic features

2. Main sources of competitive pressure and the strengths of the competitive forces

3. Driving forces

4. Market position of the rival companies

5. Competitor's strategic moves

6. Industry's key success factors

7. Industry's overall attractiveness and profitability prospects

In addition, the Hofer and Schendel model offers guidance for both the planning and activation phases of strategy (Hofer and Schendel, 1978). The varied strategic management models all include goal setting linked with the organization's mission, evaluation of strengths, and weaknesses including internal and external factors. Financial sustainability is also integrated into the models. Strategic management integrates a number of tools, including strategic mapping, SWOT (strengths, weaknesses, opportunities, and threats) analysis, and value chain analysis.

Change Theories/Frameworks

Change is a constant in today's healthcare environment. Change comes in many forms, including new treatments and diagnostics, regulations and legislation governing access, cost and quality, new health needs, and related technologies and approaches to education (e.g., those developed to address the COVID-19 pandemic in 2020 and 2021, the aging of the population, or accessing rural populations). Change produces significant challenges particularly when change is strongly linked to uncertainty. Change theory has typically explained how constructive change can take place within an organization. There are many frameworks and theories to explain change. Several that have been useful to the authors include Lewin's unfreeze, change, and refreeze as described above. In addition, the work of Kotter (2012) has contributed to understanding the process of change in identifying eight steps of change. The Conners and Smith Model, recognizes change depends on people's experiences that influence their values and beliefs, that in turn impacts action, and therefore produces the achievement of goals (Conners and Smith, 2011).

Today's guiding frameworks of change take into account challenges of uncertainty to guide us toward structures and processes that enable the creative use of knowledge by people to solve unanticipated problems. A useful framework to consider change in today's healthcare environment is characterized as VUCA: volatility, uncertainty, complexity, and ambiguity (Bennett and Lemoine, 2014).

Volatility describes the ever-changing nature of an unfolding challenge. Because of its unpredictability, situations characterized by volatility often require a broader level of preparedness. By being over-prepared or prepared for many possibilities, an organization may be better able to respond to the broad range of possible outcomes. For instance, during periods when severe weather is changing and could interfere with clinical staff either traveling to work or to their homes, precautions must be taken to ensure that a safe level of staff will be available to care for hospitalized patients. To prepare for such situations, doctors and nurses might be asked to remain overnight at the hospital in case they are needed in the morning. Extra staff might be called in early, to ensure that they will arrive on time to relieve others. In the academic setting, a clinical faculty member might encourage their students to take extra clothes and toiletries to the clinical setting when a large storm is expected to reduce the risk of students traveling in dangerous weather conditions. Ever-changing situations require preparation for many possibilities.

As it suggests, uncertainty refers to the fact that there are many aspects of the challenges faced by leaders for which we do not have enough information. For instance, when the Ebola crisis broke in West Africa (2013–2016), the medical community had very little information about the best ways to contain the spread of the virus or which drugs might be helpful to those who had been exposed. Experts conferred and pooled their information during and after the crisis. By pooling their information, they hoped it would decrease uncertainty, increase certainty, and find solutions that would limit the epidemic and support those with the disease to return to good health. Overall, the leadership strategy when addressing challenges characterized by uncertainty is to learn more about the challenge and reduce uncertainty where possible.

Complexity refers to the many aspects of a challenge that are often interrelated, and must all be addressed. For instance, when developing a program that supports staff nurses to complete small research projects on the unit, other demands for their time must be taken into consideration. Although the career ladder advancement plan may indicate that staff nurses are required to demonstrate scholarly leadership that improves patient care, the hospital's staff model is unlikely to include support for activities that are not directly related to the delivery of patient care. Even with the support of nursing leadership to engage in scholarly activities that support career advancement, the organization's financial model must somehow be addressed to allow the nursing staff to fully engage in these activities.

Ambiguity describes novel situations for which there are not clear parameters. For instance, when a school opens a new educational degree program, steps might be taken to pre-determine whether there is a level of interest in such a program but, even after demonstrating interest by way of surveys, the question remains whether qualified applicants, in sufficient numbers, will apply and commit to enrolling. When facing ambiguity, leaders need to make thoughtful observations about the relationships among factors, experiment and actively work toward plausible explanations. For instance, if the applicants do apply and are admitted, we do not know how many will actually choose to enroll (known as the yield). One strategy a leader might use would be to ask the admissions officers to enlarge the list of qualified applicants on the waitlist and hold their admissions offer until the first wave of admitted applicants returns their deposit commitments. VUCA provides a useful framework for thinking about the environmental qualities in which we experience leadership challenges and offers some direction in thinking about approaches to needed solutions.

Another useful framework for change lies in complexity science and complexity leadership theory. Complexity science is the study of adaptive systems and focuses on the patterns of adaptation and learning of the subsystems and interlocking relationships (Crowell, 2016). Appreciating that everything is related, complexity science looks to explain the processes of internal adaptations rather than impose controls on systems behavior. Complexity leadership, as presented by Crowell, requires an understanding of complexity science, a commitment to self-reflection as a tool for leading, and a commitment to active engagement. The leader undertakes actions that support the learning and adaptation of the organization.

In a detailed explanation of their Complexity Leadership Theory, Uhl-Bien, Marion, and McKelvey (2007) suggest that the goal of leadership is to foster the organizational and subgroup creativity, learning, and adaptability. The authors describe three broad types of leadership as the following:

1. *Administrative Leadership*—focused on the need for order hierarchy; alignment, and control;
2. *Enabling Leadership*—focused on creating the structures and conditions for creative problem-solving and adaptability; and
3. *Adaptive Leadership*—focused on the generative dynamics that underlie emergent change activities (Uhl-Bien, Marion, and McKelvey, 2007).

Complex adaptive systems (CAS) are interdependent agents networked in pursuit of a common goal or outcome. The CAS often emerges naturally in social systems in search of solving problems or learning and adapting. *Context* is critical to the work of the CAS as it gives rise to the persona of the CAS. Leadership is understood as behavior that influences the outcomes, as opposed to the position that a leader holds. Administrative leadership can be distinguished from adaptive leadership, the former being associated with structural and ordering work and the latter referring to leadership occurring in emergent, informal processes throughout the organization. Complexity leadership occurs in response to adaptive challenges, problems that require new behavior, learning, or innovation and not just compliance with an authoritarian dictum. Leadership refers to responses to the unknown that are ambiguous and unpredictable.

Whether referring to a group of staff assigned to a clinical unit or a department of faculty members, these groups all have resources and challenges that influence how they approach their shared work, and the results will depend on how they interact with one another, a factor largely influenced by culture.

SUMMARY

The object of the leader is to facilitate the maximum performance and effectiveness of the organization and the individuals (and subgroups) within that organization, particularly in creatively solving novel problems and learning. The context of organizational development with the accompanying theories and frameworks related to change, humanism, strategic management, and systems, provide a realistic and practical overview to understanding the challenges of leaders. The theoretical frameworks provide a historic and contextual understanding of organizations, both academic and clinical.

REFERENCES

Anderson, D. L. (2017). *Organization development: The process of leading organizational change.* (4th ed.). Sage.

Argyris, C. (1964). *Integrating the individual and the organization.* Wiley.

Bailey, Z. D., Feldman, J. M., & Bassett, M. T. (2020, December 16). *How structural racism works –Racist policies as a root cause of U.S. racial health inequities.* New England Journal of Medicine. https://www.nejm.org/doi/full/10.1056/NEJMms2025396

Bennett, N., & Lemoine, G. J. (2014). What a difference a word makes: Understanding threats to performance in a VUCA World. *Business Horizons, 57*(3), 311–317. https://doi.org/10.2139/ssrn.2406676

Beckhard, R. (1969) Organizational Development: Strategies and Models. Reading MA: Addison Wesley.

Centers for Medicare and Medicaid. (ACCESSED 2020). *NHE fact sheet.* Centers for Medicare & Medicaid Services. https://www.cms.gov/Research-Statistics-Data-and-Systems/Statistics-Trends-and-Reports/NationalHealthExpendData/NHE-Fact-Sheet

Cheung-Judge, M.-Y., & Holbeche, L. (2015). *Organization development: A practitioner's guide for OD and HR.* Kogan Page.

Colman, A. (2008). *A dictionary of psychology* (3rd ed.). Oxford University Press.

Connors, R., & Smith, T. (2011). *Change the culture, change the game: The breakthrough strategy for energizing your organization and creating accountability for results.* Portfolio Penguin.

Crowell, D. M., (2016). *Complexity leadership: Nursing's role in health care delivery.* 2nd Edition, FA Davis Co.

Follett, M. P. (1927). *Dynamic administration* (reprint 1942). Harper & Brothers Publishers.

Goleman, D. (1995). *Emotional intelligence.* Bantam Books.

Hofer, C. W., & Schendel, D. (1978). *Strategy formulation: Analytical concepts.* West Pub. Co.

Kotter, J. P. (2012). *Leading change.* Harvard Business Review Press.

Lewin, K. (1935). *A dynamic theory of personality.* McGraw-Hill.

Lewin, K. (1946). Action research and minority problems. *Journal of Social Issues, 2*(4), 34–46. https://doi.org/10.1111/j.1540-4560.1946.tb02295.x

Maslow, A. H. (1943). A theory of human motivation. *Psychology Review, 50*(4), 370–396. https://doi.org/10.1037/h0054346

May, R. (1950). *The meaning of anxiety.* The Ronald Press Company

Mayo, E. (1946). *The human problems of an industrial civilization.* 2nd edition, Harvard University.

Perlo, J., Balik, B., Swensen, S., Kabcenell, A., Landsman, J., & Feeley, D. (2017). *IHI Framework for improving joy in work.* IHI White Paper. Institute for Healthcare Improvement. http://www.ihi.org/resources/Pages/IHIWhitePapers/Framework-Improving-Joy-in-Work.aspx

Rogers, C. (1951). Client-centered therapy: It's current practice, implications and theory. Constable.

Rogers, C. (1961). *On becoming a person: A therapist's view of psychotherapy.* Constable.

Schein, E. H. (1984). *Coming to a new awareness of organizational culture.* Sloan Management Review.

Schein, E. H. (2010). *Organizational culture and leadership.* Jossey-Bass.

Scherer, J. J., Alban, B., & Weisbord, M. (2016). The origins of organizational development. In W. J. Rothwell, J. M. Stavros, & R. L. Sullivan (Eds.), *Practicing Organizational Development* (pp. 26-41). John Wiley & Sons, Inc.

Senge, P., (1990). *The fifth discipline: The art and practice of the learning organization.* Currency Publications.

Stecker, E., & Torbet, R. (2010). A 'Developmental Action Inquiry' Approach To Teaching First-, Second-, and Third-Person Action Research Methods. In S. Esbjörn-Hargens, J. Reams & O. Gunnlaugson (Eds.), Integral Education: New Directions for Higher Learning. Albany NY: SUNY Press, pp 105–126

Taylor, F. W. (1911). *Principles of scientific management.* Harper and Brothers.

Thompson, D. (2018, January 9). *Health care just became the U.S.'s largest employer.* The Atlantic. https://www.theatlantic.com/business/archive/2018/01/health-care-america-jobs/550079/

Thompson, A. A., & Strickland, A. J. (2001). *Strategic management: Concepts and cases.* McGraw-Hill/Irvin.

Uhl-Bien, M., Marion, R., & McKelvey, B. (2007). Complexity leadership theory: Shifting leadership from the industrial age to the knowledge era. *The Leadership Quarterly, 18*(4), 298-318. https://doi.org/10.1016/j.leaqua.2007.04.002

U.S. Bureau of Labor Statistics. (2020). *Occupational outlook handbook: Healthcare occupations*. U.S. Bureau of Labor Statistics. https://www.bls.gov/ooh/healthcare/home.htm

von Bertalanffy, L. (1956). *The contributions of system theory to present scientific thinking*. RIAS, Funk-Universtät.

Understanding the Elements of Organizational Life

CHAPTER 3

Organizational Culture

ACADEMIC VIGNETTE

Space is an important resource within universities and those who control space are often courted by those who want space. At Hillsman University, the laboratory spaces on the new campus are large with new and powerful hoods, natural light, and reliable generators in the event of power failures. Faculty members who are working in older labs have been lobbying the provost and leading a campaign for her support for their idea for a shared collaborative space. They have submitted white papers and held lunchtime forums to explain how their science would be advanced if their space request was granted. The requesting group has organized regular audiences with the provost and soon their request was the talk of the campus, especially when the provost began to publicly talk about the significance of the work that could take place in the requested space. Faculty in other units began asking one another how the decision about space would be made. They knew that money would need to be raised for such a massive renovation and they also knew that there were both administrative and faculty governance councils governing space.

Faculty in the school of nursing were being told that they were going to lose their wet lab spaces and that the nursing building might be torn down. As the dean of the school of nursing, you were facing angry and confused faculty members who wanted to know what was going on.

The faculty witnessing the provost's support of the lobbying group were growing angrier and angrier, but felt a collective helplessness. They approached their dean asking how this conversation about space use could be advancing outside the explicitly endorsed committee structure for space assignment. The dean invited the provost to come before the faculty and share the proposal for space to be assigned to the lobbying group. The provost accepted the invitation and came to the meeting with members of the lobbying group and shared her PowerPoint presentation, which included 55 slides. Time for Q&A was cut short, but one senior member of the faculty asked, "Has or will this proposal come before the faculty council for discussion?" to which the provost responded that she had been given authority by the president to make this decision. As they left the meeting, the faculty members could be heard saying, "It is always the same! All you need to do is lobby the provost and if you make enough noise, none of the formal channels for change are ever activated. The loudest voice wins."

CLINICAL VIGNETTE

Dr. Petty was recruited to lead the cardiothoracic surgery team. Highly regarded as a surgeon, his recruitment was considered a feather in the cap of the dean of medicine. The pressure to build a strong surgical service was great; the academic health center sought to develop a service that could attract patients from across the country. Dr. Petty's recruitment included several other team members, including three recently board-certified surgeons and two anesthesiologists who were specialists in cardiothoracic surgeries. The recruitment represented a $325 million dollar investment for personnel alone, and the medical center was committed to ancillary supports to assist with attracting patients and making sure they were in a new and comfortably appointed patient care environment.

Within a month of the initiation of the clinical services, perioperative nurses started calling in sick and three requested a transfer from the operating room to the surgical step-down units. The nursing director sought out the perioperative supervisor to explore what she knew about this situation. The nursing director was told that the nurses requesting transfer were among the most experienced and valuable and the supervisor did not want to lose them, but she could accommodate these requests if it was a necessary condition of retaining these nurses.

With further exploration, the nursing director learned that Dr. Petty and his colleagues were impatient with their new team members. They yelled and screamed at some point in every surgical case. After substantial coaxing by the manager, the clinical nurses reported that the recent uptick in harassment in the operating room coincided with the arrival of the new team of surgeons. With further prodding, the nurses acknowledged that although the organization's stated policies indicate that the members of the healthcare team respect one another and work together toward positive outcomes for each patient, the nurses who experienced the ridicule delivered by screaming surgeons saw no way to interrupt the situation. Their foregone conclusion was that doctors' concerns are treated as more legitimate than theirs, and that their concerns would be disregarded. In the worst case, their complaints could put their positions and their collegial relations at further risk. Rather than speak up collectively, these nurses solved their problems one by one, ignoring the problem experienced by many, and sought a way to improve their own working environment through transfer.

INTRODUCTION

Culture plays a major role in the influence of organizational behavior and the responses of organizations to change. Culture can be described as the shared beliefs, norms, and behavioral patterns shared by any group (e.g., a unit, a service, a family, a community, and, of relevance to our discussion, an organization). Organizational culture is a set of shared assumptions that guide what happens in organizations by defining appropriate behavior for various situations (Ravasi and Schultz, 2006). Collective beliefs undergird behavior and must be understood before organizational behaviors can be shaped. Culture is often so baked into the everyday that longtime members of the organization do not see culture; it is best seen by those new to the organization and by outsiders, for instance consumers, consultants, and new leaders and staff who enter the organization.

Levels of Organizational Culture

Schein (2010) described three levels in which culture is visible to the observer. Artifacts refer to the visible and feelable structures and processes that guide behavior. While artifacts are observable, they may not always be understood. Examples of artifacts include the physical environment, the way people behave or dress (who wears a scarf versus a stethoscope around the neck), organizational charts, and the documents that guide possibilities (e.g., Faculty Handbook or Career Ladder Policies). Other examples include the rituals observed, for instance "Nurses' Week" or the annual awarding of a "Mentor of the Year" award to a faculty member. Recognitions and objects that acknowledge and celebrate heroes, such as Florence Nightingale and Harriet Tubman, or "firsts," such as Luther Christman or Barack Obama, are also important to observers of culture. The absence of heroes that are recognized can also be notable.

Espoused beliefs and values represent a second level of culture. An organization's stated values have been described as appearing in the mission, vision, values (MVV) statement. As such, these explicit values are often revisited and serve to guide proposals for change or action. When we discuss strategic planning in Chapter 5, we note that the planning process usually begins with a review of the organization's MVV statements. Espoused beliefs can show up in statements about the signature characteristics of a school's graduates or the clinical system's commitment to be patient centric. Importantly, these espoused beliefs are sometimes in conflict with the way things work and being attuned to these conflicts will help the leader develop approaches to guiding change.

The third and deepest level of culture can be identified as the basic underlying assumptions that are foundational to an organizational culture. These beliefs are so embedded in the organization that most people never notice them. They are taken for granted and they generally do not vary from person to person or from unit to unit. For instance, a school that has few online course offerings may believe that students enroll in their school to be physically present in the classroom and that online education is inherently inferior. As part of understanding culture, the leader needs to observe, work to understand the meanings of the organization's widely held beliefs and practices, and determine whether the beliefs are working for or against organizational functionality. When cultural symbols and observed actions do not match, there is a great likelihood that there is organizational dysfunction. Even without a mismatch between symbols and actions, an organization may be dysfunctional, and as new leaders enter the organization, an opportunity to assess a culture and potentially make change is provided.

In organizations, examples of mismatches between documented values and organizational action abound. We are committed to equity but find few women and people of color in senior executive positions. We are committed to pay equity but find that the salary levels of men exceed those of women. We are committed to a diversified student body, faculty, and staff, but most of our faculty and students are white women and most staff are women from Black, Indigenous, and People of Color (BIPOC) groups. We are committed to a diverse clinical team, but the physicians are white men, the nurse practitioners are white women, and the medical assistants are black men. Our recent and growing awareness of these discrepancies has precipitated conversations about the policies within our organizations that interfere with living our aspired values. Institutional racism or structural racism and white supremacy culture are supported by values that are so embedded as to be overlooked by the majority of those within our organizations, giving rise to policies that support racism (Kendi 2019), other forms of discrimination against underrepresented groups, and unconscious bias. To affect change, these discrepancies need to be observed, measured (when possible), monitored, intentionally brought into awareness, and either improved or eliminated.

Consider: What are some of the elements of culture that are visible (artifacts) in the environment in which you work?

MODELS OF ORGANIZATIONAL CULTURE

Each organization is different in the way it organizes people and designs a model for accomplishing their mission. Organizational culture defines how an organization functions and how workers within that organization do their jobs. Some organizations are more bureaucratic or hierarchical, while some have flat organizational structures where individuals have significant autonomy and authority. Some individuals feel most comfortable in organizations that are highly structured and autocratic while others enjoy organizations that are more democratic and have greater organizational flexibility. If an individual who feels most comfortable in a highly structured organization joins a company with a high degree of flexibility and few rules, the individual may be uncomfortable at first and not have the navigational skills to accomplish the work assigned; their tenure may be short. This is the concept of organizational fit. Assessing an organization's culture prior to accepting a position is sometimes difficult, but it is especially important for the successful leader to understand and consistently monitor the culture in the early stages of the appointment. Frameworks for understanding organizational culture emphasize different elements of culture. Here we discuss two models in common use.

Competing Values Culture Model

Cameron and Quinn (2011) developed a model of assessing organizational culture by evaluating significant cultural differences that exist across the globe. They propose that organizational culture varies across two axes. This first axis describes the degree to which an organization is inward focused versus outward focused. The extreme ends of this continuum are the dichotomous descriptions: outward and inward. The second axis looks at the degree to which a culture is flexible and responsive versus stable and controlled. Again, those extremes anchor the axis and the organization's culture may fall along this axis. For purposes of illustration, Cameron and Quinn offer a two-by-two figure (Figure 3.1) in which four cultural types are described: the Clan culture, the Adhocracy culture, the Hierarchy culture, and the Market culture.

Given their position along the axes, the Clan and Adhocracy cultures are those characterized by greater flexibility and discretion. Those cultural styles do not require members to be bound by rigid rules; they may be creative and innovative in their approach to work. The Clan culture, although flexible and responsive to the environment, is inward focused in contrast to the Adhocracy culture, which is responsive to external forces. The Hierarchy and Market cultures differ from the Clan and Adhocracy cultures by their adherence to stability and control, but they differ from one another in their inward focus (Hierarchy) versus outward focus (Market).

Although most organizations have a dominant culture, Cameron and Quinn

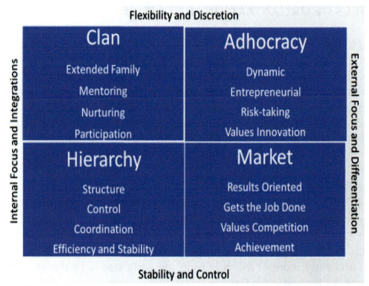

FIGURE 3.1 Cameron and Quinn Model of Assessing Organizational Culture (2011).

state that most organizations will fall somewhere along the two axes. Within some organizations, individual departments might display different culture profiles. For example, the ICU in a hospital might have a very different culture than a general pediatric unit. Their work also demonstrated that organizations featuring flexibility were generally more successful than rigid ones, as the flexible organization was able to adapt in response to changing conditions and demands. The following provides a brief summary of the four types of organizational cultures.

The Clan Culture

This culture is rooted in collaboration. Members share commonalities and see themselves as part of one big family who are active and involved. Leadership takes the form of mentorship, and the organization is bound by commitments and traditions. The main values are rooted in teamwork, communication, and consensus. This model is focused on building respectful relationships with employees, customers, suppliers, and the environment itself.

The Adhocracy Culture

This culture is based on energy and creativity. Employees are encouraged to take risks, and leaders are seen as innovators or entrepreneurs. The organization is held together by experimentation, with an emphasis on individual inge-nuity and freedom. The core values are based on change and agility.

The Market Culture

This culture is built upon the dynamics of competition and achieving con-crete results. The focus is goal-oriented, with leaders who are tough and de-manding. The organization is united by a common goal to succeed and beat all rivals. The main value drivers are market share and profitability.

The Hierarchy Culture

This culture is founded on structure and control. The work environment is formal, with strict institutional procedures in place for guidance. Leadership is based on organized coordination and monitoring, with a culture emphasizing efficiency and predictability. The values include consistency and uniformity as often seen in large, bureaucratic organizations (Cameron and Quinn, 2011).

Cooke's Organizational Culture

Cooke and Lafferty (1989) present a view of culture that draws on different dimensions. These cultural styles result from, and contribute to, the behaviors that members believe are required to fit in and meet expectations within their organization. In other words, their model emphasizes that beliefs of the orga-nization's members are critical to the development of the culture. Cooke and Szumal (2000) proposed a model of organizational culture that assumes that employees operate in a way that supports their success within that organiza-tion and assures a long-term tenure. Often these behaviors are learned from others in the organization, or the expected behaviors may be imparted in the onboarding process. According to Cooke and Lafferty (1989), the culture of an organization is the way employees behave at the workplace to ensure a stable future and growth.

Cook and Szumal (2000) describe three types of cultures commonly ob-served in organizations: the *constructive culture*, the *passive culture*, and the *aggressive culture*. Each type displays typical behaviors and rules and creates a different climate for its members.

Constructive Culture

In constructive cultures, people are encouraged to work as teams, rather than only as individuals. In positions where people do a complex job, rather than something simple, this culture has been found to be efficient. This type of organizational culture encourages healthy communication among its employees who are encouraged to share their ideas, exchange information, and discuss innovative solutions to problems that are beneficial to all. Constructive culture motivates the employees and eventually extracts the best out of them resulting in high levels of motivation, satisfaction, teamwork, and service quality. Constructive norms are evident in environments where quality is valued over quantity, creativity is valued over conformity, cooperation is believed to lead to better results than competition, and effectiveness is judged at the system level rather than the individual level. These types of cultural norms are consistent with (and supportive of) the objectives behind empowerment, total quality management, transformational leadership, continuous improvement, re-engineering, and learning organizations (Deal and Kennedy, 2000; Schein, 1992). There are four key features characterize a constructive culture:

- *Achievement*: A constructive culture helps the employees to be most effective and achieve the goals they set for themselves and the organization. People are supported to complete a task successfully by thinking ahead and planning, exploring alternatives before acting, and learning from their mistakes.
- *Self-Actualizing*: In the constructive culture, an employee stays motivated and realizes their full potential. The employee is supported in the realization or fulfillment of one's talents and abilities. People in this organizational culture demonstrate a strong desire to learn and experience things, have creative yet realistic thinking, and a balanced concern for people and tasks.
- *Humanistic*: An organization with this characteristic helps its members grow and develop. Mentoring is an integral component of this organizational culture. The organization reflects an interest in the growth and development of people, a high positive regard for them and sensitivity to their needs.
- *Affiliative*: Highly affiliative organizational cultures treat people as more valuable than things. The organization reflects an interest in developing and sustaining pleasant relationships. Employees avoid conflicts and unnecessary disputes and promote a positive ambience at the workplace.

Passive Culture

In a passive culture, people are expected to act in the ways that are defined by the norms and standards of the organization, not in the way they believe they should act in order to be most effective. People act in ways that please superiors and avoid interpersonal conflict to remain safe within the organization. Rules, policies, and guidelines are more important than the critical thinking of individuals members of the organization. There are four major characteristics of a passive culture:

- *Approval*: The individuals in the organization must seek approval from their superiors before making a decision. They are not trusted to make a decision that they feel is in the best interest of the organization.

- *Conventional*: Employees are bound by rules, policies, procedure, and standards.
- *Dependent*: Members of the organization are dependent on the decision-making of the boss and follow their orders.
- *Avoidance*: Employees suppress their own personal desires for the organization and follow the rules without question. Job satisfaction is usually low.

Aggressive Culture

In this organizational culture, competition among employees is highly encouraged. Teamwork is almost non-existent because there is a strong focus on the individual rather than the work of the group. Status and power within the organization is often seen as the most important measure of success, and expertise is often overlooked in favor of status when decisions have to be made. In these organizations, members are expected to appear confident, competent, and superior. Those who ask questions or make errors are seen as incompetent or weak. These organizations are very stressful, and often experience a high degree of turnover. There are four characteristics of the aggressive culture:

- *Oppositional*: In this culture, people are overly critical of each other, not in the spirit of improving the product or process but in trying to make themselves look better than others.
- *Power*: The search for power within the organization is the driving force for the way individuals interact.
- *Competitive*: People compare themselves to others and try to outperform their colleagues to gain more status or recognition.
- *Perfectionist*: It is expected that people will have flawless performance and people who make errors are judged harshly by others in the organization. Self-worth is associated with high achievement.

Models That Advance an Organizational Culture of Performance Excellence

Preparing for and sustaining performance excellence is challenging work. Developing a culture that will drive toward a core set of competencies of the people who work in the organization that includes trust building, high reliability organization principles, social equality, accountability structures and processes, and mindfulness is challenging work. It helps to have a structured guide for the development of such an organizational culture.

There are a number of frameworks that can be used to guide strategies and approaches for data driven decision-making, leadership, change management, organizational culture development, diversity, and inclusion. These frameworks often include the technical tools and resources for data management,

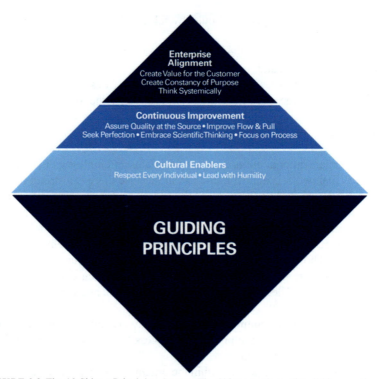

FIGURE 3.2 The 10 Shingo Principles. Source: The Shingo Institute. (http//shingo.org/model) and the Jon M. Huntsman School of Business, Utah State University (2021).

quality improvement, innovation, and evidence-based practice. Many of these frameworks will be discussed throughout this book. Ideally, the organization will establish, sustain, and advance a system for performance management excellence that will position the organization to be highly productive, competitive, financially solvent, and visionary. Two examples of models that can assist organizations in advancing a culture of performance excellence are the Shingo Model for Sustaining a Culture of Organizational Excellence and the Baldrige Performance Excellence Program. Each model identifies characteristics of an organization that can have a supporting effect or a negative impact on building a culture of performance management.

The Shingo Model provides structure on which to anchor current initiatives and with which to close gaps in working toward sustaining a culture of organizational excellence. The structure is framed within a set of guiding principles. The guiding principles are organized into three categories, Cultural Enablers, Continuous Improvement and Enterprise Alignment. Figure 3.2 identifies the 10 Shingo performance management principles that build on each other resulting in creating value for the customer.

Shingo Model Principles

1. *Cultural Enablers*: Respect Every Individual, Lead with Humility
2. *Continuous Improvement*: Assure Quality at the Source, Improve Flow and Pull, Seek Perfection, Embrace Scientific Thinking, Focus on Process
3. *Enterprise Alignment*: Create Value for the Customer, Create Constancy of Purpose, and Think Systemically

The Baldrige Excellence Framework (Health Care) (Figure 3.3) is a framework that empowers organizations to reach its goals, be more effective organizationally and more competitive in their market. Through the assessment process, organizations can identify improvement tools to assist with dimensions of the organization that need improvement. As an organization utilizes the framework, ways to build on strengths, close gaps and innovate are identified and lead to cycles of improvement.

The organization's profile provides the critical insight into the key external and internal factors that shape the organization's environment. The core values provide the foundation of the Framework. They include such areas as systems perspective, valuing people and a focus on success and innovation among others.

Each hexagon in the center of the circle, Leadership, Strategy, Customers, Workforce, Operations and Results represents a key area of all health care organizations today. The category of Measurement, Analysis and Knowledge

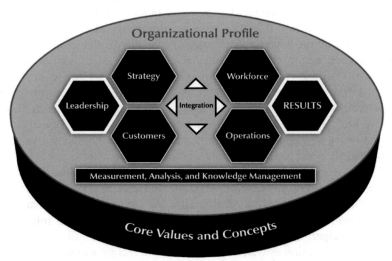

FIGURE 3.3 2021–2022 Baldrige Performance Excellence Framework (Health Care).

Management applies to all of these key areas since the measurement and analysis of data and the use of those data in decision-making are integral to all these areas of health care. Understanding organizational data and comparing it to benchmarks is the foundation for organizational improvement.

There are many models of organizational culture which examine and label approaches to describing the salient characteristics of the organization. Organizational cultures are helpful to understand so that a leader can identify those characteristics that enhance organizational effectiveness and those that impede achievement of the mission. For example, if a leader enters a highly structured organization which is characterized by competitiveness and has an embedded power structure that disempowers workers, they might have to find alternative ways to build teamwork as they begin to dismantle the challenging aggressive organizational culture.

Consider: **Are there characteristics of your organization that fit into elements of the models described here? How do these characteristics affect how you function in your organization?**

Features of a Healthy Work Culture

As described earlier, organizational culture defines how an organization functions and how workers within that organization do their jobs. No two organizations have exactly the same culture but there are characteristics of healthy cultures that are consistently seen in high functioning organizations, and the leader can be thought of as the steward of the organization's culture. There are many characteristics of a healthy work environment that seem intuitive and are evident with the opportunity to work in a healthy work culture. In healthy work cultures, employees are satisfied with, find joy in, and are engaged in their work (Perlo *et al.*, 2017). Turnover is low and when turnover is present, it results from the opportunity of members to grow professionally, and they are supported in that growth. While it is always hard to lose a valuable employee, healthy work environments celebrate the success of members of the organization who have new opportunities. Individuals know the mission and values of the organization and are productively working to achieve those goals.

Healthy work environments have a culture of mentorship that encourages people to grow, learn, and develop. Mentors can either be assigned or naturally evolve through building work relationships, but the expectation is that senior individuals reach out to support new employees or those in junior roles. Team leaders and department heads should be seen as a source of inspiration for others in the organization as well as a resource for direction and guidance on the work of the organization. Easy access to organizational leaders not only shows that the perspective of all members of the organization are valued, it reduces interpersonal conflict because all voices have a chance to be heard.

In healthy cultures, people are evaluated and rewarded for the quality of their work, not for their relationship with a supervisor or their seniority within the organization. Meaningful rewards should be given to those who have excelled in their work while avoiding the temptation to diminish the work of others by comparing them to the high performers. Each member of the organization should be recognized for their contributions to the organization and have the feeling that they are an integral member of the team. Performance evaluations are treated as opportunities for development, as opposed to routine affirmations of people disconnected from their performance.

In healthy work environments, inclusivity and differences are celebrated. Mechanisms for healthy debate are at play. Committee structures assure the active voice of the community, consumers, and all levels of employees. Policies drive equity and equality in opportunity.

Openness and transparency are often hard to achieve but are characteristics seen in most healthy work cultures. Discussing issues of work design or process among employees will result in a better outcome that is more easily adopted by the members of the organization because they had a role in its development. Organizations that are open with their employees about important issues, support teamwork, and encourage joint problem solving have employees that are more invested in their roles within the organization.

Although transparency is important, a leader needs to be thoughtful about the degree of transparency they provide in the organization as well as the timing of revealing new information. Allowing people to understand the decision-making process and the reason for decisions is important. Describing the budget and how dynamic changes in the environment or the economy can impact the organization is critical for people to understand the future threats and challenges they face.

Some of the organization's information cannot be revealed with complete transparency without violating the privacy of individual employees. For instance, labor regulations and policies prohibit disclosure of an individual's information on performance or changes in health status. Employees expect that leaders will hold certain aspects of private information confidential, such as plans for retirement or the health of family members. Although many public organizations reveal salary details, private organizations may treat this information as confidential. Divulging information that is assumed to be confidential often results in loss of trust in leaders, more conflict among the members of the organization, and results in a negative impact on organizational culture.

Finally, a healthy work culture supports and promotes a healthy work-life balance for the employees. Work-life balance has become more important in recent years for employees and as leaders in health and wellness, it is critical that wellness is supported in policies and practices. For example, expecting members of the organization to regularly work beyond their assigned hours prevents people from getting the rest they need and separation from the organization required to be effective in their role. Requiring or expecting members to respond to emails or texts when they are not scheduled to be working creates expectations that prevent people from having the focused time on family or self that every employee needs. Role-modeling and supporting work-life balance is critical for an effective leader.

Healthy cultures respond to stressful times in the lives of employees or during local, regional, national, or global crises by providing flexibility in their responsibilities if possible. For example, if a member of the organization has a sick child or is going through a personal crisis like a divorce, discussing how their job can be changed for a short period of time while they address their personal circumstances is important. Helping them to see that change is needed and the leader wants to work with them to make that change, helps employees have some control over what might feel like an out-of-control situation. If it appears the challenging situation will extend beyond the short term, leaders can show their compassion by helping the employee understand the resources they have available to them such as short-term disability or Family and Medical Leave Act (FMLA) benefits through the federal government.

There are also times in an organization's life when external factors cause significant system disruption that require a thoughtful approach that is consistent with the culture of the organization. Consider this example. An organization has a policy that employees who work at home cannot have childcare or other caregiving responsibilities during the time they are working. The culture of the organization is one of caring for employees as people and supporting them with flexibility and resources as needed. During the pandemic of 2020–2022, children were not able to attend school or daycare. Therefore, parents were working at home while their children were at home in remote learning environments. Enforcement of a work at home policy that does not allow parents to be caregivers while working during an incredibly difficult time would be inconsistent with a supportive and flexible culture of an organization. At challenging times for an organization, remembering the essential elements of the culture and acting consistent with them helps to preserve the integrity of the organization for its members.

Healthy organizational cultures do not happen without significant effort in creating a positive work environment and regular stewardship to make sure a positive culture is maintained. Using strategies of joint education activities or team building seminars, a leader can foster interdependence and a collaborative environment. While content related seminars and conferences are critical to help people see how their work is interrelated, a leader should also consider designating social time for employees to enjoy each other's company and get to know each other better. Staff wine and cheeses or lunch drop-in sessions are strategies that a leader can use to build relationships between employees that often translate into a more positive work environment.

> *Consider*: Would you describe your organization as having a healthy culture?
> Are there elements of your culture that are not healthy?

Advancing an Interprofessional Culture

As early as 2001, the Institute of Medicine (IOM is now called the National Academy of Medicine, NAM) identified medical errors as one of the leading causes of death in the US. In response to the growing problem of medical errors, the IOM explored the multifaceted role of provider practice and found that interprofessional communication and practice has a role in improving the quality of healthcare and the job satisfaction of healthcare providers (Busari, Mill and Duits, 2017). In 2011, the Core Competencies for Interprofessional Collaborative Practice were published by the Interprofessional Education Collaborative. They stated, "The goal of this interprofessional learning is to prepare all health professions students for deliberately working together with the common goal of building a safer and better patient-centered and community/population-oriented U.S. health care system" (IPEC, 2011, p. 3).

Interprofessional collaboration is when "multiple health workers from different professional backgrounds work together with patients, families, carers (caregivers), and communities to deliver the highest quality of care" (World Health Organization, 2010, p. 7). In order for providers to be able to work as a team, they need to be taught and have the opportunity to practice the essentials of team-based care. In 2009, six national education associations of schools of the health professions (allopathic and osteopathic medicine, dentistry, nursing, pharmacy, and public health) formed a collaborative organization to promote and encourage efforts that would advance interprofessional learning experiences to help prepare future health professionals for team-based care of patients and improved population health outcomes (IPEC, 2011). Individuals entering the healthcare delivery system would be prepared to work as part of a team, taking the first step in reducing fragmentation and improving health outcomes in individuals and in the community. By understanding the unique skills each member of the health team has, communication about patient care improves, healthcare costs are reduced, job satisfaction increases, and the team is able to provide an improved healthcare experience.

An interprofessional culture is not the norm in healthcare delivery models although great strides in this area have occurred in the past decade. A clinical leader has to work to develop and maintain aspects of this type of organizational culture. Building an interprofessional culture requires intention and goes beyond casual opportunities for providers from different disciplines to meet each other or discuss patient situations. Building intentional relationships is important and the first step in building an interprofessional team. Each member of the team must understand how the professional role of all the team members contributes to the improvement of care for the patient and family.

The characteristics that form the foundation for an interprofessional culture begin with the characteristics of a healthy organizational culture described earlier. There has to be mutual respect between the members of the organization, a sense of enjoyment with working together, and a commitment to the mission of the organization, which for healthcare workers is providing safe and effective care to patients and within academic settings, high quality education. Leaders will be expected to provide the team with the tools to be able to practice interprofessionally. For example, making sure the team has the ability to get important data and information through access to appropriate data bases and decision-making tools is essential. Being able to easily use the evidence is also important for fostering team-based care. Having current evidence that is easily accessible is essential for the team members to make appropriate decisions. Finally, providing access to information that is both uni-professional (focused on the individual profession), as well as interprofessional, is important to creating a culture where members feel empowered to work collaboratively based on their individual expertise.

Interprofessional practice is widely recognized for its positive impact on healthcare delivery. Nursing education leaders are expected to develop and support interprofessional models of education and practice. This may mean that the schools of nursing, medicine, and dentistry collaborate on educating their students in the science and practice of team-based care. A school of nursing in a college or university without other health professions education programs may have to collaborate with a local university that has health professional education programs or create a partnership of health professions programs focused on interprofessional education.

Nurse leaders may need to help faculty see the importance of providing students with interprofessional experiences for their development as effective healthcare providers. There are often barriers created to interprofessional learning stemming from attitudes of faculty as well as logistic issues. Logistic barriers in interprofessional education include time (aligning different academic calendars from each discipline), space (finding a space big enough to house multiple disciplines of students), curricular alignment (students in nursing learning physical assessment in the fall while medical students learn it in the spring), and faculty expertise in teaching interprofessional students. While these barriers may seem insurmountable, creativity, tenacity, and flexibility will allow these kinds of experiences to occur and our healthcare system will improve.

As a nurse leader, role-modeling inter-professionalism is important, not just because it will yield better organizational outcomes, but also because it signals that collaborative practice is valued. In clinical settings, nurse leaders who reach out to pharmacy or therapy colleagues to engage them in important organizational decisions affirms the value of that collaborative practice and the expectation that decision-making quality will be enriched. In academia, nurse leaders who build relationships across disciplines increase opportunities for shared curricula, shared resources, and the development of team science. Academic nurse leaders have a responsibility to demonstrate how nursing can be integrated into other departments and how other disciplines can inform the work of nurses. One way of creating structural inter-professionalism is for the schools to have shared faculty. Clinical and academic nurse leaders who role-model inter-professionalism will influence the culture of their organizations to develop and sustain these behaviors. Regardless of setting, understanding the organizational culture sets the stage for subsequent organizational interventions and the leader who fails to appreciate culture is at high risk of failure.

Assessing Organizational Culture

Assessment of organization culture should include measures of the business performance, critical behaviors, milestones, and underlying beliefs, feelings, and mindset (Katzenbach, Steffen, and Kronley, 2012). Managing the pace of cultural change is an important role for a leader. Measures to assess current culture and monitor change are included in Table 3.1.

TABLE 3.1. Organizational Culture Assessment Areas and Measures.

Areas of Culture to Assess	Assessment Measures
Business performance	Net income, cost metrics such as cost of agency nurses or adjunct faculty, investment in innovation, quality metrics such as patient experience and student evaluations, external rankings, vacant positions, patient and student data.
Critical behaviors	Staff respect for each other, cohesive teamwork, respect for patients/students, clinical/teaching competency, behaviors are consistent with the mission, vision and values of the organization.
Milestones	Staff meeting their targets, new policies/procedures have been implemented, new hires onboarded, and quality metrics achieved.
Underlying beliefs, feelings, and mindset	Health of the work environment, burnout measures, perceptions of how workers are valued, quality of the organization, and work environment satisfaction. What do staff value? What works in the organization and what does not? What do staff most and least appreciate about the organization? What do staff understand is the goal of leadership?

When initially assessing an organization's culture, focusing on several aspects of an organization will tell you much about the culture. Consider the following areas for assessment:

- *Onboarding process*: How is it structured? Talk to new hires and ask what their experience was and how useful it was. Was it interesting and engaging? Or tedious and boring? Did the onboarding process help new hires feel excited about being part of the organization? Is diversity and difference valued?

- *Open leadership*: Do leaders talk freely about problems? Do staff feel free to bring up concerns? Does the leadership involve employees in all levels of the organization in problem solving? Do leaders engage the people they serve in their planning and improvement work? Do the leaders know the employees they work with by name? Do they talk about innovations and new ideas?

- *Incentive system of the organization*: Are employees recognized for doing a good job? Do employees feel recognized for the work they do in both formal and informal ways?

- *Team interactions*: Do all employees within a team participate in discussions? Do employees look and act engaged in the meeting? Are team members comfortable with each other? Is respect for all the norm? (Thiefels, 2018).

Critical questions should be asked of employees and the answers should be listened to and understood. Questions about what employees like best about their job and what they do not particularly like provide useful information. Do employees see the organization as successful? Innovative? Caring? Supportive? How are mistakes handled?

Leaders often engage consultants to conduct an assessment of the culture. There are numerous firms that offer this service using their unique approach. While many large organizations have done this, it is often challenging to find the right consulting group. When using a consulting firm be clear about your goals for doing the culture assessment. Have a clear set of outcomes for the project and make certain the deliverables are agreed upon before beginning the engagement.

Culture is thought to be a major lever in affecting change in organizations. Changing culture can be difficult, but the building blocks of culture (beliefs and meaning) are essential to understanding and influencing organizational change. Understanding the dynamics and the processes of an organization are crucial for development of strategies that will assure success in the change process, which will be discussed in greater detail in Chapter 14.

SUMMARY

The culture of an organization plays a role in all aspects of its work and in the work life of the employees. Organizational culture is multifaceted and often difficult to see by those embedded in the organization. Understanding organizational culture is essential to the effective functioning of the leader and their ability to support a functional, healthy environment. A fit between the leader's values, beliefs, and the organizational culture is also critical for effective role functioning of the leader and job satisfaction. Models of organizational culture as well as organizational culture assessment help the leader obtain a clear picture of the strengths and challenges of the cultural environment.

CRITICAL THINKING QUESTIONS

At the beginning of the chapter an academic and clinical vignette were presented. Please review the vignettes to address the following the questions. The questions are specific to the vignettes.

Academic Vignette Questions

1. What aspects of culture are being challenged in this case study?
2. Are there aspects of organizational culture theory that the dean can use in working with the faculty?
3. How is the dean's role compromised in this scenario?
4. How could the dean have helped the provost before the meeting to be more responsive to the faculty issues?
5. What other actions should the dean be taking to address this situation?

Clinical Vignette Questions

1. Are there aspects of organizational culture theory that the nursing director can use in working with the staff?
2. How is the nurse's approach to solving this problem going to affect the culture of the organization?
3. How is that approach going to affect patient care?
4. How do you think the relationship between the nurses and their supervisor will be affected?
5. What will be some of the downstream organizational effects of not addressing and effectively resolving this problem?

REFERENCES

Baldrige, M., (2022). *Baldrige performance excellence framework.* Gaithersburg: NIST https://www.nist.gov/baldrige/publications/baldrige-excellence-framework.

Busari J., Mill, F., Duits, A. (2017). Understanding the impact of interprofessional collaboration on the quality of care: A case report from a small-scale resource limited health care environment. *Journal of Multidisciplinary Healthcare, 10*, 227–234. https://doi.org/10.2147/JMDH.S140042

Cameron, K., Quinn, R., (2011). *Diagnosing and changing organizational culture: Based on the competing values framework.* 2nd Edition. John Wiley & Sons.

Cooke, R. A., Lafferty, J. C. (1989). *The organizational culture inventory.* Human Synergistics, Inc.

Cooke, R. A., & Szumal, J. L., (2000). *Handbook of organizational culture and climate.* Sage Publications.

Deal, T. E., & Kennedy, A. A. (2000) *Corporate cultures: The rites and rituals of corporate life.* Harmondsworth, Penguin Books, 1982; reissue Perseus Books.

Interprofessional Education Collaborative Expert Panel. (2011). *Core competencies for interprofessional collaborative practice: Report of an expert panel.* Interprofessional Education Collaborative.

Katzenbach, J., Steffen, I., & Kronley, C. (2012). *Cultural change that sticks.* Harvard Business Review. https://hbr.org/2012/07/cultural-change-that-sticks

Kendi, I. (2019). *How to be an antiracist.* Penguin Random House.

Perlo, J., Balik, B., Swensen, S., Kabcenell, A., Landsman, J., & Feeley, D. (2017). *IHI Framework for improving joy in work.* IHI White Paper. Institute for Healthcare Improvement.   http://www.ihi.org/resources/Pages/IHIWhitePapers/Framework-Improving-Joy-in-Work.aspx

Ravasi, D., Schultz, M., (2006). Responding to organizational identity threats: Exploring the role of organizational culture. *Academy of Management Journal, 49*(3). https://doi.org/10.5465/amj.2006.21794663

Schein, E. (1992). *Organizational culture and leadership: A dynamic view.* Jossey-Bass.

Schein, E. (2010). *Organizational culture & leadership.* Jossey Bass

The Shingo Model. The Shingo Institute and Jon M. Huntsman School of Business, Utah State University. Logan, UT: The Shingo Institute, 2021. Accessed January 2022. https://shingo.org/model/.

Thiefels, J., (2018, April 24). *5 simple ways to assess a company's culture.* Engage: The Employee Engagement Blog.

https://www.achievers.com/blog/5-simple-ways-assess- company-culture/

World Health Organization. (2010). *Framework for action on interprofessional education and collaborative practice.* World Health Organization.

CHAPTER 4

Mission, Vision, Values

ACADEMIC VIGNETTE

Dr. Jane Smith is the dean of a school of nursing in a large public research university. The academic programs include a basic baccalaureate program, an RN to BS program, Masters programs in clinical practice (NP and CNS), education and administration, and both a PhD in Nursing and a DNP program. The academic programs are solid and have been for years but there has been very little attention to developing a research enterprise or to the advancement of fund-raising activities. Dr. Smith has made these two areas a priority in her role as dean.

Over the course of her tenure, Dr. Smith had the opportunity to meet a gentleman who expressed a significant interest in the school. He and Dr. Smith had developed a very positive professional relationship and enjoyed the time they spent with each other. He was an entrepreneur and had made a significant amount of money over the course of his career. His wife recently passed away, and he wanted to honor her memory with a special contribution to the school of nursing since she had been a nurse (an LPN). When discussing how he wanted to shape this legacy in honor of his wife, the donor told Dr. Smith he was ready to provide a "very significant seven figure donation" to the school of nursing, so they could start a LPN program named after her.

Dr. Smith reflected on this mission statement of the school that stated that the School of Nursing was preparing nurse leaders to transform healthcare for all and to develop new knowledge that will provide the basis for healthcare improvement. She was concerned that the development of an LPN program was inconsistent with that mission and would signal the outside community that the school of nursing was committed to this level of practice. Yet, this kind of donation could be transformational for the school and would represent the largest gift to the school of nursing in its history. In addition to funding the LPN program start up, the donor agreed to have significant funds set aside to support nursing research. To add an additional level of complexity, the university was in a capital campaign, and this gift would certainly assure the school of nursing would meet its goal. She talked to her executive council to obtain their opinion.

CLINICAL VIGNETTE

Dr. Sally Jones is the newly hired CNO and vice president for patient care services at a large metropolitan hospital. She was recruited for this role and was excited by the diversity of patients that rely on the hospital. The majority of patients are underrepresented minorities and the quality of care they receive is equal to other hospitals in the region and nation. In the first few weeks of her tenure with the hospital, she noted that the nursing service unit did not have a mission, vision, or value (MVV) statement. Although the hospital had statements she believed were appropriate, the statements targeted the institution and she believed that addressing nursing was also important. In one of her early one-on-one meetings with the CEO, she shared her desire to work with the nursing leadership and other hospital stakeholders to define a MVV statement for the nursing service unit.

Her CEO indicated that she was not supportive of a separate statement for nursing, believing that separate MVV statements would be divisive. In contrast, she asserted that all employees could be directed by way of the institutional MVV. She shared that she was afraid of showing favoritism to nursing and did not want stakeholders in other departments spending their time involved in a nursing project or feeling that their unit should develop their own MVV. The CEO pointed to the metrics that show the nursing staff were providing the high-quality care to underrepresented minority patients that the institution holds as part of their values.

When Dr. Jones mentioned this to her nursing leadership group, about half of the members felt it was critically important that the nursing service department have their own MVV statements and half felt that "they are doing just fine" and why do they have to take on this additional work.

INTRODUCTION

Mission, vision, and value (MVV) statements are core elements of every organization and provide the foundation for much of the work of the organization. They provide direction for the organizations and a focus for the work of the employees. They also set the tone for the aspirational goals of the organization. The authority to set the organization's strategic mission and vision may rest with the top leadership with input of the board of directors or trustees. Before a process to develop a MVV begins at whatever level in an organization, it should be clear who is responsible for developing and ultimately approving the MVV.

The Importance of Mission, Vision, and Values

The MVV can enhance employee engagement, set a direction for the organization, be used as a tool in decision-making about resource allocation, and inform the external world about the who, what, why, and how of the organization. Organizations that do not have MVVs do not know where they are, where they want to go, or what they aspire to. Yogi Berra, a famous baseball player and manager, was well known for his "Yogi-isms." One of his Yogi-isms was, "If you don't know where you are going, you will end up someplace else." MVVs are the guides that tell us what an organization is focused on accomplishing (mission), what it aspires to do (vision), and the values that undergird both. MVVs statements represent the reason that everyone "gets up each morning and goes to work." Therefore, the MVV statements must have meaning for each person in the organization to continue to inspire them. This means that the MVVs must reach the strongly held beliefs at an emotional level. It is useful to keep in mind that nearly all people enter a health career because they are driven by the desire to help others. Recognizing this is important in developing the MVV statement. Every employee should be able to proudly state the organization's MVV statement.

MVV statements that are well worded, with substance and meaning, can have both tangible and intangible benefits. Tangibly, they identify essential services, describe the fundamental purpose of the organization, and define its core and enduring principles. On the intangible side, they unite staff around a common spirit of service and professionalism (MacLeod, 2016). The MVV statement sets out the organization purpose and meaning and points it in the right direction. Rather that detailing the products and services the organization provides, the MVV statement lays out the reason why these products and services are provided. These three documents, collectively, give focus and direction within the organization and to its employees, and provide a commitment by the organization to the external community.

Consider: **Find your organization's MVV statements. Do these statements provide a sense of the purpose and meaning of the organization? Are they accurate?**

Mission

Stephen Covey (2004) wrote that your mission statement becomes your constitution, the solid expression of your vision and your values. Mission statements answer the question, "Why do we exist and why are we important?" In taking Covey's questions further, Hull (2013) proposes that a mission statement should answer the following:

- What do we do?
- How do we do it?
- Whom do we serve?
- What value do we bring?

The mission addresses the inner core of the organization's existence. For example, a hospital's mission would not just be to care for patients, because it does not address the key questions a mission statement should include. Rather it might include a statement about increasing access and affordable care through community outreach programs to the underserved population so they can live a healthy, engaged life. A mission statement will often be a succinct statement about the organization's impact. For example, "serves as a center of excellence for healthcare," "to make cancer history," or "develop leaders that will transform healthcare for all." A mission statement is a summary of the aims and values of an organization. It clarifies for the external community the essence of your business.

The mission statement is important to several constituencies because it tells them what you do and why it is important. The first constituency is the employees. Employees want to know what the work of the organization is, why it is important and how what they do furthers the mission. They want to understand where they fit in the mission. The translation of where they fit is the responsibility of the leader. A second constituency is the people the organization serves, its customers (students if an academic organization and patients and families if a clinical organization). Customers want to know what the healthcare organization or academic program is committed to. Finally, external partners want to know what the organization values are in order to make a judgment about a partnership. For instance, if a hospital has a clear mission to serve underserved populations, community service agencies supporting low-income populations may be more interested in partnering than if a hospital has a mission of providing the most up to date technology to their patients.

Vision

Leadership and Vision

The vision for the future is what a leader brings to an organization. New leaders are expected to have a vision of what is possible for the future and to reinvigorate or renovate an organization. The vision reflects the future aspirations of the organization. It is the "why" that Simon Sinek talks about in terms of the first work that leaders should do. While some leaders envision the "what" and the "how" of an organization, wise leaders focus first on the why (Sinek, 2009).

A leader's vision needs to touch an emotional chord with individuals in the organization. Getting to the emotional level is more effective in generating passion for the work of the organization than having a fact-based vision of the future. Healthcare providers have an emotional commitment to help people and make the world a better and healthier place. In order to sustain passion for one's work, an emotional connection to the vision for the future needs to generate that passion. A quote from Sinek summarizes this idea. "If you hire people just because they can do a job, they'll work for your money. But if you hire people who believe what you believe, they'll work for you with blood and sweat and tears" (Sinek, 2009).

A vision needs to couple the emotional buy-in with a need. The need creates the passion, especially when individuals feel that they are contributing to something important. Needs can be identified from several sources. One of these sources is to listen to the customers. Measuring patient and family experience of care is a beginning attempt to understand their needs. Knowing how patients perceived their care experience can inform the leadership about opportunities for improvement and strengths of the organization. Identifying business opportunities goes beyond collecting and analyzing required measures. It means taking the time to do focus groups or just asking people engaged in the service what might be missing.

A source of information to inform a vision is following the trends in healthcare. Healthcare is complicated, and we often do not know what policies may be in place for the long term or what advances in diagnostic and treatment modalities will evolve. However, several trends in healthcare are important to watch including:

- Reorganization and consolidation of healthcare
- Value driven payment
- Cost containment efforts
- Access to healthcare for both primary and specialty care
- Technology and artificial intelligence
- Consumer demands for accountability
- Care coordination
- Interprofessional care teams
- Issues of racial equity
- Consumer empowerment
- Healthcare disrupters

In academia, trends to watch include:

- Models of education—online/blended/in-person, full-time/part-time
- Student demographics
- Curricula—new programs/revised programs
- Regulations on licensure/certification/accreditation
- Enrollment projections/demographic trends
- Approaches to clinical education
- Issues of racial equity
- Changes in the healthcare system and changing roles of nurses

Trends in healthcare and academia provide leadership with the foundation for envisioning the future and provide the spark that will help define the work of the organization. Another source of information about needs and opportunities that informs the vision is the organization's competitors. Is there an opportunity for a new program that may not have been launched by competing nursing schools? Is there an opportunity for a women's health clinic to address issues of maternal and infant mortality and morbidity? A great source of new ideas is the identification of gaps in education or service based on personal experience and observation. Whatever the source of information about a need, the need to be addressed is the "why" of the organization and should be reflected in the leader's vision.

When your customers are your students, it is important to develop mechanisms for input from this important constituency. Developing an opportunity to hear from students in informal settings or through anonymous data collection allows the leader to see the organization through the eyes of the end user. This gives a perspective to creating the vision that cannot be accomplished without this information. Other constituencies that are important sources of information for the academic leader as you develop an organizational vision are employers, alumni, and community leaders.

If your customers are patients and families, critical review of patient satisfaction data will provide the context for creating a vision for improvement. Data from employees, payers and stakeholders will provide additional information a leader can use to create and refine a vision for the organization.

Writing the Vision Statement

The vision statement identifies where the organization wants to be in the future. Vision is different from mission in that vision is a statement for the future while mission reflects the present life of the organization. A vision statement is an aspirational statement made by an organization that articulates what they would like to achieve. Furthermore, the vision guides the direction of the organization's efforts (Wright, 2018). Many vision statements include three characteristics:

- It is motivational, hopeful, and realistic.
- It defines a dream. What the organization will look like several years from now.
- It includes the behaviors that you hold yourself to that will not change (Boardsource, 2016).

The work of creating a vision for an organization may get lost in the eagerness to define the mission and objectives. It is important that the work of creating or revising the vision is done in collaboration with the employees of the organization. Being inclusive encourages employees to feel that they are part of the organization and engaged in work that moves the organization toward the future. The vision of an organization can be inspiring and energizing when individuals come together in a shared understanding of how they contribute to a preferred future. The vision provides guidance for the mission and will help leaders and employees see what type of future their organization will create through its mission or purpose. A vision statement for a healthcare organization might be, "Be at the forefront of medicine by fostering a culture of collaboration, pushing the boundaries of medical research, educating the brightest medical minds, and maintaining an unwavering commitment to the diverse community we were created to serve." For a school of nursing, a vision statement might look something like, "Our graduates improve the health of populations across the globe through the application of scientific knowledge and a commitment to health and social equity." A vision statement can include several aspirations or just one.

Consider: **Have you ever been involved in writing or revising the vision for your organization? What aspirational elements of the organization did you consider in the context of the environment?**

Values

The final foundational document of an organization is the statement of the core values. The values of an organization serve to describe how the organization will behave while accomplishing its mission. They serve as a moral compass or north star for the organization. When considering the development of core values, the organization might ask itself: "What values are unique to our organization? What values should guide the creation of our organization? What conduct should our employees uphold?" The values statement defines what the organization believes in and how the organization will act, even in difficult situations. For example, an organization might be tempted to take a large donation from an individual who made the majority of his/her money in an industry that has a negative impact on health. Accepting the donation could be useful to the organization and perhaps even enable them to do work that is very important to the health of the population served. However, accepting the donation would violate the core values of high-quality healthcare for all and protecting the rights of the underserved for which the organization stands. Knowing the core values and using them to guide decision-making is critical for the organizational leader.

Values such as quality, caring, pursuit of excellence, respect for human dignity, inclusion, and honesty are examples of values that are closely aligned with nursing and support the goals and priorities of the nursing profession. While these values are highly regarded as critical in the healthcare domain, they are just words on a page if they are not reinforced at every level of the organization in both attitudes and actions. For example, if a value of the organization is inclusion, this value should be seen in the day-to-day operation of every level of the organization's work (recruitment, hiring, pay, promotions, space, etc.) If the CEO is not inclusive in their decision-making processes, the employees cannot be expected to embrace this value in their work.

Aligning Nursing Mission, Vision and Values with Organizational Goals

Healthcare organizations and universities are highly complex and are often organized in silos for what is perceived as maximum efficiency. Each unit of an organization could have their own MVV that drives the work of that unit. This occurs more often within universities than within healthcare organizations. For example, a school of nursing in a university will often have a MVV statement that drives the MVV of the school. They should be aligned with the larger MVV statement of the university and are frequently displayed prominently on the university website. Perhaps the frequency with which this occurs in the academic setting is due to the uni-professional nature of a school of nursing and the explicit focus in academia on education, research, practice, and outreach.

Although having a unit based MVV is not as frequently seen or clearly defined in the hospital setting, it is important for the nursing service to have its own MVV statement. Aligned with the organizational MVV statement, a nursing service MVV statement will communicate nursing's core purpose in the organization and establish a unified sense of professional direction for the staff (MacLeod, 2016). The organizational and unit statements should enhance one another.

It is widely recognized that nursing and nurses are the key drivers for patient satisfaction in hospitals and are responsible for many of the quality and safety initiatives that impact patient care. It is also well recognized that nursing is the largest cost center in the hospital and when there are financial pressures, nursing is where many hospital administrators go to find relief from these pressures. Establishing MVV statements for the nursing service department helps to set a solid base for why nursing is critical to the organizational mission and provide the foundation for resource allocation decisions.

The process for establishing or revising the MVV statements for a nursing service department starts with engaging support from senior management. Helping senior management see the benefit of having a visible and engaged nursing service department in supporting quality patient care is a critical first step. By engaging a diverse set of ideas and opinions, nursing leaders must develop the MVV statements in such a way that they are in line with and compatible with the MVV statements of the organization. Having the nursing service MVV statements support and enhance the statements of the organization makes visible, the critical alignment of nursing within the organization (MacLeod, 2016).

Consider: **How do the MVV become integrated into the daily work of the members of your organization? Do you see your organizational leader referencing the mission, vision, or values in their communications with the members of the organization?**

Academic-Practice Partnerships

Academic-practice partnerships that develop the capacity and infrastructure to create and solve problems is significant for the future of nursing practice innovation, education, and science. The opportunity to advance the alignment between academic institutions and health systems with the potential to create knowledge and use evidence to assure high quality patient care outcomes was detailed in a publication from the American Association of Colleges of Nursing (AACN, 2016). The report proposed a blueprint for academic nursing that embraced a transformation in the way education is conceptualized. This strategic approach centers on the need to create stronger partnerships across the healthcare delivery, education, and research enterprise. The imperatives listed in this blueprint include six pillars: (1) embrace a new vision for academic nursing, (2) enhance the clinical practice of academic nursing, (3) partner in preparing the nurses of the future, (4) partner in the implementation of accountable care, (5) invest in nursing research programs and better integrate research into clinical practice, and (6) implement an advocacy agenda to support a new era for academic nursing.

The third imperative calls for the development of academic-practice partnerships across institutions and may prove to be the most powerful approach to creating a nursing workforce across systems and populations who are expert clinicians, providers, leaders, and scientists. The potential for health system nurse executives and academic nursing deans to create a joint vision and mission for nursing is exciting. It offers the potential to collaborate across systems to strengthen the nursing curriculum that enhances student preparation for clinical practice and enhances the ability of clinicians to participate in the development of evidence based approaches to clinical practice innovation. It also partners nurse leaders from the clinical and academic environment to develop transformative strategies to enhance infrastructure, patient care, technology, performance, decision-making, and clinical research. It has the potential to address social determinants of health disparities though innovative community outreach. It also has the potential to create learning labs across institutions for rapid cycle innovation.

All of these current and future innovations, along with the most creative and visionary strategic plans, will go unrealized without astute financial planning. A good strategic plan should incorporate the finances required to realize the vision. The executive team with input from internal and external stakeholders, will need to use the institution's mission, vision, goals, operational assessment, and productivity targets to create a financial plan. This includes developing the organizational budget, monitoring the day-to-day utilization of fiscal resources, and modifying organizational goals and objectives based on variance analysis and productivity measurements. The data used by the leaders to modify goals, strategies, and tactics should generate ongoing modifications at each level of the organization. Managers are responsible for the organizational goals, strategies, and budget specific to their area of responsibility. In most organizations, managers are charged with developing unit or department-level goals, strategies, and budgets and are held accountable for ensuring that the programs stay within those fiscal projections. Managers are also ultimately responsible for performance and productivity, both of which are major drivers of financial stability. It is critical that managers partner with those they manage to co-create a culture of inclusion, respect, and meaning for all so that organizational goals are shared by all.

SUMMARY

The MVV statements provide the true north for organizations as they navigate both the challenging and less challenging times in the organization's life. They should be reviewed periodically, often in conjunction with the strategic planning process. Organizational leaders should talk about the MVV statement regularly and describe ways the concepts have been used to guide decision-making. By making these documents visible in the work of the organization, the leader fosters a sense of true ownership and inclusion by others in the organization.

CRITICAL THINKING QUESTIONS

At the beginning of the chapter an academic and clinical vignette were presented. Please review the vignettes to address the following the questions. The questions are specific to the vignettes.

Academic Vignette Questions

1. Should the School of Nursing start an LPN program and if they did, what do you think would be the consequences?
2. Does the inclusion of dollars for nursing research in the donation influence the decision? If so, in what way?
3. Where could Dean Smith go to get support or direction in making this decision?
4. Should the Executive Council of the School make the decision or is their role advisory?
5. If the decision is not to start the LPN program, how does Dean Smith salvage her relationship with this donor?

Clinical Vignette Questions

1. What points should Dr. Jones use to make the case with the CEO that the nursing service department should have MVV statements?
2. How can Dr. Jones enlist the support of non-nursing hospital leadership to convince the CEO that nursing service department MVV statements are important for the hospital?
3. How should the leadership team's opinions factor into this decision?
4. Are there data points (internal or external) that would be helpful in making the case with the CEO?
5. What professional decisions does Dr. Jones have to consider if the CEO continues to prevent the nursing service department from having its own MVV statements?

REFERENCES

AACN (2016) A New Era for Academic Nursing. American Association of Colleges of Nursing. https://www.aacnnursing.org/Portals/42/Publications/AACN-New-Era-Report.pdf

BoardSource. (2016). *Elements of a vision statement*. BoardSource. https://boardsource.org/resources/vision-statement/

Covey, S. R. (2004). *The 7 habits of highly effective people: Restoring the character ethic* ([Rev. ed.].). Free Press.

Hull, P. (2013, January 10). *Answer four questions to get a great mission statement*. Forbes. https://www.forbes.com/sites/patrickhull/2013/01/10/answer-4-questions-to-get-a-great-mission-statement/#3696d37767f5

MacLeod, L. (2016). Aligning mission, vision, and values: The nurse leader's role. *Nurse Leader, 14*(6), 438-441. https://doi.org/10.1016/j.mnl.2016.09.005

Sinek, S. (2009). *Start with why: How leaders Inspire everyone to take Action*. Penguin Publishing.

Wright, T. (2018, May 1). Good vision statement examples. *Cascade Strategies*. https://www.executestrategy.net/blog/examples-good-vision-statements

CHAPTER 5

Creating the Future Through Strategic Planning

ACADEMIC VIGNETTE

You are the Assistant Dean for Strategic Development for your school and part of your job is to complete a new strategic plan for the school. The current plan will be completed by the next academic year. Your school has 80 full time faculty, 20 staff, many part time and clinical faculty, and over 1500 students. The previous strategic plan goals were to: (1) increase enrollment (enrollment increased from 1000 to 1500 over 4 years); (2) be ranked in the top 25% of schools (your school is now ranked number 22, up from 42); (3) increase research funding (research funding has doubled to include $3 million in NIH grants; and (4) achieve 10-year recognition from the accrediting agency (this has been completed). You know that to create a strategic plan, everyone needs to participate and consider trends in nursing education, clinical practice, and changes in the broader environment including economic, political, and social changes. Your job is complicated because the university is also engaging in a strategic planning process. The one element that is clear is that the mission and vision statements will remain the same for the university and the school. The mission and vision statements are:

- *Mission*: To prepare students to be excellent clinicians, advocates, educators, and leaders to advance high quality, patient centered care that is evidence-based and to create a caring, just, and compassionate health system that is based on innovation and research.
- *Vision*: To improve the health of all through education, research, and innovation and create strong partnerships to do this work.

You understand that since the previous strategic plan goals have been met,

79

the faculty don't seem to have the level of commitment that you know is important. You have heard faculty say we are already successful, and the work of strategic planning will distract us from our important work. Your goal is to engage the school community in the creation of a strategic plan that clearly links to the mission, vision and values (MVV) of the university; to inspire faculty, staff, and students to fully participate in the learning process; and to lead the nation in nursing education.

CLINICAL VIGNETTE

You are the Associate Vice President for Nursing at your 800-bed hospital. The newly appointed Vice President for Nursing has asked you to lead the strategic planning efforts for nursing. Seven years have passed since the last strategic plan was completed and since then, there have been significant leadership changes in the organization; no new plan was developed during the seven-year interval. Turnover rates for nursing staff are higher than the national average; however, no exit interviews have been completed in the last seven years. Given the significant turnover rates, the nursing staff has expressed that they feel overwhelmed. You are concerned about how to engage the staff in the strategic planning process, anticipating that they might see the expectation as adding to their growing responsibilities. You know you need to develop the plan and need the nursing staff to engage in the process. You recruit a small group of leaders who understand the importance and are willing to be the core group implementing the process. Nursing has mission and vision statements that will guide the development of the strategic goals:

- *Mission*: To provide excellent nursing care compassionately to all people in our care.
- *Vision*: To advance health for all patients, families, and communities we serve through evidence-based care, innovation, and research, and to engage in continuous quality improvement in partnership with patients and colleagues.

You are very aware of the ever-changing healthcare environment, especially the increasing pressure to reduce costs and the changing expectations and related demands of consumers. The hospital is under a great deal of pressure to improve the patient experience and readmission scores to be more competitive; you know nursing is central to both of these improvements. Your first step is to begin to communicate to staff through a variety of venues that a strategic planning process is starting and that their input is essential. You are also transparent in stating your goal that the strategic plan is intended to create a better work environment for all.

INTRODUCTION

A strategic plan is essential to the success of an organization, particularly in industries such as healthcare and higher education, in which change is a constant. Strategic planning highlights the priorities for the organization's work and guides goal setting and direction of resources. A plan identifies the actions to be undertaken, leading to goals the organization aspires to accomplish. Strategic planning provides a roadmap for where you want to go and how you will get there. A strong plan inspires community members to make changes in strategic areas needed to improve the value of the organization and improve its products including academic programs or healthcare services. Notably, plans often consist of activities and goals that evolve as conditions change, goals are met, and new challenges emerge. The ongoing evaluation and update of strategic plans helps to support its evolution, as well as to encourage the organization's further efforts by recognizing the accomplishments already attained.

Strategic planning is not busy work. While there is often groaning about strategic planning, it can be one of the most meaningful activities (if not the most important) for an organization. When a new or updated strategic planning process is announced, sometimes people respond with comments like, "what is the point" or "it is so tedious." Limited enthusiasm may result if the leadership of an organization fails to link the activities of the strategic plan to the work people actually do and the desired outcomes. The leadership challenge in strategic planning is to create a plan that defines goals to meet the future (not the present) and includes everyone in the organization.

The rapid rate of change in healthcare requires that you, as leader, keep a constant eye on strategic directions and related planning. In the recent past, it was common for organizations to create five-year plans, a time interval now considered to be too lengthy. In today's world, the time frame is often shortened to three years with annual reviews for adjustment. The COVID-19 pandemic has starkly illustrated how essential it is for ongoing strategic planning. Anything that had been planned prior to the pandemic was changed, accelerating some activities (e.g., online educational delivery formats or increased use of virtual meeting platforms), and slowing down others (e.g., travel abroad trips for healthcare delivery or medical tourism). Both clinical and academic institutions have faced shifts in revenues that required changes in the annual and projected budgets. Beyond the pandemic, changes to available technologies and revised contracts with bargaining units will influence the activities and goals set out in a strategic plan. Further, academic and healthcare organizations often require that subunits revise their plans to better address the plans of the parent unit (e.g., school of nursing accommodating to the university plan, or the nursing department aligning with the health system's plan). Each of these examples argues of the ability for plans to serve as dynamic roadmaps for strategic change. This chapter will build on Chapter 4, MVV, and will focus on the steps that are needed in a strategic planning process once the MVV have been established.

Consider: **What is your experience with strategic planning? What role did you play? Was the process useful? Did the organization consider the strategic plan static or did they revisit it on a regular basis?**

Understanding Terms

Strategic planning employs commonly used terms. Terms are often used interchangeably and often without precision. The following provides a summary of definitions we will use in this chapter related specifically to strategic planning.

- *Goal*: A major outcome or destination to be achieved that is consistent with a MVV of an organization. A goal can be short, intermediate, or long term. Goals provide more detail to the vision of an organization yet are broad statements for the future.
- *Objective*: Provides in general the answers to the questions of how much and when. They provide the details to the goal and should be specific, measurable, achievable, and timely.
- *Strategy*: Provides the general approach to achieving the objectives. It answers the question of how we are going to achieve our goal.

TABLE 5.1. Example of Strategic Planning Terms.

Term	Academic Organization	Clinical Organization
Goal	Develop and offer an online Doctor of Nursing Practice Program	Nursing will advance translational research
Objective	Secure $500,000 to start the program within the year	Each nursing unit will develop one research project each year
Strategy	Explore outside funding as well as institutional support	A research nurse will be hired with the main role to teach and support research on each unit
Tactics	Submit grant to Health Resources and Services Administration for one million over three years to develop the DNP program for the next submission cycle	The research nurse will establish educational sessions for nurses interested in research
	Create a budget that shows return on investment (ROI) of the program to the University leadership for approval by the next University board meeting	The research nurse will work with each unit to develop a research project

- *Strategic planning process*: The process of an organization in defining their objectives and priorities and aligning those with MVV and resources.
- *Tactic*: Is the specific way to accomplish the strategies. A tactic provides the detail of what exactly needs to be done to implement the strategy.

Table 5.1 provides examples of the terms defined above that are relevant to academic and clinical organizations.

OVERVIEW OF THE STRATEGIC PLANNING PROCESS

To anticipate the impact of actual or probable change in healthcare, strategic planning encompasses the integration of purposeful development or refinement of the organization's mission, vision, goals, strategies, priorities, and metrics that are central to the dynamics of an organization. Strategic planning is a critical component of any organization and, if taken seriously, evaluated, and updated regularly, will make a considerable difference in the success of the organization. There are many elements in developing a strategic plan that will guide the organization and its people toward its mission and vision. The success of a process for strategic planning will depend a great deal on the ability and commitment of leaders to engage the organization's members, its customers, partners, and community members.

We will begin by setting a framework for how to think about the process. Organizations approach strategic planning in a variety of ways depending on their structure and leadership. An organization with multiple divisions, departments, sections, units, and locations may approach strategic planning as a centralized responsibility creating a specific roadmap for each of the organizational units. An example of this model is an organization that develops a "corporate" level mission and vision including the "why do we exist" question with value statements, goals/objectives, and strategies and tactics for each of the units within the organization. A decentralized model common to clinical and academic organizations is to create a strategic plan at the organizational level and then have each specialty or department within an organization create their specific plan. Within a clinical organization, the services might be the cardiac surgery service, nursing, the emergency services, and special care units to name a few specialties. Within an academic institution it may be the different schools or departments that comprise the institution. The plan of each individual unit will be closely aligned to the organization's overall plan.

The strategic planning process may take different forms. Some organizations use the terms goals and objectives interchangeably. Some leave the detailed strategies and tactics to unit or department level teams. Evaluation may be driven by specific metrics and others will create qualitative approaches to outcomes. The approach matters and the specifics of the approach should be aligned with the complexity of the organization. What matters most about the process of strategic planning is that an organization, big or small, clearly understands the business that they are in, what they want to accomplish, how they will accomplish it and how they know whether they succeed. In defining the desired outcomes, it is critical to understand and appreciate the needs of the customer.

A strategic plan is intended to set the organization apart from others who share a similar business. Having a competitive advantage is critical to the success of an organization. Healthcare and education are both highly competitive. Competition is driving health systems to be seen as a high-quality provider. Patients often have a choice of providers even though there continue to be limitations based on access, insurance and cost. Insurers are also becoming more discriminate in the providers that they recognize with many insurers having preferred provider partnerships. In academics, universities compete for the top scientists and brightest students. Scientists compete for grants based not only on their research but on the organization's ability to support the research enterprise with appropriate grant management, lab space, access to mentors, etc. It is essential that the strategic plan enable the organization to create a competitive advantage. The plan needs to inspire the internal workforce, and it must also inspire key stakeholders and customers.

Strategic Planning is a Team Effort

Our focus will now take a deeper dive into each of the steps of the planning process, including linking the mission and vision to collecting information, assessing strengths and weaknesses, establishing goals and priorities, creating a timeline and implementation plan, and evaluation. It would be a wonderfully easy world if leaders could review their strategic plan and all that needs to be done is to present the plan to their team and their team members would eagerly endorse it and enthusiastically engage in implementation. Reality is a bit different. The reality is that for a strategic plan to be successful, all parties need to be engaged in the development of the plan. Everyone has an opinion or perspective about future directions so that the organization can fulfill its mission and vision. A leader will need to let go of controlling the outcome of a planning process in order to integrate the thinking and ideas of all stakeholders.

Getting buy-in from the highest-level leader or a board of directors is crucial at the beginning of the process. It is important to understand the range of tolerance for change of the leaders, the willingness to commit resources to fulfilling the plan, and the level of support for moving forward. To provide the support needed, it is essential for the leader to understand how the process will support the overall vision and mission of the organization.

To think that everyone will be enthusiastic about the process of strategic planning or the outcome is to deny reality of human nature. What enables individuals within an organization to embrace the process and outcomes? Simply put, it is the leadership. If leaders do not value and participate in the process it is unlikely results will follow. In the clinical setting, the leader's ability to engage staff in the process of designing their preferred future will define the effectiveness of the strategic planning process. Strategic planning has the potential to enable the transformation of nursing education if it tackles some of the challenges that schools of nursing face including having sufficient high-quality clinical placements. Both clinical and academic institutions have the daunting challenge to redefine, and in some ways rebuild, their business models with the challenges presented by the pandemic. Being mindful of new ways of teaching, learning, and providing care, such as expanding telehealth, are critical to pivoting and creating a new plan.

It is important to listen to those who disagree, as they often have very important observations to add to the discussion. However, open disagreement must be managed. There are levels of disagreement ranging from mild disagreement, to not happy but will go along with the process, to outright hostility and sabotage. In the latter situation, the leader has three choices: (1) engage the person to see if it is possible to sway them to support; (2) minimize the impact of negativity by restructuring job responsibilities; or (3) work toward removing the person from the team to either a different area of the organization where the fit may be better or toward termination. In all cases, trying to engage the person should be a first step. Leaders are often rightly reluctant to terminate employment of someone. However, a leader cannot have a member of the organization overtly working to undermine their new vision. Just one person can create a dysfunctional environment and derail movement toward the vision. In thinking about the behaviors that appear to interfere with progress, as the leader, it will be helpful to consider the theories of change described in Chapter 14. When resistant behaviors are viewed through the lens of change, they can help you understand the barriers you, as a leader, need to lower or, conversely, the driving forces you need to strengthen. This will be described in greater detail in Chapter 14.

Often leaders look forward to engaging in a strategic planning process and may also feel pressure to quickly move to action. Competitive organizations have limited tolerance for slow moving processes; however, the time it takes to recommit to the organization's mission and vision and get buy-in from all levels of members is time well spent. Communicating the plan for the process, the importance to the future of the organization, and the value of everyone's input will be important first steps. When necessary, this process can be fast-tracked. The initial process of providing information and creating dialogue usually can be done within a fairly short time frame and can begin with the launch of the process. The launch should start with an all person meeting or several meetings to recognize people working different shifts. Food is always good at a meeting even if it is donuts and coffee. The entire leadership team needs to be on board and enthusiastic. It helps to let everyone know when the vision phase of the path forward will be complete. A leader and their team will need to help each person in the organization understand how they can contribute to the vision and therefore the planning process.

Consider: **In your own experience, who were the members of the core team for a strategic planning process? What additional teams were created to do the work of process? What do you think are the challenges of creating multiple teams to address specific issues of the planning process?**

Steps in the Process

Understanding the process and structure of strategic planning is a prerequisite to setting the direction and outcomes of an organization. Equally important is to assure alignment around authority and ownership of strategic planning. Although there are many different approaches and frameworks used in creating a strategic plan, as noted above, we will discuss the steps that are generally used in a strategic planning process. The steps of the planning process include:

- Develop/review the MVV statement (addressed in Chapter 4)
- Plan for data collection and analysis
- Assess strengths and weaknesses, internally and externally (risks and opportunities)
- Develop goals and objectives, aligned with MVV
- Determine strategies and tactics
- Create a timetable and evaluation metrics
- Implement
- Evaluate.

The important point in creating a framework for strategic planning is to be clear about what needs to be accomplished, how it is to be accomplished (for instance, who will be responsible to do the work), when will the plan be implemented, and what are the important metrics for success. Strategic planning can be engaging and fun, but complexity can bog it down. Although widespread staff involvement in the process provides an opportunity for everyone's voice to be heard and expertise to be contributed, it is critical that the number of people involved in the process not derail the process. One effective strategy is to empower a core group responsible for developing and guiding the strategic plan, and periodically bring together a larger group for review of progress and to offer feedback and input. Opportunities for providing anonymous feedback electronically or use of a suggestion box may be valuable. The power differentials that are inevitable with organizations (e.g., faculty to staff, or nurse

administrators to medical assistants) can limit community members from offering honest feedback or innovative ideas. Anonymity can enlarge the opportunities for everyone to contribute.

Collect and Analyze Data

After reviewing and recommitting to the MVV as described in chapter 4,
the next step is to identify the key members of the data team. In a large organization that has technology and data teams, key members will include at least
one member who is knowledgeable about the databases and can run analyses
needed for the planning process. It will also be useful to have a leader knowledgeable about previous strategic plans and the outcomes related to the data
plans. Another important member is a person who is directly involved in the
day-to-day working of the organization at a direct clinical or teaching level.
Finally, having an administrative person who knows the details of running the
organization is critical. For smaller organizations, the team could be a three
member team including the administrative leader with knowledge of the data
collected, a clinical or academic leader and a faculty or clinical staff member.

Data are critical to knowing where the organization is to determine where it
wants to be. Data that are relevant to strategic planning can be either internal
or external to the organization. Depending on the size of the organization, large
organizations will likely have a more robust capacity to collect and analyze
data than smaller organizations that have limited capacity and limited data. Regardless of the size of an organization, no one ever feels they have enough data
or that the data is exactly what they need to make decisions. Data collection
and analysis should be driven by the mission and vision of the organization as
well as by the data that is part of the everyday evaluation of the organization
and its activities.

Data that are readily available will provide the baseline of information to
inform leaders of where the organization is currently. It may be useful to organize the data into a table to reflect the name of the data; who "owns" the
data in terms of who collects, stores, and analyzes the data; the frequency of
collection; and what the data measures (outcome, process, procedure). Organizing data in this way will help determine gaps related to evaluating current
activity reflecting the mission and vision. See Table 5.2 for an example of how
to organize data.

Sources of data internal to the clinical organization could include quality of

TABLE 5.2. Organization of Data Sources.

Name of Data	Owner of Data	Frequency of Collection	What is Measured

care data such as patient experience or never events, readmissions, administrative data related to staffing, finances, and patient demographic information. The data could be for the overall organization and for specific clinical units. Measures required by payers including private insurers, Medicare, Medicaid and the Child Health Insurance Program require specific measures to be reported that are useful in the strategic planning process. For educational institutions, data could be related to student numbers such as numbers of applicants, admissions and matriculants, course evaluations, finances, and outcomes of student success such as pass rates on the NCLEX or other licensing and certification exams as well as employment information. The data collected for the *US News and World Report* rankings provide useful internal data for the planning process.

In addition to the internal data, external data are vital. Sources of external data include journal articles, government reports, and data sets available to the public (federal, state and local), data from professional organizations, reports available from foundations, such as the Commonwealth Fund, the Robert Wood Johnson Foundation, and the Kaiser Family Foundation. In addition, there are sources of data from "futurists" that forecast trends in healthcare. The possible sources of external data can be overwhelming and require careful thinking about what data is relevant to the strategic planning process based on mission and vision, and a previous strategic plan if there is one.

Although there are numerous sources of external data, examples useful to strategic planning for clinical organizations include the Centers for Medicare and Medicaid (CMS) Medicare compare sites for hospitals, nursing homes, home care and other organizations (CMS, 2021a). Leaders can use the compare sites to assess their performance in specific clinical areas, as well as patient experience compared to other organizations in their region that are competitors, and also at the state and national levels. In addition, CMS has numerous reports that can provide national, state and local data related to their oversight of the Medicare, Medicaid and Children's Health Insurance Program (CHIP). The CMS Innovation Center provides information about new models and strategies being implemented and tested that can be used to know what is new in the service delivery (CMS, 2021b).

The Agency of Healthcare Research and Quality (AHRQ) has several databases that issue reports from the Health Care Cost and Utilization Project (H-CUP), Medical Expenditure Panel Surveys (MEPS), and the US Health Information Knowledgebase (USHIK) (AHRQ, 2021a). AHRQ provides infographics that summarize trends and briefs that provide a concise summary of current state and trends. In addition, for leaders to stay up to date on clinical quality data, AHRQ has available a weekly summary of new information related to clinical care and issues a report annually on health disparities in the US, the most recent one being the *2019 National Healthcare Disparities Report* (AHRQ, 2021b).

Clinical sites will need to know data relevant to current and future staffing that may be available through state workforce centers. In addition, the Department of Labor and the Department of Health and Human Services provides data related to different professions and provides projections of supply and demand. As noted, there are many sources of data and the noted sources above are examples.

Examples of external data that may be useful to academic leaders include the student data published annually by the American Association of Colleges of Nursing (AACN), and also the National League for Nursing (NLN). There is also information related to pass rates of NCLEX licensing exam by state and institution as well as accreditation status information by institution from Collegiate Commission on Nursing Education (CCNE) and the NLN Commission for Nursing Education Accreditation. The *US News and World Report* rankings of nursing programs and institutions provide useful comparison data. This information provides competitor data for universities, colleges, and departments of nursing. In addition, the data relevant to clinical organizations, both clinical and workforce numbers, is also relevant to educational programs.

Although there is much data available, data useful to strategic planning might not be available, internally or externally. If this is the case, required data will need to be defined and collected if possible in order to fully move forward. For academic institutions, data that might be critical could include a summary of grants written (not just those funded), faculty publications, information about the work environment and faculty, student and staff satisfaction, or the type of community service provided by students and faculty. For clinical organizations, data that might be important could include research conducted, number and type of quality improvement projects completed and the outcomes of the projects, staff that have completed an undergraduate or graduate degree. There are, of course, many more types of data that could inform strategic planning that could be part of the data collection.

Being thoughtful about the analysis of the data requires the strategic planning data team think through the questions that need to be answered to inform the planning process. Data are only useful to the extent that they address the issues important to the process. This requires asking the questions: What data do we need? What analysis of data do we need to inform the strategic plan? How can we show the results of the data in a useful way to enhance the understanding of the data? What process should we use to create agreement about interpretation of the data? These are not easy questions and reflect the need to have both data analysis expertise as well as clinical expertise to be able to interpret clinically the meaning of the data.

Consider: **Who within your organization would be responsible for the data collection and analysis for a strategic planning process? What critical data might be relevant to a strategic planning process in your organization?**

Assess Risks and Opportunities

One of the ways a leader can collect information on the organization and the external environment in the process of establishing a vision is through a SWOT analysis. SWOT stands for strengths, weaknesses, opportunities, and threats, with strengths and weaknesses focused on the internal environment and opportunities and threats focused on the external environment. The SWOT analysis is a structured way of determining areas for organizational development, for the use of resources and areas in which the organization needs improvement. It can help identify gaps in data that may need to be collected for further exploration before a decision can be made related to a plan. In addition to informing the vision of an organization, the SWOT informs the strategic plan by helping to identify areas that the organization can build on and what it needs to be aware of in terms of barriers to success. See Figure 5.1 for an example of the SWOT framework.

When assessing strengths, ask questions such as: What do you do better than anyone else? What makes your organization better than those that do something similar to you? What do you do that is different from competitors? Issues to focus on when determining weaknesses include the organization's areas for improvement and areas in which your competitors do better than you. Reviewing internal and external data is critical. Benchmarking yourself compared to others will provide important information about gaps. Another important area to explore that could be either a strength or weakness is financial resources. Do you have funds to invest or not? In the post pandemic environment, many institutions have worked with fewer overall resources.

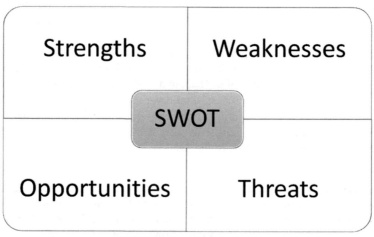

FIGURE 5.1 SWOT Framework.

Opportunities center on trends in the marketplace, changes in technology that affect your business and demographics, population profiles, and social patterns that your organization is poised to address. Threats are those external factors that have an opportunity to derail your organization. In academia, the reduced number of high school graduates nationwide has threatened the existence of many small colleges and universities. In healthcare, bundled payment or value based payment models might have a negative impact on cash flows. Thinking about issues, such as obstacles the organization faces, competitors and changes in governmental programs will help identify the threats to the organization.

Once the members of the organization have brainstormed the four areas of the SWOT, the analysis continues with identifying priorities in each of the categories. By using this approach you can create a vision that distinguishes the organization from its competitors by capitalizing on strengths, addressing weaknesses and managing the threat in the environment.

Consider: **What are the strengths and weaknesses of your organization? What are the major external threats and opportunities?**

Establish Goals and Objectives

Goals and objectives provide information about the envisioned future, what you have set your sights on achieving. Goal statements are broad and are coupled with objectives that are more specific and measurable. For instance, your organization whether clinical or educational may have a goal to increase diversity of the staff. This provides staff a general understanding of one important area to move toward. The objectives related to this goal will provide more detail in terms of what it will look like, such as the organization will increase minority staff by 20% within two years. The following sections provide a more in-depth exploration of goals and objectives.

Goals

Leaders must set goals and priorities to move forward with the strategic plan. The challenge in today's environment is that goals and priorities may need to change based on changing internal and external environments. New leaders are often brought in to shake things up or to implement a new mission and vision. The expectation is that they will do this quickly. A leader may be moving an organization forward in meeting their goals and vision and a single event, such as a change in the CEO or a pandemic, can create significant challenges or stress in the organization. We have seen significant and rapid changes to organizational goals with the impact of the pandemic. However, other changes such as a new hospital being built by a competitor, a change in reimbursement rules by CMS, or severe budget cuts to an academic program may create a need to rethink goals and priorities.

The rapid changes also include new treatments, mergers and partnerships, use of big data, and the increasing use of artificial intelligence. These changes can happen very quickly and will very likely require changing goals and priorities. Healthcare and health professions education are competitive environments requiring rapid responses to opportunities and threats. Organizations that are nimble in redefining goals and priorities are those that will likely remain viable and thrive. An example is the evolution of on-campus to technology-mediated nursing education programs. Programs that have not made this transition have limited opportunity for growth and access to top faculty. Being constrained by geography can be a threat. In the clinical area, telemedicine programs provide opportunities for efficient service to populations who cannot access services in their home community. Those academic institutions that moved to online learning and clinical organizations that had moved to telehealth options were better able to meet needs of students and patients during the COVID-19 pandemic. Technology also provides for the opportunity to connect with exceptional clinicians and providers that would not be possible without technology. Trends provide the information for the vision that then drives the setting of goals and strategies.

While there are many challenges affecting the development of goals and priorities, there are three important considerations:

- Goals and priorities need to be aligned with the culture of the organization reflected in the mission and vision;
- There needs to be adequate return on investment (ROI); and
- Goals and priorities need to be evaluated frequently and changed based on an internal and external environmental scan.

Goals define what is to be achieved within the organization's mission: "excel as the national model for innovation in data science," "embody a culture of respect, integrity and diversity," or "function at the highest level of accountability and effectiveness." Priorities are those actions and initiatives that will have a greater impact and should be on the top of the list for goals.

Goals and priorities need to be aligned throughout an organization. The goals and priorities are based on the culture of the organization, past experiences—success and failures, results of a SWOT analysis and estimated ROI (*see* Chapter 8). The culture of an organization is a critical consideration to setting priorities. The culture reflects not only mission, vision, and goals but also underlying beliefs, assumptions, values, and ways of interacting. This contributes to the unique social and psychological environment of the organization and the unwritten rules of the organization. It is the "personality" of the organization.

Some organizations are very risk averse and have limited tolerance for what might be considered a high-risk goal and priority even if it is consistent with the vision statement of the organization. Others may have a culture of innovation with a high acceptance of failure. Leaders are faced with the challenge of working within an organizational culture and working toward change of the culture as needed to move the goals and priorities forward. Leaders who are new to organizations have a particularly significant challenge to understand the personality of an organization in all of its unique ways of working. A new leader needs to have a go-to person who can help explain the unwritten rules and expectations in order to have a successful planning process. Not understanding the culture of an organization for leaders new to the organization often does not end well for the leader.

A new leader needs to take time to understand the culture of an organization before moving forward with a new set of goals and priorities. The upside of having leaders who have experienced the culture from within is that they may more easily be able to bridge the current and future culture more easily. The downside is that leaders who have been within a culture may be unintentionally limited in their thinking about what could be possible and lead within the context of an existing culture that may not position the organization to respond to opportunities and challenges. See more about organizational culture and change in Chapter 3 and Chapter 14.

It is important that all members of the organization share a common set of values and beliefs to support behaviors that lead to the desired results. Within a system context, the quote by Edward Deming applies to culture, "every system is perfectly designed to get the results it gets." One could alter this quote by saying "every culture is perfectly designed to get the results it gets."

Adequate ROI

For organizations to remain viable, financial sustainability is a must. Any new endeavor that might be part of the strategic plan will need to draw on existing resources or create new funding streams to support it. If the activity uses existing resources, there will need to be a decrease or elimination of resources for another activity. This is when defining priorities becomes essential. Leaders are constantly confronted with tradeoffs often involving very difficult decisions. Those decisions are based on what will best prepare the organization for the future, is most consistent with the mission, and is most likely to be successful. More detailed considerations of ROI are considered in Chapter 8.

Frequent Evaluation of Goals and Priorities Based on External Scan

As noted above, the healthcare environment is changing rapidly with new models of service delivery, value-based payment programs, expectations related to quality of care, technology advances, and diagnostic and treatment advances. These changes challenge both the clinical and academic leaders. The external changes require constant vigilance of the relevance of the goals and priorities. The strategic process does not begin and end but is ongoing to continually scan the environment for changes that will affect the goals and priorities.

Create Goals and Objectives

Goals and specifically the accompanying objectives, should be measurable, time specific, and reflect the desired change in the organization. One rubric for developing goals and objectives is SMART (Doran, 1981). In the literature SMART is referred to both as goals and objectives. If using SMART, the goals and objectives should meet the SMART criteria of:

- *Specific*—Targets an area, population, process that can be clearly defined.
- *Measurable*—Can be quantified to know when achieved.
- *Achievable*—Can be accomplished even if it is a stretch
- *Relevant*—Adds value to the organization and consistent with mission and vision.
- *Timely*—Can be achieved within a time frame to support organizational change.

In addition to SMART goals and objectives, there is the rubric of DUMB goals (dream-driven, uplifting, method-friendly, and behavior-driven) and objectives.

Setting goals and objectives using DUMB is intended to expand a vision and support great creativity and risk taking. The criticism of SMART goals is that they keep organizations within their comfort zone because people define goals and objectives that they can meet. They may limit the real potential of an organization. However, SMART goals integrate measurement into the process that is more specific about outcome achievement. SMART and DUMB are not exclusive and can complement each. DUMB goals are:

- *Dream-Driven*—What do you wish for? Defining a goal that is important at a very deep and emotional level and is transformative.
- *Uplifting*—Does this goal create a positive feeling and sense of excitement?
- *Method-Friendly*—Are there methods and processes who can make this happen? What is a natural part of the organization that can take on the dream-driven goal?
- *Behavior-Driven*—What do people in the organization do that can support the goals?

Goals and objectives define the work that needs to be done in a way that is detailed enough to create an understanding of how a goal will be met. Each goal will likely have several objectives to show how the goal will be attained.

Consider: **Based on your response to the above question about the SWOT, what are two goals that you would identify that are relevant to your organization for nursing?**

Determine Strategies and Tactics

Once the goals and priorities are established, the strategy and tactics for achieving each goal needs to be established. Members of the organization with differing expertise need to be part of creating the strategies and tactics because having different areas of expertise enhances creativity and are critical to figuring out how to achieve the goals. The likelihood of the overall plan being successful is heightened when the people responsible for executing the tactics help define them. Strategies should be specific enough to guide the work and answer the following questions:

- What processes need to change?
- What resources are necessary?
- What skill sets are necessary?
- What infrastructure changes are needed?
- What systems or system changes are needed?

Strategies can be long term because the specific tactics may require significant time to accomplish or short term because the work required can be completed quickly. Each tactic should include a timeline that is realistic such as, "Establish a training plan for all faculty in the use of online educational technology by the end of fall semester," "Implement the new policy on hand hygiene for all nursing staff by October 30," or "Evaluate the effectiveness of the training plan for discharge planning by June 30."

Leaders often confuse strategy and tactics. While strategy is the approach to attain goals and objectives, tactics are statements that detail how each of the strategies will be accomplished. There is a saying, "Think strategically, act tactically." Tactics are the specific ways we are going to implement the strategy detailing how each of the strategies will be accomplished. Multiple tactics are generally needed to effectively accomplish a strategy. Table 5.3 provides an example of how goals, objectives, strategies and tactics are aligned. Note that Table 5.3 includes only one example of each component and in reality, there would be several objectives, strategies and tactics. Also, there is no one right way as to how the components are written as long as there is alignment, and each component provides greater specificity as you move from goal to tactic.

TABLE 5.3. *Examples of Strategies and Tactics for Academic and Clinical Organizations.*

Strategies and Tactics	Academic Organization	Clinical Organization
Goal	Expand online educational opportunities	Reduce nosocomial infections on all units.
Objective	Offer 3 continuing education opportunities (within 12 months)	Increase hand washing though a multi-pronged effort. (begin within 1 months)
Strategy	Identify faculty interested in online learning to form a core group of faculty to develop online continuing education programs (within 1 month)	Develop and implement a comprehensive educational program to reinforce handwashing (within 2 months).
Tactic	The instructional design director will develop and conduct learning opportunities for the core faculty to develop skills in creating high quality online learning (within 2 months)	The Director of Nursing Education will work with the Office of Quality and Safety to implement a comprehensive hand washing educational effort using multiple modes of delivery including online information, required attendance at webinars, posters hung throughout the clinical area as reminders and other formats. (begin within 2 months)

Pacing and Timelines

"Timing is everything" is an overused saying, yet true for leaders contemplating change. Timing and pacing are not simply time management, it is planning the timeline for change. A major reason for failure of new initiatives is change battle fatigue (Gleeson, 2017). Organizations often try to implement too many changes in too short of time. If one change fails, a cycle sets in that lays the groundwork for future failures. While there are other issues that relate to implementation failures, timing and pacing of change is critical to success.

At times, sudden and rapid change is needed which is extremely disruptive to the organization. For example, when the coronavirus pandemic of 2020 hit, hospitals had to make dramatic and substantive changes in operations to prepare for the influx of COVID-19 positive patients. Academic programs had to pivot to a fully virtual delivery of all nursing education. These kinds of changes are necessary and are recognized as short term until a crisis is abated. Long term change can be planned for, and the pace managed. Change that happens quickly or change that happens too slowly can be detrimental to the performance of the organization. Managing the rhythm and pace of change is done by examining both the internal and external factors affecting the adoption of the change.

When leaders have an idea that they are passionate about, the tendency is to want to move forward quickly and get to the action stage of implementation. Leaders may also get pressure from higher-level leaders for quick action. However, knowing the culture, the type and impact of more recent changes will guide the decision to move forward or pause moving forward with the idea. The strategic plan also signals the community that changes will be initiated and gives them a timeline to adapt to the anticipated changes. The identified priorities determine which changes will be done first and which will come later in the plan. The leader has the responsibility for determining where in the timeline of implementation each goal will be addressed.

When setting the timeline and pace of implementation, a balance needs to be struck between the urgency of attaining the goals with that of maintaining stability and awareness of change fatigue. Healthcare provides the challenge of continuous and often intense change. The context of the strategic planning process can occur while extraordinary change is taking place in the environment. The impact of the changes should be reflected in SWOT.

There are multiple internal factors that a leader should consider in managing the pace of change. For instance, a hospital that just launched a new integrated medical record might need a little time getting used to that system before another new electronic database is introduced. Similarly, in the academic setting, there might be a period of time before launching two new academic programs. It is important to consider the following in creating a timeline for plan implementation:

- What is the change fatigue level of the organization?
- How have members of the organization experienced past changes?
- What is the level of urgency in terms of mission of the organization?
- Has the leadership team been stable?
- Is it difficult to get the leadership group engaged with the idea?
- What is the recommendation of the leadership group in terms of timing of implementation?

How do leaders know how fast or slow to go in accomplishing a change? What is too fast or too slow? If a leader goes too fast, they can often leave the members of their organization behind. The members of an organization may not feel part of the change and the leader is left trying to justify why the change is important. Moving too fast can also result in errors that are difficult to correct once they happen. If the leader goes too slow, the members of the organization lose interest in making the change. According to Kotter (1996), the sense of urgency can be lost. Most leaders err on the side of going too slow, especially those in healthcare and higher education, because slower change is safer, less disruptive, and less stressful. A leader must recognize the risks of moving slowly include losing a competitive advantage in the environment.

Striking a balance on the right pace of change requires the leader to be a thoughtful and receptive listener and an astute and keen observer. By being open to the messages, both overt and subtle, that the members of the organization are giving, the leader can make adjustments to the pace of change to more closely fit the needs of the organization. There must be time to lay the groundwork prior to implementation. This may include reworking budgets to ensure adequate resources for the plan, hiring people with specific skills, or reorganizing the work teams. The more critical the need for change, the more compressed the time frame. Ideally, for a non-urgent change implementation, giving employees time to understand and have feedback is critical. Staff will benefit from having time to learn new strategies and habits and this does not happen quickly. Support for staff might come in the form of new resources, professional development, or a reward system. Continuing communication with all members of the team is essential for the leader to have a deep understanding of how the change is affecting the organization.

Implement the Plan

Implementing the strategic plan after doing the data collection and analysis, identifying strengths and weaknesses, establishing goals and objectives, creating strategies and tactics, and establishing a timeline is probably obvious. Why do all of the work of developing a plan if it is not going to be executed? Implementation is largely defined by the goals and objectives and action plan in terms of identifying the person responsible for specific aspects of the plan, following the timeline and measuring desired outcome. The challenge of implementation is for staff to see the work of the plan as central to their responsibilities and integrated into their daily work. Implementation is not something done on the side. It is not something outside of the usual work. It needs to become part of the usual work. Everyone in the organization should take the implementation of the strategic plan seriously, as if their job depends on it. The level to which an organization's people embrace and participate in the implementation process is what creates a strategic plan that can stimulate excitement, innovation, and outcomes (Evans Inc., 2020).

There may be added time demands as the implementation process begins, but over time, the work of the plan should be less of an add-on and more integrated. Accountability is a key factor in the implementation phase. The role of the leader is to be accountable for having the resources and expertise needed to successfully implement the plan. The leader is also the "go-to" person to help problem solve as needed and to support and recognize the work that is being done. Establishing a structured accountability is necessary for success. The individuals assigned to oversee the specific goals need to know when they

TABLE 5.4. Action Plan Template.

Goal	Resources Needed	Begin Date	Due Date	Complete Date	Person Responsible	Notes

report on progress, what they report, how they report and where they report. The accountability process to be successful needs to be structured, focused, consistent and visible.

Below are some examples for each of the elements of accountability of implementation.

- *When*: Once a month and when there is a significant problem or success, more often, less often
- *What*: Metrics related to the specific goal, barriers encountered, additional resources needed, and team functioning in achieving the goal etc.
- *How*: Verbally, written document, email summary, text and web-based accountability documentation
- *Where*: Private meeting with leader, team meetings, committee meetings, newsletters, and electronic communications

An action plan includes the following elements: goal, resources needed, date begun, date due, date completed, person responsible, and notes that provide clarifying information. See Table 5.4 for an example of an action plan template.

There will be adjustments to the strategic plan based on the challenges encountered during the implementation process. The changes required should be those that reflect more effective and efficient actions to achieve the goals. There may be a need to change the goals (though rarely) based on major changes within the organization such as a new CEO taking charge and having a different vision for the organization, or external changes such as a changing market based on an innovation or a pandemic!

Consider: **What is your experience with the timing for strategic planning and implementation? Did you have enough time? Did the implementation conflict with other changes happening simultaneously?**

Evaluation of the Strategic Plan

There are two important levels of evaluation of a strategic plan. The first level is to evaluate the plan itself. There are several criteria that can be considered:

- Is the plan aligned with the mission, goals, and values of the organization?
- Is the plan realistic in that it can be done in the time frame allotted (most of us underestimate the time it will take to accomplish goals)?
- Do you have the resources needed to execute the plan? Resources include both funds and expertise that is needed to accomplish the plan. If your plan includes developing a DNP program, do you have DNP faculty who could do this? If you are going to open a nurse run clinic is there a nurse to lead this effort? Are there funds in the budget to cover new positions of consultants needed to achieve the goals?
- Is the current organizational structure going to support the plan? If not, what needs to be changed?
- Are policies in place (or soon to be in place) to implement the plan?
- Is the right person responsible for the action plan and results? Do you need an experienced person or is there an opportunity to develop leadership capabilities in others?
- Is the plan balanced so that the goals reflect a broad picture of the organization and is not top heavy in addressing a narrow part of the organization's work? For example, if a strategic plan focuses primarily on the undergraduate programs of a school of nursing, the graduate programs may be unintentionally compromised. In a clinical setting, focusing on patient experience could compromise other important care issues.
- Is the strategic planning document clear and easily understood? It will be useful to provide a summary document. An infographic could be constructed to reflect the plan so that employees can quickly understand the plan.

The second level of evaluation focuses on the progress toward attaining the goals. The evaluation plan is developed during the planning process and is often altered during implementation if the original evaluation plan does not provide the necessary information or new data become available. The evaluation should identify movement toward the goals noting successes that the leader can share throughout the organizations. Quick wins can keep staff engaged in working toward fully achieving the goals. It is useful to have a visual that depicts the progress toward the goals that can be shared and seen by the whole organization community. The visual should be easy to see, colorful, and convert the goal into a picture of the actions to be taken leading to achievement of the goal. Illustrations that are often used include a picture of climbing a mountain, running along a path, or a thermometer as in Figure 5.2. The visual as in Figure 5.2 can provide important feedback about the progress of the work and serve as a motivator for the members of the organization. A specific person needs to be assigned to keep the visual updated and milestones need to be celebrated.

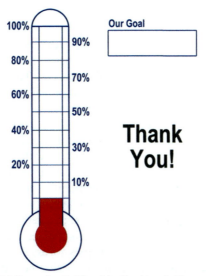

FIGURE 5.2 Example of a Visual for Tracking Achievement a Goal.

Measuring the progress toward each of the goals requires defining metrics accurately and monitoring progress at pre-identified times. Measures for the evaluation should be specifically linked to each of the goals separately and include short- and long-term measures. Measurement of impact should include feedback from target populations, and workers to assess their perceptions of the impact. The evaluation plan will likely include measures that already are being collected by the organization, either as part of an internal monitoring system or because they are required for accreditation and/or payment. Using existing measures can reduce the resources needed to execute the evaluation plan. There should be specific time frames identified for the collection and review of data related to the goals. Attainment of the goals will likely proceed along a defined timeline and knowing if there is movement toward the goal is important in making mid-course corrections. Was the patient experience metric moving toward improvement? Was student feedback about the ease of the application process improved? The vision speaks to the end point of a path forward, the goals and priorities make more specific the vision, and the only way a leader knows if there is movement toward the is through measuring the goals.

If there is not a positive movement toward achieving goals, it is important to identify barriers that are faced in the achievement of goals. An example of a barrier might be having a goal of increasing the number of underrepresented minorities succeeding because resources were not allocated to achieve the goal. Knowing the barriers to achievement of goals is critical to being able to address them over the course of the strategic plan.

SUMMARY

Strategic planning is a critical process for leaders of organizations to employ. The process should include all members of the organization and be built on teamwork to move through the process. The core competency of leaders of strategic planning is communication and particularly listening. If members of the organization do not feel listened to, they will resist participation in implementing the plan. Terms commonly used in strategic planning include goal, objective, strategy, and tactic. The strategic planning process involves several steps with the first being to review the MVV of the organization. Collection and analysis of informative data are essential to assessing the strengths and weaknesses, as well as opportunities and threats. Based on data reflecting the internal and external environment, goals and objectives are developed that drive change in the organization to meet new challenges or better address current challenges. Once the goals and objectives are clearly defined, strategies and tactics are identified. Strategies are essentially what will be done to achieve the objective and goals, and tactics are how the strategies will be implemented. As the plan is being implemented, both formative and summative evaluations will provide information about progress. It is important to note that with the rapidly changing healthcare and educational environments, strategic plans are a living document and will need to be revised often. A strategic plan is never done.

CRITICAL THINKING QUESTIONS

At the beginning of the chapter an academic and clinical vignette were presented. Please review the vignettes to address the following the questions. The questions are specific to the vignettes.

Academic Vignette Questions

1. How will you manage the faculty perception that strategic planning is not necessary given everyone is doing a great job?
2. What process will you use to engage all faculty and staff in the strategic planning process?
3. What data related to assessment of the school will be useful to inform the work on a strategic plan?
4. Give an example of a possible goal and related objectives, strategies and tactics related to the Academic mission and vision.
5. For the example of a goal in question 4, how will you evaluate progress toward achieving this goal?

Clinical Vignette Questions

1. What potential effects do the leadership changes have on strategic planning?
2. Who are the constituencies that you need to engage in the process? Your staff? All nurses? The vice president for nursing's leadership team?
3. Who will you want on your strategic planning core team? What factors will you consider in selecting the members?
4. What would be the major challenges in a position with the responsibility of improving quality in a large organization with a diverse line of business?
5. How will you evaluate progress toward the goals of the plan? What will your dashboard of progress look like?

REFERENCES

Agency for Healthcare Research and Quality. (2021a). *Data*. Agency for Healthcare Research and Quality. https://www.ahrq.gov/data/index.html

Agency for Healthcare Research and Quality. (2021b). *2019 National healthcare quality and disparities report*. https://www.ahrq.gov/research/findings/nhqrdr/nhqdr19/index.html

Centers for Medicare and Medicaid. (2021a.). *Find and compare nursing homes, hospitals and other providers near you*. Medicare.gov. https://www.medicare.gov/care-compare/

Centers for Medicare and Medicaid. (2021b.). *The CMS innovation center*. Centers for Medicare & Medicaid Services. https://innovation.cms.gov.

Doran, G. T. (1981). There's a S.M.A.R.T. Way to Write Management's Goals and Objectives. *Management Review, 70*,35-36.

Evans Inc. (2020). *Strategic planning by Evans Incorporated: A human-centered innovation solution*. Evans Consulting. https://www.evansconsulting.com/wp-content/uploads/2020/02/Evans-Human-Centered-Strategic-Planning-whitepaper.pdf

Gleeson, B. (2017, July 15). *1 reason why most change management efforts fails*. Forbes. https://www.forbes.com/sites/brentgleeson/2017/07/25/1-reason-why-most-change-management-efforts-fail/?sh=63ec83e546b7

Kotter, J. P. (1996). *Leading change*. Harvard Business School Press.

CHAPTER 6

Governance and Structure

ACADEMIC VIGNETTE

Dr. Michael Garcia has served as Dean of the School of Nursing in upstate Kentucky for three years. He has a relatively small faculty focused primarily on baccalaureate nursing education although plans are being developed to add two new degree programs, a master's degree focused on preparing nurses for a role in nursing education and a Doctor of Nursing Practice degree focused on advanced practice. With the challenge of preparing for the upcoming changes, Michael decides he needs to engage the faculty in more strategic roles including sharing decision making responsibilities. Michael attends several academic workshops on faculty governance and decides to move ahead and establish a faculty governance model and structure. He proposes this idea to the faculty at a faculty meeting and is pleased that they are eager to take on this role. While Michael has some knowledge of faculty governance, he has not experienced it himself. Based on the two workshops he attended on faculty governance he moves ahead to establish a faculty governance committee. Michael appoints three members of the faculty to develop the structure for faculty governance. After four months the three faculty bring their plans to the full faculty. Michael is somewhat alarmed that the plan for faculty governance was not shared or discussed with him ahead of the faculty meeting nor was advice sought from other members of the faculty. Their proposal transforms most of the responsibilities for faculty hiring, performance reviews, and promotions along with the management of school resources. These responsibilities are all delegated to a faculty governance committee. Michael sees a significant shift in power and authority from the Dean's office to the faculty. He is unsure how to express his concerns over the process and plans without seeming to "take back" power and authority from faculty who are enthusiastic about the assignment of new powers and authority.

CLINICAL VIGNETTE

Dr. Eliza Evans has been recruited to the Board of Trustees of a mid-size health system located in a county that serves a population of just over 500,000 people. The Chevy Hills Health System is one of three health systems within the county and is considered the primary provider of trauma care. Eliza is the Dean of the School of Nursing at Lincoln University, the only university in the county with a school of nursing. She was recruited for the board position by the Chief Nursing Officer of the Chevy Hills Health System. Eliza has not had experience in corporate board governance but has been interested in gaining experience, so she eagerly agreed to join this board. Eliza's orientation to the Board of Trustees consisted of a dinner with the members of the Board and was given a board manual that provided background on the Chevy Hills Health System. Neither the current board members nor the CEO discussed with her the role of governing the health system as a trustee. The Chief Nursing Officer of the Chevy Hills Health System was pleased to recommend her to the Board of Trustees, but did not discuss the role of the Trustees or expectations for board members. At her first board meeting, Eliza was asked to chair the committee responsible for evaluating the health system's CEO. Eliza was concerned about taking on this important role as a new board member, particularly after learning that the board had not evaluated the CEO's performance in the past five years. She asked the Board President for guidance and was told to develop a report that highlighted his activities. Eliza was uncomfortable with this approach but moved ahead with the Board Chair's request. She talked with each board member about the CEO's performance but received few specifics. Eliza's discomfort increased as she realized that the board overall had limited knowledge of the governance responsibility of a corporate board of directors.

INTRODUCTION

This chapter explores the development of a leader's role in governance and examines why structure is such a critical dimension in guiding excellence within organizations. We will explore those governance and organizational structures that promote clarity, order, and lead to excellence in performance. The environments where leadership is practiced may be very different but similar principles apply. In this chapter, we will examine the leader's role in the complex environment of governance and the essential role of creating, maintaining, and moderating an organization's structure and governance within health systems and academic environments.

While this chapter focuses on governance and structure within health systems and academia, it is important to recognize that governance and strategy are critical to any organization that strives for excellence. Therefore, learning from leaders in a variety of environments is important. For example, two recent books on leadership that provide examples of significant governance challenges include Doris Kearns Goodwin's book "Leadership: Lessons from the Presidents for Turbulent Times" (2018) and Jim Mattis' book on his long leadership career in the Marine Corp and as Secretary of Defense (Mattis & West, 2019). Doris Kearns Goodwin examines the leadership of four presidents: Abraham Lincoln, Theodore Roosevelt, Franklin Roosevelt, and Lyndon Johnson. Her curiosity about their ambition to lead and the impact of adversity in each of their lives vividly presents how personal ambition and intellect shapes exquisite leadership but also extraordinary challenges. Jim Mattis writes a vivid account of the challenges of leading in multiple roles within the highly complex environment of the military in peacetime and in conflict. His experiences as a military leader, four-star general, and as the Secretary of Defense are examined through the lens of three types of leadership: direct leadership, executive leadership, and strategic leadership. He examines the critical aspects of structure and governance that enable competence among individuals, promotes a bond and caring among people, and strengthens conviction in what an organization stands for and why. He writes about the creation of organizational structures that require leaders to have a clear conviction about what the leader and organization stand for, an understanding of one's strengths and weaknesses, a focus on continuous evaluation of strategy, the building of confidence and the willingness to take risks, debate ideas, and examine one's own behaviors.

These stories offer insights into how these leaders created processes and rules or norms that determine the direction of an organization. While the context of governance is different for different organizations, every organization has its unique history and culture, governance is critical to the effectiveness of the organization.

Consider: **What have you learned about governance of organizations in either your current role or in an academic program? How does governance of your organization affect your day-to-day work?**

Clarifying Decision Authority and Boundaries

The basic premise of governance within an organization is to assure there is clear accountability for organizational performance, structures and policies for decision-making, and financial oversight at all levels of the organization that enables leaders to lead with purpose. It would be difficult to participate in a governance role without authority for decision-making. It would also be difficult to create an avenue for developing strategy without decision authority.

Authority is a key requirement in defining roles, responsibilities and clarifying decision authority. Within organizations, particularly large complex organizations, boundaries in decision authority may be perceived as limiting. However, establishing boundaries for roles and responsibilities is critical for freeing up team member energy and enabling a focus on their responsibilities. A boundary essentially defines where one's responsibilities begin and end in relationship to others. Establishing detailed roles and responsibilities helps to prevent conflict. A job description is an important tool that should be explicit about the boundary of decision-making authority. However, it needs to be flexible enough to provide growth and opportunity without interfering with roles and responsibilities of other team members. There will always be some overlap areas and those will need to be monitored and clarified consistently.

A management position, whether at the unit or department level or as a senior executive of a health system or within an academic institution, should come with clear expectations of the role to establish authority including reporting relationships and responsibilities for performance appraisal and for providing feedback on a regular basis. Clarity about how work is structured within the organization is critical. For example, are you responsible for developing your own workplan or is your work plan assigned to you? Are you part of the team that develops the strategic plan for the organization? Strategic planning is a useful process for not only setting much of the future work of the organization, but also designing an organization's future. The opportunity to serve in a capacity that involves strategic planning is an important milestone in leadership, giving the leader insight into and influence over the future of the organization.

Creating the Structure for Governance

Structuring an organization so that it has a clear strategy for how it operates and how it designs its vision and mission is critical whether we are talking about a clinical or academic environment. There are multiple ways in which health systems and academic organizations define themselves and how they clarify decision-making and reporting relationships. Most organizations reflect one of three basic designs: functional, divisional, and matrix. These designs form the structure for governance of the organization. The functional design (Figure 6.1) is the most traditional and organizes work based on similarity of function. For instance, a hospital may have all nurses in the nursing unit, all physicians in their unit, all IT people in the technology unit and all finance people in their unit because of their similarity in work. Each unit would have a manager that has expertise in the work being done. Decision making is often centralized and hierarchical.

Organizations defined by divisions rather than departments are structured by the specific services or products they provide. In a hospital the services provided could be radiology, home nursing care, intensive care, medical care and

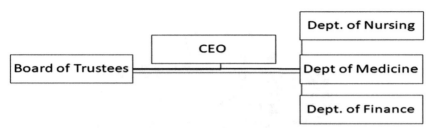

FIGURE 6.1 Functional Design with leaders reporting to the CEO and who are responsible for similar disciplines and clinical services.

others. Each division is given the authority to develop the plans for how to best provide those services at the division level. The communication usually flows up and down with the division director communicating with the executive officer and vice versa thereby providing a more decentralized process.

An example of divisional design (Figure 6.2) is nursing and medicine each having their own finance, marketing, human resource and administrative staff. Academic divisions are generally structured by the academic levels such as the undergraduate or graduate division each having their own support staff. The Dean or CNO often serves in a facilitative and problem-solving role working to bring the faculty and staff to consensus.

A matrix organization (Figure 6.3) tends to be somewhat of a hybrid of functional (similarity of skill set) and divisional (similarity of product or service). A matrix design enables individual skills to cross boundaries leading to more innovation and distribution of talent across product or service lines. A matrix organization has a structure in which employees report to multiple individuals across the organization depending on the skill similarity or the product. This structure is more flexible and generally more innovative. There is the "hard" line and "dotted" line for reporting. While there are benefits of a matrix organization, the challenge is to assure that employees know who to report to and for what. To support creativity and productivity, a matrix organization needs to clearly communicate and monitor how responsibilities are assigned,

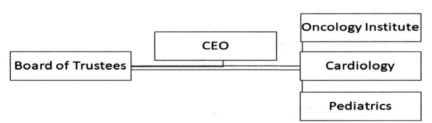

FIGURE 6.2 Divisional Design with leaders reporting to the CEO and are responsible for departments or divisions based on a type of service rather than a specific discipline.

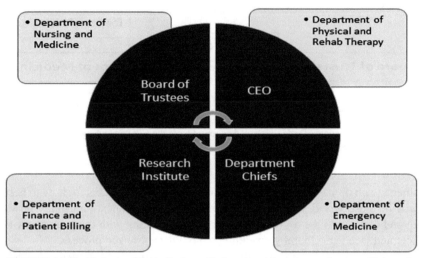

FIGURE 6.3 Health System Matrix Design with department leaders reporting to multiple senior leaders depending on the situation.

how evaluations are accomplished and how salaries and other incentives are decided.

Leaders often inherit the structures they will be overseeing. You can see how this could be a challenge for leaders who have experience with one type of organization model and transition to a different type. If the leader is a "top down" manager, they may have difficulty providing the flexibility that comes with a matrix organization. The opposite is true for a leader who has experienced the benefit of more flexible and open decision-making who then joins a faculty who are used to "following orders." It often comes down to how an organization and its leaders can best fulfill its mission with the potential need to re-organize.

Each of these governance models will typically utilize organizational charts to clarify not only the roles of individuals but whom they directly report to and what other reporting relationships they may have. In a functional design that tends to be hierarchical, reporting relationships are generally up and down the chain of command. In matrix organizations reporting may be to more than one individual depending on the work they are doing, the teams they belong to and the flexibility an individual has in designing their own work assignments.

Practicing Governance

The various ways of constructing decision making and reporting structures allow an organization to create the type of environment that will best serve its vision and mission. However, the structure does not change the nature of the role of governance either at the top level of the organization or throughout the organization as in the case of shared governance. Governance is both a process and structure that guides the core values, mission, and aspirations of an organization and assures that the organization creates a culture of quality, sound policy, financial responsibility, community engagement and orientation to achieving the mission. The opportunity to apply leadership knowledge and skills to governing requires a strategic and informed approach so that the nursing leaders successfully participate in governance with a well-developed set of skills. The cultivation of these skills occurs through education and/or experience and is critical to advancing policy that will drive evidence-based quality care. Finding opportunities for leadership should be strategic so that early successes pave the way for more challenging opportunities. As nurses develop leadership skills and begin to cultivate and seek opportunities for advancement participating in governance and policy through joining association and community boards and committees is useful. Nurses have long served in leadership roles within their own professional associations that provides excellent opportunities to "govern" within organizations that we understand.

Drenkard (2015) discussed opportunities available for nurses to influence policy at a local or state level through board service for associations, community based not-for-profit organizations and professional societies. This article clearly describes the necessary steps to gain access to these opportunities and points out the challenges including access to board leadership opportunities, the skill to govern and set policy, the challenge of taking on an elections process if required, the commitment required and the ability to influence are important skills for governing successfully.

Think of Dr. Michael Garcia's dilemma in creating a faculty governance structure within his organization. Neither he nor his faculty have significant experience in creating a governance structure. Dr. Garcia moves forward with the development of a structure, yet he has not taken the critical step of immersing himself and his faculty in the concept of faculty governance and how it can facilitate excellence within the organization. He, the faculty and staff need to understand that it can also create power struggles if not managed well.

Consider: **What is the governance structure of the organization where you work? Is there a shared governance model bringing together management and workers? How do you participate in governance? How have you prepared yourself to participate in governance?**

Working in Concert

Who likes going to a meeting? The truth is that many meetings created for the purpose of communicating information and solving problems fall short of this goal. Why? Often the answer is that meeting management is an important skill but leaders do not always take the time to develop the art of "the meeting." First, the value of a well-managed meeting is that individuals who are responsible for assuring quality, safety, satisfaction, and high performance on a day-to-day basis need a safe place to try out ideas, discuss current challenges, and learn from others. Leaders need a team they can trust with the opportunity to offer support and ideas to colleagues. Governance cannot succeed without the development of trust among the leadership team members to facilitate systematic strategic planning and action. A few rules can help leaders have consistently effective meetings of their leadership team:

1. Set a tone for the meetings. This should be a time for sharing among the leadership team. It is important that each team member trusts that they will be heard and that the conversations are confidential. An agreement about how healthy debate and conflict resolution should be determined and routinely revisited in addition to other meeting ground rules. The leader needs to monitor the interaction and tone of the team meetings and intervene if the conversation goes off topic or becomes disruptive. The team needs to support one another and offer ideas, not criticism.

2. Meetings should be scheduled at a time convenient to team members. The leader in charge and the leadership team should decide on the frequency, day and time of management meetings and stick with it. There are always exceptions given the needs of the organization, but in general if everyone can agree on a meeting time and place, each member is accountable for attending.

3. An agenda for each meeting is essential so the team knows what to prepare for and what materials to bring to the meeting. Agenda setting by the team can be done at the end of each meeting to facilitate and plan for the next meeting.

4. In most cases, meetings should be kept to an hour or hour and a half. It encourages people to be concise in their conversations. Longer meetings do not increase the quality of meetings.

5. Stick to the agenda. Everyone coming to the meeting knows what the agenda is and should be prepared for the conversation and strategy planning. When the discussion wanders off, particularly if the discussion is dominated by one person, the rest of the team may lose interest.

6. Make time at the beginning of the meeting to briefly touch base with how

the team is doing. This is a good time to celebrate the efforts of the team and share good news and accomplishments of team members.

7. Assume that each of the leaders has something to share or a concern to discuss. The executive can accommodate this by going around the table and asking, "what's up?" This avoids a one-sided conversation. Make room on the agenda if a problem needs immediate attention from the team.

8. Utilize the leadership meetings for briefings. This assures that the team receives important news and can start to work together if there are problems to solve or good news to share. If one of the leaders misses that meeting where critical news is shared, the executive should always follow up with that individual. However, avoid making the meetings about "news" that can be shared in other ways.

9. Wrap up meetings with topics for the next agenda.

If management meetings are defined by their support, problem solving and celebration, team members will make them a priority.

Shared Governance Models

While the governance structures of health systems and universities are similar to those in the non-health care corporate sector, a model for assuring that the professionals within the organization participate in governance is known as "shared governance." The focus of this governance model is to bring together managers and employees to create strategic direction, set priorities, plan and develop policy for the organization through shared decision-making. Shared governance is intended to bridge the "us" vs "them" thinking between management and the workforce. Engaging professionals in the governance of the organization is a best practice that can result in both a positive work environment and quality outcomes.

The term governance is generally used when describing how an organization oversees and assures a set of operational and strategic goals, However, it does not necessarily consider the role of the workforce in the actual day to day delivery of the vision and mission. While this may be assumed, those who produce the outcomes may not have the opportunity to participate in shaping the strategies of the organization. This is at the heart of Magnet designation, a certification process for health systems developed and operated by the American Nursing Credentialing Center. Within academic organizations there is a similar philosophy for sharing governance which emerged in the early 1970s. As is true with many systems of ensuring that management succeeds with its mission and goals, traditional governance structures may constrain the workforce in unintentional ways. Sharing the development and evaluation of the processes and outcomes of governing is at the heart of shared governance because it embraces participatory leadership and focuses on empowering others to lead.

Structural empowerment is one of the key characteristics of Magnet recognition along with transformational leadership, exemplary professional practice, the use of new knowledge, innovations, and improvements, and empirical outcomes   (www.nursingworld.org/organizational-programs/magnet/magnet-model). The expectation of Magnet is that strategy, operations, resources, clinical approaches, and practice plans are managed through shared governance both at the hospital level and/or in multi-hospital systems. These models include system CNOs, individual hospital CNOs and councils populated by staff and management nurses. Clear communication, peer mentoring and frequent interaction through councils can create a culture that encourages nurses to take on responsibilities for practice decisions, outcomes, quality and safety.

Health systems that include multiple hospitals and clinics are particularly suited to a shared governance model and the span of control for a senior nursing leader may include engaging other system leaders. Often shared governance at one hospital is linked to the other system hospitals through a system wide council. The council may also involve academic institutions that are partnered with one or more of the hospitals within the system. In these large multi-system organizations, individual hospital chief nursing officers are responsible for providing leadership within their own system; they are also charged with the responsibility to align their mission with other system hospitals. This responsibility requires a leader who is flexible enough to adopt new ideas from others to assure that the entire system operates in concert with one another.

Schools of nursing that want to apply similar characteristics to their own governing processes also use the term shared governance. Empowering others to lead is at the heart of shared governance including preparing faculty to take part in decision-making and participation in directing efforts that are oriented toward specific goals of the organization. Shared governance is often operationalized using councils or committees that take on certain aspects of decision making. Committees within schools of nursing are likely to oversee the development of the school's curriculum, advise on faculty promotions and tenure decisions, review and manage the discipline of students, and participate on university wide faculty senate committees. More so than traditional hierarchical governance models, shared governance is very much relationship focused. Individuals within a shared governance model must develop the capacity to create a common purpose, setting the vision and mission of the school, participate in strategic planning, create models for the distribution of work, and the development of strong open relationships among faculty, staff, and leadership.

The literature contains many examples of positive outcomes from shared governance both in schools of nursing and health system settings. Benefits of shared governance include increased job satisfaction, higher productivity, independence, and engagement along with positive coworker relationships (Owens *et al.*, 2018).

Board Governance

All organizations need a process and strategy for accomplishing their vision and mission. In most organizations a designated board has oversight of a select set of high-level responsibilities in addition to setting the vision and mission. The board may include consumers of the organization's services, community members, employees at various levels and individuals external to the organization who can provide the knowledge and expertise to drive priorities, strategic decisions, and philanthropic funds to support the mission. For-profit organizations include stockholders and industry leaders. A board's authority and responsibilities generally include hiring and evaluation of the chief executive for the organization, setting corporate policy and strategy, finance, risk management, compliance, quality, planning, credentialing, employee satisfaction and overall outcomes. Boards may choose to delegate some of these responsibilities to the top level executives, but the ultimate responsibility for accountability and performance rests with the Board.

This set of responsibilities, known as "governance," is designed to assure that the organization is operating within a model that has system level oversight and accountability. According to Deloitte and Touche LLP (2013) the operating model for governance includes the following components: development of policies and procedures, oversight of CEO performance and responsibilities, assuring the appropriate talent is available to lead the system, setting the organization's culture and assuring appropriate infrastructure. Each of these components enables the board to provide oversight to the organization, establish board and management committee structures, organize a reporting structure, assure management accountability and authority, establish, and review performance measures and implement compensation and incentive systems.

It is critical that the members of the Board of Trustees are clearly oriented to their oversight role even if some of the responsibilities are delegated. Boards should regularly review and update their understanding about the terms for board members, and committee responsibilities. Within health system boards, members are often involved in the nomination of new board members, oversight of quality and safety, community benefit, investment and finance, and patient experience. Expectations of board member engagement must be clearly articulated and reviewed regularly along with clarity about what competencies are valued in a board member. For example, board members should have talent in quality and safety, systems thinking, interpersonal skills, and commitment to the mission of the organization. If a CEO does not use their Board of Directors to guide the above expectations, the organization will be at risk of failing at regulatory compliance and creating effective strategy and financial stability. In addition, oversight of executive performance may be compromised. An excellent reference for a new member of a board of trustees is "Framework for Effective Board Governance of Health System Quality," a report from the Institute for Health Care Improvement (Daley *et al.*, 2018).

It is important to understand the difference between the terms "board of trustees" and "board of advisors." As described above, a board of trustees is charged with guiding corporate decisions, tracking performance, setting policy, and providing oversight among other responsibilities. They are decision makers at the highest level of the organization and although they do not run the day-to-day operations, they are ultimately responsible for assuring that the chief executive does so. On the other hand, a board of advisors is responsible for providing advice and feedback within an organization. For example, schools of nursing reside within universities which have a board of trustees providing high-level policy and oversight. However, a school within the university may want a mechanism for alumni, community members, corporate leaders, etc. to provide advice and counsel to the dean on the school's strategic plan, development, and future trends. A board of advisors can be very influential and helpful in guiding policy and assisting in predicting future ventures. However, they are only as effective as the chief executive/dean makes use of them and by developing a board that is knowledgeable about the business of the school and its vision.

Consider: **If given the opportunity to serve on a Board of Advisors or Board of Directors, which would you prefer and why? How might you seek a board role? Would you consider seeking a mentor who could guide you in board governance? Why or why not?**

Governance is critical in assuring that organizations have structures and processes in place that guide, monitor and improve work including appropriate roles and responsibilities of individuals and teams who carry out the work within organizations. Organizations that do this best have established a connection between the organization's strategy and work process performance. Organizations that do not think like a system and do not use strategy to direct the priorities and work processes of the functional units leave their employees operating in the dark and the talent and energy of precious human resources are wasted. Talented individuals my then feel apathetic and joyless in the workplace leading to less creative and effective organizations.

Staying on the Good Side of Power and Authority

It is an honor to be selected to lead or participate in the governance of an organization, whether as a member of the Board of Trustees or Board of Advisors, appointment as the top executive or as a member of a leadership team. Accepting such an appointment and honor can bring exceptional rewards. Most of these rewards involve seeing others succeed and the organization thrive. Governing and managing organizations, developing, and executing strategy, mentoring teams and leaders is a privilege that can bring incredible satisfaction. It can also be incredibly challenging. Organizations are complex beyond belief and a successful leader is one who recognizes these challenges, manages within a complex environment and above all values their colleagues and the mission and vision of the organization. No one succeeds alone. No one can foresee every circumstance. No one can solve every problem. No one should celebrate alone. Leading is a gift and learning to lead is hard work.

SUMMARY

In order to govern an organizational structure a built-in system for oversight of policies, finance, mission, quality, safety, community engagement, and a commitment to the organization is necessary. A system of governance is essential for achieving the mission of quality and safety, financial solvency and overall performance excellence and there is no more critical environment than within health care and within academic settings that educate the future healthcare workforce. The structure of governance demands a high level of commitment from those whose role is to govern. The delivery of high quality and safe care within a health system and the delivery of exemplary knowledge and science within academic environments is dependent on oversight by individuals who understand the role of governance and the structures necessary for quality and safety and assuring high quality performance.

There are many opportunities for nurses to learn and practice governance. Gaining basic knowledge about governance is available through a number of nursing organizations and the placement of nurses on boards is an important mission of the American Nurses Association, the American Academy of Nursing, the Nurses on Boards Coalition and many others. It is critical knowledge for all nurses.

CRITICAL THINKING QUESTIONS

At the beginning of the chapter an academic and clinical vignette were presented. Please review the vignettes to address the following questions. The questions are specific to the vignettes.

Academic Vignette Questions

1. Propose several alternate strategies that Michael could have taken in approaching the topic of faculty governance for the School of Nursing?
2. What strategies could have been used to engage the faculty in planning for faculty governance?
3. Given Michael's concerns about the faculty's approach to a governance model, how could he have evaluated and responded to the faculty's plan for governance?
4. Would you advise Michael to accept and support the faculty plan?

Clinical Vignette Questions

1. What early warning signs could have helped Eliza take a more strategic approach to joining this board.
2. What alternative approaches to the CEO evaluation would provide more benefit to the organization, the CEO, and the Board of Trustees?
3. What key responsibilities should Eliza be aware of?
4. How might Eliza have prepared herself for the board role in advance of her first board meeting?

REFERENCES

Daley, U., Gandhi, T. K., Mate, K., Whittington, J., Renton, M., & Huebner, J. (2018). Framework for effective board governance of health system quality. IHI White Paper. Institute for Healthcare Improvement. http://www.ihi.org/resources/Pages/IHIWhitePapers/Framework-Effective-Board-Governance-Health-System-Quality.aspx

Deloitte and Touche LLP. (2013). Developing an effective governance operating model: A guide for financial services boards and management teams. Deloitte Development LLC. https://www2.deloitte.com/content/dam/Deloitte/global/Documents/Financial-Services/dttl-fsi-US-FSI-Developinganeffectivegovernance-031913.pdf

Drenkard, K. (2015). Influencing and impacting the professional through governance opportunities. *Nursing Administration Quarterly, 39*(1), 38-43. https://doi.org/10.1097/NAQ.0000000000000085

Goodwin, D. K. (2018). Leadership: Lessons from the presidents for turbulent times. Penguin Random House.Mattis, J., & West, B. (2019).

Mattis, J., & West (2019) Call sign chaos. New York: Random House.

Owen, D. C., Boswell, C., Opton, L., Franco, C., & Meriwether, C. (2018). Engagement, empowerment, and job satisfaction before implementing an academic model of shared governance. *Applied Nursing Research, 41*, 29-35. http://doi.org/10.1016/j.apnr.2018.02.001

CHAPTER 7

Using Policy to Guide Practice and Operations

ACADEMIC VIGNETTE

Dr. Frances Manon is the new Dean for the University of Dover School of Nursing and is busy getting to know the university and the faculty and staff along with their priorities and concerns. When she was hired into the role, the President of the University shared with her that the School of Nursing needed a review of its policies and procedures as several faculty had voiced concerns about equity, course assignments and the process for promotions. Dr. Manon is planning for a school wide strategic planning session as a way of reviewing current plans for the school and to test how open the faculty and staff were to change. Meanwhile she has been reviewing past documents related to policies and procedures for the school. To her dismay, she discovered that there was no strategic plan, the policy manual was ten years old and written guidance for promotions was absent.

Prior to the strategic planning session, she holds individual meetings with the senior faculty to get a sense of how to approach an overhaul of the policy manual and their thoughts about where to begin with guidelines for promotions within the school. What she discovers from these conversations with senior faculty is that their knowledge of how to develop and utilize policy is limited and she detects reluctance to set guidance in writing for promotions and other actions such as course assignments. She begins to develop an agenda for the strategic planning meeting that includes a discussion about updating policies and how to assure that faculty and staff are engaged in the process.

CLINICAL VIGNETTE

Eastern Health, a large urban multi-hospital health system, has recently initiated the process for Magnet designation. Nursing leadership was fully committed to the process and the benefit it would bring Eastern Health. The Board of Trustees for the health system was supportive of the venture and willing to invest in the process of improving the work environment and establishing the health system as a top performing system for clinical outcomes. The Sr. Vice President for Nursing and Chief Nursing Officer, Dr. Abebe, had met with the Board of Trustees on several occasions to discuss the process associated with achieving Magnet designation. She explained the requirements including transformational leadership, structural empowerment, exemplary professional practice and new knowledge innovations and improvements (American Nurses Credentialing Center Magnet Recognition Program, 2018). Dr. Adebe was confident that Eastern Health had the system in place and practice excellence they would need for Magnet, but she was unsure whether they had a robust enough program to generate new knowledge innovations and improvements across the system, particularly the involvement of nurse clinicians in research to enhance their practice.

After consulting with the nursing leadership across the health system, Dr. Adebe approached Dr. Martin, the Eastern University School of Nursing Dean, to discuss developing opportunities for nursing staff to engage in research. The two leaders had partnered in several educational related initiatives and had a strong relationship. After three months of dedicated effort, the two chief nursing leaders and their respective senior leaders had designed a program that would pair nurse scientists within the academic setting with unit leaders in the health system to develop clinical studies that would increase the research knowledge of the staff nurses and develop the evidence they needed to solve several unit-based concerns about patient safety. Jointly they developed a policy that described their vision for research engagement, the shared responsibility across the two organizations, the outcomes they wanted to achieve and the roadmap to get there. This policy presented the framework and direction for establishing a research partnership to enhance the excellence of both organizations. It also laid out the specific roles each organization would take, the oversight for the day-to-day research projects, the sharing of expertise and funding, and the management of resulting publications.

INTRODUCTION

Chapter 7 introduces policy decision making as a critical responsibility of every leader in every organization because of the impact on the lives and well-being of people in the organization and those served. Many aspects of health systems and academic institutions rely on policies to guide how to approach a multitude of opportunities and challenges. We generally think of policy as a tool to structure laws and the associated regulations. One definition of policy making is the formulation of ideas or plans that are used by an organization or government as a basis for action and decision making (Collins English Dictionary, 2020). The simplest way to think about policy is that it provides guidance to groups, institutions, governments, and populations on how to clearly set a roadmap for managing and/or responding to the work of the organization as well as problems and opportunities.

In health care, we are guided by federal, state, local and institutional policies that address issues related to the three major areas of public concern: access to health care, quality of care and cost. In the US, cost and quality have been perhaps the strongest driver of policy. We see this currently in the focus on value-based payments for care linking quality to payment. However, there are many policy issues that relate to health that include basic "rights" such as equal access to high quality health care, housing, nutrition, public safety, health prevention programs and allocation of public services (water, clean air, roads, etc.). Laws or regulations include information about standard approaches to address issues or problems to be solved or prevented. Generally, laws define the policy approach and regulation provides the information about implementing the policy.

Policy making occurs at many different levels including the federal, state, local, and organizational level. Healthcare systems develop policies that relate to clinical practice, program development, the management of risk, finance, and people. Academic institutions develop policies to address student, faculty and staff issues as well as the operations of the institution. At the end of this chapter, you will have an opportunity to critically think about the questions related to the case studies presented above.

The Power of Policymaking at the Institutional Level

Policy making is a powerful tool to establish a way of addressing a problem. The best policy making process is informed by evidence. If developed in a strategic way, policy can be utilized to assure quality and reduce risk within health related environments and to define operational changes. However, policy making at all levels can be a very messy endeavor because of the influence of stakeholders who hold varying opinions, have conscious and unconscious bias, and who may win or lose something they value when policies are created or changed. When policy is approached in a strategic and evidenced based manner it is likely to solve or prevent problems. However, the importance of policy may be overlooked as a source of evidence informed action.

At its most basic, institutional policy guides action through the setting of "rules" about how different situations and practices should be managed or performed. It may also set guidance about how to approach decision making, problem solving, priority setting or manage conflict. Policy sets "best practices" when it is derived from evidence, although policy is most certainly influenced by culture, organizational priorities, finance, and values, mission, and vision.

If you scrolled through policies related to health promulgated by congress, state government, health systems, or academic institutions, you would no doubt find inconsistencies in policies around a specific problem. There is often a lack of clear evidence that a problem requires a policy solution. Kingdon (1995) recognized the situation of "policy looking for a problem." The idea is predicated on a phenomenon in policy making where an idea for a policy is ahead of the problem to be solved. For instance, a school of nursing may identify a problem of too few tenured faculty and believe this could be solved with a policy. The policy for tenure is often developed at the University level, perhaps by a faculty senate with members being drawn from all schools across the university. The school may address the issue of a limited number of tenured faculty by developing a mentoring program for faculty to prepare them for tenure. The school response is an action and not a policy to increase the number of tenured faculty. Many issues can motivate the development of institutional policy, but the problem to be solved must be clearly identified and amenable to a policy solution, otherwise developing a policy is a waste of time.

Consider: Is it difficult to distinguish between a policy, a law, or an employee manual? It can be challenging and doing a little practice could be helpful. Start with your own institution or university. Track down the manuals used by the organization and see if you can distinguish among them in terms of laws, policies, or employee/student handbook. It is unlikely that you will find a "law" within a university or health system, but you should be able to find a policy manual or an employee handbook.

Policy Making Process

Creating effective policy can be mediated in part with a clear pathway for the process of policy making. That pathway should include a series of steps which apply to both policy development and policy revision. While the policy making process has largely been identified with government decision making, the same process steps apply to organizational policy making. The process begins with a clear understanding of the problem or potential problem to be solved or mediated. Every problem does not need a formal policy, but systemic problems that have serious consequences for quality, safety, and patient, provider and employee satisfaction do require system solutions. However, policies are not always driven by problems. Often a policy is set in motion to support excellence and strengthen the workplace environment. For example, a health system that decides to seek Magnet status is knowingly adopting policies and standards that guide how excellence is achieved and maintained. Either way, the development of a policy should always begin with a thorough analysis of what is to be achieved and what specific action will address the problem. Figuring out the actions often requires a rigorous policy analysis process.

The steps related to policy decision making for institutions is very similar to that used for legislation and regulation at state and Federal levels. Having a systematic method of creating or changing policy will heighten the likelihood of the desired outcome. There are several formulations of the specific steps in the policy making process all including the following (McLaughlin & McLaughlin, 2018):

- *Identify and define the problem.* This is the most important step in the process. Everything else follows from how a problem is defined. Consider why it is important to create a change. Are patients or staff members identifying a problem? What is being done currently to address the concerns or contribute to the problem? Analysis of the problem to understand the contributing factors is critical.
- *Formulate a policy.* What are the inputs and outputs related to the issue of concern? Who is doing what? Several steps need to be taken. Map out the existing processes that yield the current outcome. Knowing the specific factors and process steps contributing to the policy problem can most easily be identified using a process map. Generate a list of solutions/strategies based on evidence related to the issue of concern and choose the most likely to be successful alternatives. Choose not more than 2–3. The list of possible solutions can be done using a number of techniques such as convening a group who have varied expertise related to the problem and simply brainstorming possible solutions. Another method is to explore what other organizations have done to address the problem.
- *Assess the internal and external factors that will affect policy options selection.*
    - —*Review the literature and other sources of information for data related to policy options.* Evaluate the fairness, impact on quality, engagement of employees and other impacts of the proposed solutions. Consider both qualitative and quantitative data. This topic is covered in more detail later in the chapter.
    - —*Consider stakeholder influence.* Table 7.1 is a stakeholder table related to a clinical nurse leader proposing a policy to address the issue of nurses on medical surgical units not having timely physician response related to changing patient conditions. The policy proposal that best fits the problem was to integrate nurse practitioners into the nursing staff of the medical surgical units. This is the first hospital in the region to propose employing acute care NPs. While this grid may look different

in different states and regions, it helps to identify and clarify the groups that may need attention in "selling" the policy.

—*Consider the technical and economic feasibility.* Economic feasibility is a factor that can powerfully sway a decision to adopt a policy. The return on investment must outweigh the cost either in terms of dollars or prestige that translates into dollars. However, even the most financially solid policy proposal for an organization may threaten specific groups within the organization such as physicians who may see a threat to billing for visits. In addition, a financially feasible proposal may run into very strongly held beliefs such as who provides the best quality of care. The technical feasibility relates to this proposal being implemented. Are there enough nurse practitioners to recruit to positions and what institutional credentialing processes would need to change to support the inclusion of nurse practitioners.

—*Select the best policy option.* Deciding on a policy that will guide action should only be made after all the possible alternatives have been discussed. Weigh the qualitative and quantitative data for each of the options, the stakeholder support, financial and technical considerations and choose the preferred policy and begin the process of information dissemination. There are usually multiple ways of addressing problems, however, a policy is intended to assure that a consistent and evidence-based solution is selected.

- *Implement the policy.* Know who supports the policy of choice and who opposes. Understand the reasons for opposition to the policy and create a plan to move the policy forward. Decide on the steps, timeline and who will do what to implement the policy.
- *Evaluate the policy.* Both the process of developing the policy as well as the outcome will need to be examined.

The steps noted above include a clear definition of the problem, challenge or opportunity that needs to be addressed, evidence that policy is the correct pathway to a solution, and information that can inform policy options. Individuals affected by the policy should be involved in its development. Understanding

TABLE 7.1. Stakeholder Assessment.

	Low power	High Power
Low Interest		CEO Heads of non-clinical departments
High Interest	State NP Association Board of Nursing Nursing staff	Medical Staff State Medical Society Chief Financial Officer

of the literature and research on best practices related to the problem is critical. Knowing what has been successfully tried or failed is also essential to the process. Evaluation is a critical step to assess whether the policy achieves the desired goal. If it does not, the policy will need to be revised. When a policy is formulated based on factors not related to the problem, the policy will fail to produce the desired outcome.

Leaders within an organization need to actively participate in some if not all facets of policy-making including direct engagement in setting policy, developing the specifics for how policy is carried out, communicating policy to others, mediating policy changes or educating about policy. Nurse leaders are responsible for policy decisions, not just politicians, boards of directors, and senior officials. Most of us are engaged in policy creation in some capacity within an organization. It is a critical factor in assuring that organizations perform to the highest level of competence, accountability, and safety.

Health care and education are highly regulated environments in part because there is significant risk associated with both. If educational programs fail to adequately teach students and if practicing nurses do not provide an expected standard of care, patients may be seriously harmed or die. Regulation guides the healthcare environment including the design of the clinical environment, standards that guide a clinician's practice, rights of patients, and finance and payment practices. These policies take the form of standards of practice for clinicians based on the evidence for best practice. In addition, regulation provides guidance to health purchasers, health payers/insurers and health systems, as well as rights of patients and consumers. Regulation also guides academic institutions in terms student financial aid, housing requirements, learning environments and financial stability.

Clinical and academic organizations generally implement policies through establishing rules, processes, and procedures. Rules to assure safe practice within a hospital could include nurse/patient staffing ratios, performance appraisals, hiring practices, guidance on continuing education for providers, specific practice standards that guide clinical procedures, and medication administration. Academic policies are often implemented for credentialing, requirements of clinical experiences, research, licensing requirements, state specific scope of practices laws, and university policy on curriculum and the conferring of degrees.

Evidence Informed Policy Development

It is important to consider in more depth the role of evidence in policy making. Within the profession of nursing, we understand that the overarching driver of expert patient care, safe environments, and optimal clinical outcomes is the evidence-based standards and processes that guide the clinician's practice. This is supported by the expectation of ongoing education, supervisory support, high functioning clinical environments and the support of leadership including executive management and health system trustees.

The decision about when policy is needed begins with identifying a problem to be solved or prevented. For example, within a health system the trigger may be efforts to increase safety and quality related to an increase in patient falls or medication errors. In an academic environment it may be the result of a drop in the number of RN graduates who pass the NCLEX or the need to increase the quality of research grant proposals. In both environments, sensitive policy issues may be driven by concerns about sexual harassment, discriminatory hiring, and other socially unjust workplace practices as well as scheduling and staffing and workload.

To augment the policy process noted above within the step of formulating a policy, it is critical to focus on either accessing or evaluating the evidence base to inform policy decisions. While evidence is not the sole, nor perhaps a significant determiner of the selection of a policy, evidence is important. Loversidge and Zermehly (2019) have recognized that there are factors beyond evidence that contribute to policy decisions. They use the term evidence informed policy to describe the role that evidence plays in developing policy. Adapting the evidence based practice work of Melnyk and Fineout-Overholt (2015), Loversidge (2016, p.17) defines evidence informed policy as "combining the use of the best available evidence and issue expertise with stakeholder values and ethics to inform and leverage dialogue toward the best possible health policy agenda and improvements". While evidence is important to informing policy decisions, there is always a context that includes political and belief systems of stakeholders. Understanding context is important in considering factors beyond evidence that go into policy decisions and includes:

- Acknowledging the boundaries of the use of evidence in policy making
- Recognizing the rapidly changing, and politically charged policy environment
- Acknowledging a global standard that has emerged for health policy (Loversidge and Zermehly, 2019, p. 15)

It is important to differentiate policy making from politics. Politics can be defined as the activities associated with the governance of a country or other area, especially the debate or conflict among individuals or parties having or hoping to achieve power (Oxford Dictionary, 2020). This compares to "a course or principle of action adopted or proposed by a government, party, business, or individual" (Oxford Dictionary, 2020). The connection between policy and politics is that a policy is adopted or rejected within a political context.

While we think of politics as being within the purview of government, organizations can be hotbeds of politics. Stakeholders have differing perspectives of how an organization should be run. Physicians may "lobby" for additional equipment for procedures whereas nurses may "lobby" for better staffing resources. Within academic organizations the Dean for the School of Nursing will be lobbying the administration for funds to develop a DNP program whereas the Dean for the Law School may lobby for the same funds to expand their program. The lobbying efforts usually come down to resource allocation. What are the priorities of the organization and how and to what degree will they be funded?

Evidence informed policies and their specific actions, laws or regulation will help create the best solutions to a problem focused on improving the education of students and the care of patients. However, because of stakeholder influence, the policy with the strongest evidence may not move forward and it may be the next best policy option. For all nursing leaders, evidence informed policy development should be a core area of responsibility with the requisite knowledge to use the policy process to enhance the outcomes of practice, education, and research. This requisite knowledge when it comes to policymaking must include the foundation of evidence-informed policy making.

Selecting or developing evidence-informed policies that are likely to be effective within a health system or academic environment requires a thorough review of what has caused the need for a new or more effective policy and what is likely to be effective in solving a problem or enhancing success. "Evidence-Based Policy: A Practical Guide to Doing it Better" refers to this as "effectiveness prediction" (Cartwright and Hardie, 2012). The evidence for a potential policy should support the "prediction" that the policy will work within a specific environment and that the evidence supports the prediction. The guiding question is: given the problem or opportunity, what specific evidence is available that predicts the selected policy will improve a problem or enhance a high performing individual or team?

Review and Update of Policies

Policy is dynamic. It is created to guide decision making and actions and must be relevant to the problems and opportunities it was designed to impact. All policies need to be reviewed on a regular basis to assure that the problems or opportunities they were designed to address have in fact occurred. How do we assure that policy remains relevant to the situation it was designed to guide? The Pew Trust in collaboration with the MacArthur Foundation began a project in 2014 titled the Pew-MacArthur Results First Initiative that recognized the importance of examining current programs addressing policy related problems. While their focus was on government programs, their approach is clearly relevant to organizations and includes three basic steps (Pew-MacArthur, 2018): (1) Create a comprehensive list of currently implemented policies related to specific issues; (2) Assess which programs are most likely to be effective; 3) Use findings to inform programmatic, policy, and funding decisions.

Every organization has many policies in place to address issues and it is often not clear how effective those programs may be. Periodically stepping back and evaluating them based on rigorous research will help determine which programs are effective. Specific questions that apply to the review include: (a) Does the policy align with the original intent? (b) What was the problem/s or opportunities the policy was intended to address? (c) Does data suggest that the policy was effective in addressing the problems? What are the metrics? (d) Does the policy need to be continued, revised, or eliminated? (e) Does the policy create barriers to social justice or action to reduce structural racism or racial policies? Policy can provide leaders with levers to guide practice, decision making, patient safety, clinical outcomes, technology, staffing, the utilization of types of staffing.

Once the details of the policy are developed, it should be added to the policy manual and shared with faculty and students. There is a similar process for developing policies within a health system that assures the policies for guiding patient care are at least evidence informed, available to all care providers and are updated on a regular basis. Within nursing, the chief nursing officer and management staff are generally responsible for guiding this process for nursing staff. In a shared governance model, clinical policy making is central to the function of the governance model. An example of this is the Johns Hopkins Hospital/Johns Hopkins Health System Corporation Employee Handbook. They have developed employee handbooks for union and non-union employees. These handbooks include the organization's mission and core values along with a system map of the individual organizations that are part of the university and health system. The handbook describes the system's purpose, culture, and basic requirements such as licenses and certifications, performance management, employee rights and responsibilities, discipline steps, HIPAA, workplace violence, disaster planning and many other topics. It is a comprehensive guide to the system's policies (hopkinsmedicine.org/human resources/_doc/employee_ handbook_non-union-non-represented.pdf). This policy manual is not a guide to care procedures which are specific to the different professions within the system.

Another good example of policy guidance is found in the Columbia University School of Nursing policy and procedures manual (https://www.nursing.columbia.edu/students/policies-and-procedures). Included in the manual are policies related to professional integrity, academic ethics, academic related violations, behavioral and professional related violations, among others. The policies and procedures cover a range of situations where guidance for both faculty and students is critical such as satisfactory academic progress, grading, academic review, probation, leave of absence, testing and exams, social media policy, plagiarism, falsification of records or credentials, and many others. Policy needs to be relevant to the current needs of a practice or education environment and as new evidence that guides practice changes, so must the policies change.

Practical Matters

How does one get started? Engaging in policy is essential to the development of strong and strategic systems and innovation in practice and education. Unfortunately, for many of us our exposure to policy development is often limited and we think it is something that politicians do. Leadership requires strategic thinking and the ability to guide practice and education using evidence informed policy. These are "must have" skills. One way to gain experiences for exposure to policy development is through service on a board of directors. One of the most important responsibilities of a board is overseeing policy development and assuring that the execution of policy throughout a system is based on evidence. Small or large, corporate or community based, board service is one of the best places to learn about policy and how to apply policy to a system. However, there are many opportunities within an organization to engage in the policy making process. Serving on institutional committees, actively leading or participating in shared governance structures and management decisions provides many opportunities to practice policy making skills. You could also identify a policy in your institution that has been implemented and track the history of the policy and how it became part of the institutional context.

Some possible areas to explore in the clinical setting include digging into policies that may limit nurse's autonomy, control over practice, decision making or actions. Also, what policies govern hiring nurses? Are there policies related to associate degree prepared nurses compared to bachelors prepared nurses? In an academic setting, policy issues to explore include policies related to shared faculty governance, admissions criteria for students, and faculty tenure and promotion. An example within academic settings relates to student cheating. Faculty members need guidance on how to approach cheating that will avoid, as much as possible, concerns about arbitrary decisions and unfair consequences for students. The policy needs to guide both student and faculty, and staff behavior so that students know the consequences and faculty know how to prevent or manage cheating among students. The policy could include: managing the testing environment to reduce the opportunity for cheating, reducing the likelihood that tests could be obtained and circulated among students, defining a process to investigate a cheating incident and the establishment of a committee to oversee and make the decisions about evidence of cheating and the assignment of consequences.

Consider: **An interesting cross cutting issue is one of covid-19 vaccinations. What was the policy process used in your organization to define the requirements related to vaccination? How was this determined and who had the loudest voice? How was it communicated and implemented?**

SUMMARY

The development and utilization of policy and the "practice" of politics are very different, yet highly dependent on one another. There are opportunities for nurses to participate and contribute to the development of policy at all levels and take part in the deliberation of how policies may solve problems and generate new innovative programs for society. The deliberative process in applying a policy to solving a problem or guiding action often requires inevitable compromise. We do it every day in our own environments as we bring our clinical skills to innovate new solutions for our patients and in the academic environments as we seek new strategies for research, teaching and practice. Each action is necessary for the creative process of solving problems or creating innovation. Policy-making is critical not only to the process of governing, but also to improving environments where individuals and populations can thrive. Think of the major problems we have yet to solve; racism, poverty, equal access to care, education, discovery of new life saving treatments, climate change and so many other challenges. Think of how nurses could change the world if we all engage in the work of policy development and mastering the politics of compromise!

CRITICAL THINKING QUESTIONS

At the beginning of the chapter an academic and clinical vignette were presented. Please review the vignettes to address the following questions. The questions are specific to the vignettes.

Academic Vignette Questions

1. What key actions would need to occur to enable faculty and staff to gain confidence in participating in an update of the policy manual?
2. Because the faculty's knowledge of developing and using policy is limited, how might Dr. Manon approach an overhaul of their policy manual?
3. How would you assign faculty and staff members to the different components of creating policies that ensure quality education for students?
4. How might you utilize policy for teaching assignments, promotions, and tenure?

Clinical Vignette Questions

1. What outcomes of creating a research program within Eastern Health would Dr. Abebe identify for the partnership with the school of nursing?

2. How might Eastern Health engage clinical nurses and stimulate interest in the development of the research projects?
3. What policies would be important to the success of this initiative in both the health system and the school of nursing?
4. What types of oversight would the two leaders want to employ to assure that the partnership garners the intended outcomes?

REFERENCES

About Magnet (nursingworld.org), American Nurses Credentialing Center Magnet Recognition Program. (2018).

Cartwright, N., & Hardie, J. (2012). *Evidence-based policy: A practical guide to doing it better*. Oxford University Press.

Collins English Dictionary (2020) Collins.

Kingdon, J. W. (1995). *Agendas, alternatives, and public policies*. Little Brown.

Loversidge, J. M. (2016). An evidence informed health policy model: Adapting evidence based practice for nursing education and regulation. *Journal of Nursing Regulation, 7*(2), 27-33. https://doi.org/10.1016/S2155-8256(16)31075-4

Loversidge, J. M., & Zumehly, J. (2019). Evidence-informed health policy: Using EBP to transform policy in nursing and health care. *Critical Care Nurse, 39*(5), 81.

McLaughlin, C. P., & Mclaughlin, C. D. (2018). *Health Policy Analysis*. (2nd ed.). Jones and Bartlett Learning.

Melnyk, B. M., & Fineout-Overholt, E. (2015). *Evidence-based practice in nursing and health care: A guide best practice*. (3rd ed.). Lippincott, Williams, and Wilkin.

Oxford Dictionary, 2020, Oxford University Press.

Pew-MacArthur. (2018). *How to use the results first program inventory*. Pew-MacArthur Results First Initiative. https://www.pewtrusts.org/-/media/assets/2018/04/rf_program_inventory_factsheet_v4.pdf employee_handbook_non-union_non-represented.pdf (hopkinsmedicine.org)

CHAPTER 8

Financial Resources

ACADEMIC VIGNETTE

You are the director of the advanced practice registered nurse (APRN) programs that incorporate certified registered nurse anesthetists, family, adult geriatric, and pediatric nurse practitioner programs and several certificate programs. The programs have been ranked in the top 25 in the country and are critical to the mission of the school to prepare a workforce to care for vulnerable populations. You have a total of 500 students. Your university has been sharing the changing financial picture due to the COVID-19 pandemic with the loss of revenue estimated to be over $100 million. The dean of the school of nursing has asked you to reduce your budget by 10% for the coming year. The reduction comes on top of a reduction of 5% reduction prior to the COVID-19 pandemic. With the previous 5% reduction, line items such as travel, subscriptions, and other expenses, were either greatly reduced or eliminated. All of the APRN programs have maintained their enrollment and therefore their financial base. The programs had moved to online education prior to the pandemic and the students have been able to maintain their clinical placements. Other programs in the school of nursing are less financially stable. You have six open full time faculty positions (nearly 20% of positions) that you are currently recruiting. While the faculty and staff have readily taken on an additional workload given the reduction in faculty and having faculty ill with COVID-19, they are feeling burned out. You have promised them for which the open positions would be filled as soon as possible. You could meet your 15% reduction by not filling three of the open positions but you are worried about your faculty and staff and your promise that help was coming. You are faced with a situation in which there is not an easy answer.

135

CLINICAL VIGNETTE

You are new to your leadership position. In your previous position, your set of responsibilities included being accountable for the work that those who reported to you were assigned to do. You were involved in hiring and firing people who were your direct reports. You were given a budget each year, but the vice president of nursing, the chief finance officer, and your manager determined the number of positions and overall budget for your unit based on past budgets and current productivity metrics. You had no input into creating your budget as that has been done at the higher level, the level you are at now. You are feeling unsure about how to go about developing budgets for not just the previous unit you were in charge of, but five other units now within your sphere of responsibility as well. You now understand that there was a cost overrun for your units during the past two years and now each of the units you manage will have a 10% cut in their budget. While you know budgets will be cut, the leaders of each of the units have let you know they are understaffed and have begun to lose some of their best people because of the stress of ever increasing workloads. In addition, the patient experience metrics have declined for each of the units. To add to your concerns, you realize that budgets determine not only staff resources but also space, equipment, support for professional development of staff and other critical resources. You know you need to establish the priorities for what you want to accomplish. You have the challenge of managing your constrained resources and achieving the organization's priorities.

INTRODUCTION

The opportunity to provide leadership in an organization comes with the responsibility of managing the resources of that organization. Some leaders, such as a school of nursing dean, will have the responsibility for the entire organizational budget, while others might have responsibility for one dimension or program of the overall budget. Regardless of the size and scope of their financial responsibility, the leader needs to have a full understanding of the key drivers for resource development and allocation: (1) the process and principles of financial decision-making; and (2) management of budgets within organizations.

WHY FINANCIAL RESOURCE MANAGEMENT IS IMPORTANT

The budget is a representation of the organization's plans and priorities. In quality improvement, we say what is measured matters. From a financial standpoint, what is funded matters. Both the mission and the budget provide focus and direction to the organization. It communicates primarily to the people who make up the organization a shared understanding of the organization's intended direction. The budget tells the employees that, as an organization, we value a certain set of priorities because this is where we are putting our resources. An example of the messaging that a budget gives an organization can be seen when strategic priorities are highlighted for funding. Often a strategic plan is a multiyear document with many goals that require financial resources. If a leader clearly signals that one of those initiatives will be funded in the first year, it tells the members of this organization the initiative is of particular value to the organization and its future and sets the direction for the organization for that year.

One of the most important influencers of the budget process is the institution's character which is influenced by the organization's history, culture, administrative structure, and operating climate. A small private college will have a very different approach to the budgeting process than a large public university. Similarly, a religiously affiliated hospital, which is part of a large health system, will approach their budgeting process differently from a small, independent community hospital. The budgeting process is influenced by the population served, the stakeholders that are represented in the budgeting process, and the constituencies that need to approve the budget. Understanding the organizational culture will help leaders effectively develop and manage budgets in a way that is congruent with the organization approach to budgeting and consistent with its mission and values.

The kind and level of involvement of organizational stakeholders are part of the institutional character of an organization. In some organizations, especially those with shared governance, the budgeting process includes stakeholders such as faculty, staff, students or clinical nurses, and technical staff on a clinical unit. In other organizations, the budgeting process is much more of a top-down activity with the leadership team of the organization having the full responsibility for its development. However, the budget is developed, it is important that the leader share the principles included in the budget with the community it affects. If there are parts of the budget that have been significantly reduced, a separate conversation with the affected individuals before the budget is shared publicly is important. Similarly, if there are additional resources included in the budget to do a specific project or add capacity to a program or service, that should be shared with the affected individuals as well, prior to any public meeting. The leader should try to make sure that there are no surprises in the budget since that will create distrust of the leaders and the budgeting process.

Consider: **What is your experience with budgets? Is the budget process transparent in your organization? Does everyone have access to budgetary information? Are you part of the process? In what way do you participate?**

WHAT DRIVES FINANCIAL DECISION-MAKING

Financial decision-making is based on priority goals that are being or have been established. Resources may be needed to improve internal efficiency based on the results of a gap analysis, or for investment in internal or external opportunities. The challenge for leaders is to establish a timetable for the goals recognizing that some goals may need to be funded in future budget cycles.

The most important document that drives financial decision-making in an organization is the organization's strategic plan. Consider the purpose of a strategic plan. (See Chapter 5 for in depth understanding of the strategic planning process). The Balanced Scorecard Institute (2020) states that, "strategic planning is an organizational management activity used to set priorities, focus energy and resources, strengthen operations, ensure that employees and other stakeholders are working toward common goals, establish agreement around intended outcomes/results, and assess and adjust the organization's direction in response to a changing environment." If the institution plans effectively, it will be clear what budgetary decisions need to be made. By funding the goals in the strategic plan, the leader is creating the coherence between the goals and objectives the organization has identified as important and the resources needed to achieve those goals. The importance of linking the budget with the strategic initiatives cannot be overstated.

Consider the following example. A school of nursing might spend a whole year in defining their strategic plan. Multiple groups of stakeholders meet over the course of the year to define the important strategic goals that will take the school into the future. The stakeholders identify five goals, each with five to six strategic initiatives with accompanying tactics that will help the organization reach its goals. At the end of the strategic planning process, the budgeting process begins. Funding of the strategic initiatives in the plan tells the organization that the leader is committed to creating a common goal that all members of the community can work toward. It also lets the stakeholders know that their work in creating the plans for the future was valued. This strategy gives the leader a chance to demonstrate to the organization that the budget and the strategic plan are aligned.

Consider a different scenario. Stakeholders in a large clinical department spend several months working on creating a strategic plan for their future. After a review of clinical data, the stakeholders determine that an important goal for this unit would be to work on reducing the number of surgical site infections. As they reviewed their clinical data, they determined that their rate of surgical infection was higher than any other post-surgical unit in their hospital, yet their patient population was not unique. At the end of their strategic planning process, the budgeting process begins. The leader decides to allocate additional resources to a program focused on recognizing and treating elderly abuse and reduce the allocation of resources to those programs that would reduce the incidence of surgical site infection. This decision leaves the members confused about the organization's important priorities and unclear about how to focus their energy and their work. In addition, the stakeholders that gave of their time and expertise are left wondering how their work contributed to the future of the organization.

While the strategic plan provides the roadmap for the resource decisions in an organization, it is important to recognize that organizations need to be flexible and able to change in the face of external and internal forces. It will be impossible to design a strategic plan for every situation that could arises over a one-, two-, or more-year time frame. That is why a strategic plan needs to be flexible and changeable in a rapidly changing environment. A strategic plan is the organization's best assessment and plan at any specific point in time. Unforeseen challenges and opportunities will arise and the leader needs to assess their importance and how funding them will affect the original goals. Being flexible and responsive to important opportunities is a critical element of financial decision making.

Managing the budget requires the leader to examine priorities and determine which ones will get the limited funding that is available in most organizations. In determining where resources can be obtained, it is important to recognize that resources can be found in both the revenue and expense side of the ledger. Either revenue is increased, or expenses decreased. For example, the strategic plan of a college of nursing calls for the addition of a new pediatric nurse practitioner program. There are no new resources in the university for the addition of new programs, so the dean begins to look at the current portfolio of programs in the college. On close examination of the budget and analysis of cost per student, she finds that a small neonatal nurse practitioner program is undersubscribed and high cost. By moving on the processes to close the neonatal NP program, the dean can find the resources within the college to open a larger and more cost-effective pediatric NP program. She works with the neonatal faculty to get them on board to teach in the pediatric program. If a leader is willing to be open to new approaches of budget management, budget efficiencies can be found in many places within the budget including existing programs that are not cost effective, bloated administrative costs, and inefficient operational processes.

Consider: **Does your organization's budget reflect its mission and vision? Will the budget help your organization achieve its mission?**

NUTS AND BOLTS OF A BUDGET

Operational budgets reflect both income/revenue and costs/expenses. Income for clinical organizations is mostly from patient care revenues, which include direct payment by patients and third-party payers such as private insurers and governmental programs such as Medicare, Medicaid, and CHIP. Clinical organizations may also have income from grants, contracts, or gifts. Income for educational institutions are primarily tuition dollars, state funds for public institutions (although these have been reduced substantially over the past decade), grants, gifts, and (for some institutions) clinical income such as from nurse run clinics.

An operating budget is done on an annual basis and addresses the day-to-day running of an organization. A capital budget is done separately and reflects long term investment and may extend five to ten years. The types of capital investment often include real estate, technology, and machines. Capital budgeting is both a financial commitment and investment decision intended to increase profitability or extend the work of the organization consistent with the mission, vision, and goals. Examples of a capital investments for clinical organizations include building a new hospital and buying a new MRI machine to enhance care and increase market share of patients. An academic organization capital budget could include buying land to extend the campus or building out a high technology simulation lab for a school of nursing.

Fixed and Variable Costs

The cost side of budgets are generally considered within the context of fixed and variable costs. Fixed costs are those that are constant regardless of the output of services or goods. Fixed costs include rent, insurance, property tax, and cost of personnel that are essential to the basic business. Fixed costs represent the majority of an organization's budget and can be 80% or more of a budget.

Fixed costs are often used in doing a break-even analysis for an organization. The break even analysis is establishing the amount of income that is needed to cover fixed costs. For instance, an educational program will need to meet certain requirements established by the institution and accreditation for space, faculty, equipment, and other inputs regardless of the number of students. A break-even analysis would be based on the amount of tuition dollars and therefore number of students and course credits per year needed to exactly cover the fixed costs. A similar break-even analysis would take place for adding a clinical service (e.g., home care). The issue would include what number of patients with a specific type of payment (given different payer rates for care, with Medicare paying about 70–80 cents on the dollar) would be needed to cover the fixed costs of offering a home care service that meets CMS certification requirements.

Variable costs change with output. Variable costs are directly tied to the number of patients cared for or students enrolled in an academic program. Variable costs include any costs associated with the number of students/patients served beyond the fixed cost. Examples include needing to increase staff in a hospital for an infectious disease outbreak such as managing the needs of coronavirus patients or adding adjunct faculty to teach if there is a large student increase. A variable cost is any cost associated with additional services provided beyond the fixed break-even cost.

Direct and Indirect Costs

Costs can also be considered in terms of direct and indirect costs. Direct costs are those that are the result of providing a specific good or service. In a clinical setting, direct costs would be the costs associated with patient care including nursing salaries and supplies. In an educational organization, an example of direct costs is faculty salaries. Indirect costs are those costs that are necessary to run an organization but cannot be linked to a specific product or service within an organization. Indirect costs include utility costs, administration, research offices, facility maintenance, and information technology. These services are used by all parts of an organization and cannot be attributed to a single unit.

The importance of direct and indirect costs is seen in how the indirect costs are managed and assigned to different budgets. The indirect costs related to any organization need to be covered. Some organizations assign a rate for indirect cost coverage to the subunit of the organization. For instance, in an academic institution, a school of nursing may be charged a rate of 50% by the university to cover the organization's indirect costs. The indirect cost can be calculated by multiplying the total direct costs by 50%. This cost is then factored into the school of nursing's overall expenses. A budget with direct costs of $5 million dollars would then have indirect costs of $2.5 million for a budget total of $7.5 million. Agreements can often be negotiated to reduce indirect costs.

Institutions that receive federal grant funds through the National Institutes of Health submit, on a periodic basis, estimates of indirect costs that become a rate that the institution will receive with any NIH grant as the percent applied to the direct costs. The range of indirect costs varies with institutions and has been as high as 100% of direct costs. It is important for leaders to know what their direct costs are and the basis of the organization assessing an indirect cost rate. As noted above, there is often room to negotiate some indirect costs to be considered direct costs and therefore reduce the indirect rate. This may be particularly important with grants that carry limited indirect costs. In starting a new program, a leader will want to negotiate reduced indirect charges related to the program to give the program time to become financially sustainable. Relief of some indirect costs are often the difference in the financial success of new programs.

Frequently Used Types of Budgeting

Leaders also need to be familiar with the type of budgeting process used by their organization. There are four basic budgeting processes used by organizations. These are activity-based, incremental, zero-based, and value-based budgeting (CFI, 2021). Organizations may go from one method of budgeting to another based on the needs of the organization—whether to more tightly control costs, or to assign costs and income to specific units of production.

Activity-based Budgeting

This type of budgeting is a complex method that involves a deep understanding of the activities that carry a cost that go into the goods or services provided. It is usually intended to identify unnecessary steps or inputs that can be eliminated from the costs of the production of goods or services to create more efficiency. This method of budgeting requires research and analytics in order to understand the cost of the inputs and the processes involved. It is focused on reducing costs as much as possible to be more competitive while maintaining or expanding income in order to increase profits. An example of activity-based budgeting would be a chief nurse needing to budget the cost of a home care service. Costs of activities that go into the home care service includes the service delivery by a provider (there may be several different types of providers including nurses, physicians, OT, PT, and social work), transportation, equipment, insurance, and others. The costs will depend on the type and the amount of service projected. By doing the analysis for activity-based budgeting, it may show that transportation and provider costs related to home visits could be reduced, creating greater efficiency for both patients and providers, by using telehealth monitoring to substitute for some percent of home visits.

Incremental Budgeting

This type of budgeting is commonly used and based on the previous year's budget plus adding or subtracting small amounts to each budget line. Incremental budgeting assumes that the activity for the next year will be very similar to the current year. For instance, if a school of nursing has offered a family nurse practitioner program and the enrollment has been stable with the only change being salary increases, the budget for the program will look like it has in the past with the addition of funds to the personnel line to address the salary increases. A clinic will know how much is spent on rent and utilities from the previous budget, and will incrementally add a small amount to recognize inflationary increases in the costs. While incremental budgeting can be done reasonably quickly and provides operational stability, the drawbacks can be substantial. One disadvantage is that incremental budgeting can stifle creativity by continuing to allocate all of the resources to the known goods or services.

Then, there are limited or no funds to create a new initiative. Incremental budgeting can also create cost creep with little additional value and no incentive to look for efficiencies. This type of budgeting is sometimes used after going through a zero-based budgeting process or activity-based process the previous year when budgets have been deeply vetted.

Zero Based Budgeting

Unlike incremental budgeting, zero-based budgeting does not consider the previous budgets. The budget starts from scratch and includes an assessment of the activities that are essential to the organization in reaching its goals. It provides a fresh look not only at priorities, but also the necessary inputs to produce a good or service. Zero-based budgeting creates greater efficiency than incremental budgeting and can better support innovation because of the efficiency and the elimination of non-productive activities. However, zero-based budgeting often comes to similar bottom lines as incremental budgeting. For organizations that use incremental budgeting, any new activity or program starts with zero-based budgeting.

Value-based budgeting

This budgeting type has organizations consider if each line item in the budget is of value to the customer, other stakeholders, or the organization. Is the cost aligned with the mission and vision of the organization? Budgets of any organization can have costs that at one time may have provided value, however, over time with changes in technology and mission those costs are no longer aligned with the goals. For example, if a health system decides that its mission is to strengthen its community outreach, it will need to expand the budget for programs that reflect the value of community partnerships and likely eliminate other costs.

It is important to note that while distinct approaches to budgeting can be defined, any given budget process uses several types in constructing the overall budget. Incremental budgeting could be used for the majority of a budget, while assessing the alignment of the budget with the values of the organization. Most budgeting processes of large organizations also include start- up of new activities using zero-based budgeting.

In addition to understanding budgets, leaders need to know how financial data are collected, reported, and used. There are many types of budgeting software available. Leaders should know the software program that their organization uses to understand the collection and reporting capability. Generally, each large unit in an organization has a finance person that reports to the overall organization's financial office. Smaller organizations may have a single finance person or office manager. Whichever is the case, leaders will greatly benefit by having a collaborative working relationship with the finance staff. While understanding the capabilities of budgeting and financial monitoring software programs is important, the responsibilities of leaders is to be financially responsible for the most effective allocation of resources to do the best job possible.

Consider: **What type of budget method does your organization use? Do you think it is the most useful approach to budgeting for the needs of your organization? How does the nursing budget fit into the overall organizational budget?**

LEADING IN A RESOURCE CONSTRAINED ENVIRONMENT

One of the most challenging aspects of leadership is leading within constrained resources. Budget reductions become a cyclical event in nearly all healthcare related businesses caused by changes in reimbursement policy, change of ownership, need for high-cost investments, and competition that may reduce income. At times the need to reduce costs may come suddenly or they may be planned over time as the organization evolves. Budget cuts often affect nursing and patient care positions in acute care more than any other non-hospital-based service area because nursing services make up the largest cost. Nursing and patient care services departments have been considered a cost center in hospitals and budgetarily they appear as a cost.

However, changing the perception of nursing as a cost is critical to recognizing nursing as the reason people come to hospitals, so it is the service that is the basis for income. Advanced practice registered nurses are perceived differently because of the ability to bill for services. There have been many situations where the cost effectiveness of midwives, nurse practitioners, certified registered nurse anesthetists and physician assistants are incorporated into a service area because of their cost-effectiveness, ability to generate income and improve patient outcomes (McCleary *et al.*, 2014; Yox and Stanik-Hutt, 2016).

A resource constrained environment requires very close attention to the strategic plan and goals. The strategic plan is work that needs to be accomplished. Because of unanticipated changes such as a pandemic, there may be a need to prioritize the goals or establish a different time frame for achieving the goals. A situation may arise in which the limitations on resources are so severe that a leader may determine that the cuts in funding will cause an unacceptable decrease in the quality of education or clinical services. In this type of situation, the leader will need to make an ethical decision about the likelihood of influencing the necessary change and based on that decision, stay, or go. Some of that decision may be based on assessment of the need to see an organization through a challenging time and the likelihood of improvement in the availability of resources.

ORGANIZATIONAL INVESTMENT DECISIONS

Making a case for investment dollars can be applied to either internal or external funding opportunities. Organizations have different timeline views for making decisions about investing resources. Some organizations prioritize a short-term view in which the return on investment needs to be within a year or two. Many for-profit healthcare organizations have investors that expect a quick return on investments. Publicly traded companies live by their quarterly report on earnings that get highlighted in the news, especially when there is a significant increase or decrease in earnings or there is a gap in projections compared to the actual earnings. Emphasis on quarterly reports puts pressure on organizations to have a short term return on investments. Some organizations take the long view and are willing to invest in mid-term or long-term results recognizing that meaningful investment decisions take time to produce a return. While there may be a predominant investment timeline strategy, most companies employ both long- and short-term strategies.

Investment decisions are complex and involve a number of considerations on the part of organizational leaders. A major challenge for investment decisions is to address the future and not the past, align with the organization's strategic goals, and be financially sustainable. Too often leaders respond to a need or opportunity based on what is happening currently or in the past. For some healthcare organizations, investing in something based on data from a year or two prior which may be too late to create a meaningful return in the future. For instance, using technology two years old in order to save costs will miss the opportunity to have a machine based on the latest technology providing more accurate diagnosis of a breast mass, with the result being that women choose to go elsewhere for their mammogram. The organization may have saved costs but lost revenue.

Every investment decision should be aligned with the strategic goals of an organization. The investment should move them toward fulfilling their goals. Clearly there are many ways of meeting organizational goals, and leaders need to prioritize their goals for investment and analyze the costs/benefit or return on investment on funds allocated. Cost/benefit analysis includes the tangible costs, intangible costs, and benefits of an investment and is therefore a more in-depth analysis of a potential investment whereas return on investment is based largely on the tangible costs and benefits such as personnel costs, space, and equipment. Intangible cost may include costs related to enhancing the image of the organization, improving the star rating of a hospital, or improving patient experience.

Sustainability usually means that the investment produces a financial return that sustains the activity at least covering direct and indirect costs. However, sustainability does not necessarily mean that it produces a profit. There may be a strategic reason to provide ongoing support to an activity even if it is not profitable, such as improving the quality of care or education, meeting the demands of a new regulation, or improving the reputation of an organization. Some benefits of an investment may not be quantifiable in a usual budgetary way and the investment may then be sustained through profits from other areas of the organization.

Investment decisions by organizational leaders require leaders to be well informed about the budget trends of the organization, past investment performance and the details of how resources are deployed. Nurse leaders need to be at the table for these discussions and decisions and understand that vying for internal resources of an organization can be an emotionally charged experience. While leaders of various units are expected to collaborate and work together for the good of the organization, when it comes to internal resource deployment, the resource pie is only so big and leaders compete for resources for their organizational units. It is normal for any leader to be disappointed if their department or unit was not allocated the investment funds they worked hard to get. It is critical to then focus on future budget cycles by regrouping and re-strategizing about how to best put the request forward.

FINDING RESOURCES BEYOND THE OPERATIONAL BUDGET

Internal Resources

Finding resources to fund new initiatives or priorities is often a challenge for a leader. Funding sources can be internal or external to the organization. There are three primary sources of internal resources for new goals and priorities as discussed below.

1. *Repurpose current resources.* To find major funding within an established budget, revising the responsibilities of the current workforce is one way. Revision of responsibilities may be done within current job descriptions. However, there may be a need to reorganize the workforce, creating new job descriptions and organizational structures in order to match skill sets with work to be done. Working with human resources is essential for a reorganization. If the organization is unionized, it is essential to work with union leaders. A reorganization will cause considerable anxiety and this work should be done with transparency and completed as quickly as possible. Some re-purposing can be done in small ways, such as re-allocating travel funds, limiting the cost of travel nurses or adjunct faculty,

and many other ways of finding funds without making changes in actual staffing full time equivalents (FTEs) or role responsibilities.

2. *Use investment funds from within the specific organizational unit.* This may be more common in academic settings than in clinical settings. Many leaders have access to investment funds that are put into a special fund for specific purposes of investing in innovation and professional development activities. The investment funds are usually intended for new projects, goals, and priorities, but can also be used to temporarily support an activity or service that is in between funding from outside sources. In this case, the likelihood of future outside funding needs to be reasonably high.

3. *Request investment funds from the organization.* Making the case for resources within the organization can be challenging. Usually, the situation includes units competing for a fixed amount of resources. The department of medicine may want more physicians and the department of nursing more nurses. Both academic and clinical organizations may have an innovation fund that nursing can apply for. Success in obtaining these funds depends on the availability of investment funds, the quality of the argument for additional investment, the perceived likelihood for success, political power, and the fit with the organization's goals and priorities.

External Resources

External sources of funding are more challenging since the funds are controlled by external individuals or organizations. Too many leaders go after external funding for projects that have little relevance to their goals, and it distracts from moving forward with their priorities. Outside resources are usually pursued for the following reasons:

- Funds to support a specific activity that is part of the organization's goals and priorities
- The desire for prestige that comes with outside funding
- Pressure to bring in any funding

It is most useful for a leader to go after external funds when they are aligned with the goals and priorities of the organization.

External sources of funding are usually grants, contracts, or gifts. Grants and contracts require an organization to have the capacity to manage the requirements related to accepting the grant and reporting process. A grant is a sum of money that is given to an organization to fund an idea or a project. Federal grants can be complicated and having a grants office is necessary, as well as having a principal investigator knowledgeable about the responsibilities. Grants from foundations are generally less cumbersome in requirements. To get a grant from a foundation, it is useful to develop a relationship with a program officer or someone within the foundation. Foundations tend to fund people they know will deliver on the work to be done. Some foundations will only fund people and projects they invite for funding, others will accept applications in response to a call for proposals. There are many foundations that fund only local initiatives and there are a few foundations that are national in scope such as the Robert Wood Johnson Foundation, Kellogg Foundation, Commonwealth Foundation, and others. Foundation grants often will fund indirect costs but at a level much lower than the NIH research grants, often at the 10% to 12% rate if at all.

A contract is similar to a grant but in a contract, the funding agency defines specific deliverables that must be completed in order for the organization to receive payment. It will be important to have a clear picture of the deliverables and the understanding of who on the team can complete the work before entering into a contract. Contracts often do not allow for an indirect cost rate to be included. To address this, costs that are often considered indirect such as rent are included in the budget as a direct cost. It is always important to know the payment restrictions.

Many organizations in which nurse leaders work are considered 501(c)(3) organizations. This designation is given to nonprofit organizations that have been approved by the Internal Revenue Service as a tax-exempt, charitable organization. In addition to being exempt from federal income tax, these organizations can be the recipient of tax-deductible gifts from individuals. In the clinical setting, a large number of donors are grateful patients. Often patients will go home and realize that the care they received was high quality and had a significant impact on their recovery. They decide they want to give a gift to the unit to support the nurses or nursing care provided.

In the academic setting, the largest group of donors are the alumni who realize that their life has been forever changed from the experience they had during their academic program and are moved to give back. Many leaders in academia have, as part of the job responsibilities, the requirement to engage people who want to provide financial support to nursing. For example, the dean of a school of nursing is usually expected to spend a considerable amount of their time on philanthropy. Philanthropy is based on developing relationships with key constituents who have the funding capacity for big and small gifts to the organization. Understanding the major constituencies of an organization and the principles of philanthropy will be essential for a leader of an organization.

Gifts can come into an organization as restricted or unrestricted. Restricted gifts are those in which the funds can be used only for the activities defined by the donor. For example, a donor might give a restricted gift to a community health center to be used exclusively to support continuing education for the nurses in that center. Just as you need to make sure that grants and contracts are aligned with the organization's mission and goals, restricted gifts should also be accepted only if they advance the strategic priorities of the organization. Restricted gifts are designated to be spent in certain ways, such as for scholarships or faculty support, or for cancer care or health promotion screening. If a donor wants to fund a program that is not consistent with the goals of the organization, the gift becomes a burden and will often divert the organization from its intended goals.

Unrestricted gifts are given to an organization without any requirements of how they can be used. However, the funds are used, it is important to keep the donor informed of how the donation was spent, the impact of the donation on the organization, or on the individuals it supports. Stewardship of gifts, restricted or unrestricted, is an important practice for keeping the donor engaged and excited about the organization. Donors want to know if their funds are being used as intended and what the benefits are.

Being open and aware of non-monetary resources is important. These contributions could include a person with a specific skill may be "loaned" for a project without any cost to the project. Another example is the donation of supplies or equipment that would be cost prohibitive for the organization to purchase. While a person's time is money, and supplies and equipment certainly have a cost, there is no cash transfer with these types of gifts.

Other non-financial sources can be garnered from partnerships. The first step in building a partnership is to identify a stakeholder who shares a common goal or interest. It may work best if the leader has worked with this potential partner and knows them to be trustworthy or the person has a well-known trustworthy reputation. The partnership must produce a win-win. The plan will need to clearly define what the win is for each party. A partnership will not work if there is not something gained by each party. It is critical to have a very clear agreement as to how any revenue associated with the partnership will be shared. Money often complicates perfectly good partnerships that are based on non-financial outcomes.

Too often, one party may try to get more than agreed upon. If this happens, the partnership is greatly jeopardized if not completely fractured. Partners need to agree on the metrics used in evaluating the outcomes of the shared goal and the benefits. Being able to see what has been accomplished through the partnership will provide momentum for its continuation. Finally, a partnership needs to be based on consistent, transparent, and clear communication around the shared goals.

The Process to Seek Internal and External Funding

The ideal beginning of the process of seeking funding is to have a conversation with the person who has control over the funds. This is an opportunity to elicit interest. In addition to sharing your ideas with the funder, you want to listen carefully to the priorities and passions described by the funder—whether the CEO of an organization or outside funder. If there is no interest in the idea during the first conversation, figure out how to re-package your idea in a way that would be a better fit with the interests of the funder. Many leaders fail to realize that the funder, whether internal or external, wants to invest in projects that will further their goals and priorities. Helping the funder see the match between the organization's needs and the funder's goals and priorities is a critical first step.

Investors, whether internal or external, also want to know why a leader thinks they will be successful in meeting their goals. This often comes down to having a track record of success. Highlighting prior successes is often helpful. It is also helpful to communicate that the workforce is on board and ready to move forward and that there is a well-developed work plan with metrics built in to provide feedback about progress at various stages of work. Metrics related to the outcome of the investment are critical. Metrics should be based on usual financial metrics, specifically return on investment, as well as the metrics that the organization uses to measure outcomes. These are also key performance indicators (KPIs) defined as, "a set of quantifiable measures that a company uses to gauge its performance over time" (Surdez, 2018). These measures are specific to organizational goals and strategies. KPIs should adhere to the SMART goals for establishing measures being specific, measurable, attainable, relevant and with a defined time frame as described in Chapter 5.

If there is interest, a written proposal is the next step. Often a brief one- to two-page statement provides the summary of the project. This provides an overview that busy people can see at a glance. Some external and internal funders may require a full proposal as the first step. A summary and full proposal usually includes: (1) a clear statement of the goal; (2) how the investment furthers the mission of the organization; (3) the actual resources needed; (4) the expected return on investment; (5) statement (ideal if there are data) supporting the potential for success; (6) metrics to be used in evaluating the outcome of the investment. The full proposal will have much detail. Large organizations may have a unit specifically designed to write grants that can be very useful in pursuing external resources especially from federal, state, or local agencies and foundations.

Having a clear statement of the goal is often a challenge. The statement needs to be brief yet compelling and complete. For instance, a leader requesting more internal resources may start a goal statement by saying, "we need more nurses to provide better care to patients." While this may be true, a more compelling statement that includes outcome information might be, "We have a serious problem on medical-surgical unit A. Our patients are telling us they are not satisfied with our care, our patient experience metrics have significantly decreased. That unit has experienced a higher patient to nurse ratio than other units that have great patient experience metrics. Adding x number of nurses will improve our patients' experience of care. We want all of our patients to be able to count on the high quality of care which is our vision."

Linking the investment request to the overall vision and priorities of the organization is a way to provide context for the proposal. In the above example, if the organization's vision is to provide consistent high-quality care, linking to the patient experience metrics will be useful. It is important for top-level financial decision makers to understand the context of the request. Relating the request to overall organizational priorities makes it easier for them to understand how the funding will benefit the organization.

The actual amount of the resources requested will need to include specifics. It is usually reasonable to start with the overall amount of the request and then go into the more detailed request especially the larger ticket items. A leader needs to be ready with the full budget before going into any budget meeting that involves an investment request. Since most organizations are concerned about financial viability, the financial return on the investment is critical. Organizations go through cycles of less investment and more investment depending on the profitability of the budget year. If there is an expectation of a return on investment, the greater the return (as well as being consistent with overall organizational priorities), the greater the likelihood of being funded.

Consider: **In a resource constrained environment it is often necessary for a nurse leader to access internal and external resources. Reflect on a need that requires you to convince the CFO or financial manager that they should give you additional resources to complete something. How did you convince them to invest in your project or program?**

RETURN ON INVESTMENT (ROI)

ROI is the profit (or loss) from an investment and is a critical consideration in making an argument for funding. Even though a vision statement and element of a strategic plan may include providing access to care for a specific population, a goal of starting a community clinic is going to need to have a business case and ROI is a key element of a business case. A business case is intended to provide information to a decision-maker about the financial aspects of a goal or project in determining whether the investment is a prudent use of resources. ROI is often used as the basis of a business case because of its simplicity. The calculation is:

$$\frac{\text{Gain from Investment} - \text{Cost of Investment}}{\text{Cost of Investment}} = \text{ROI}$$

ROI is reported as a percent of the net income divided by the cost. The higher the percentage (or ratio) the greater the return. The simplicity of the calculation provides a way of exploring multiple options and assessing the projected investment and return.

An example of ROI is an academic institution having a vision to improve the health of children living in rural areas and considering starting a pediatric nurse practitioner program or expanding the family NP program. There are not sufficient resources to do both. The leadership team has financial data from other schools for developing a PNP program, and the biggest additional cost is faculty. The calculation for investment would include PNP faculty costs and tuition income being generated. In calculating the ROI for the PNP program, assume one additional faculty is needed with a cost of $100,000 salary and 25% cost for fringe benefits for an annual cost of $125,000. There would be one year for developing the program prior to the admission of students. Assume the pediatric program has 10 students per year. The tuition is $1000 per credit (it is a private nonprofit institution), with an average of 24 credits per year for two years, for a total of 48 credits. The alternative is to expand the family NP program by 10 students. This could be accomplished by adding 10 students at the next admission cycle. There is an FNP faculty teaching in the undergraduate program who could be reassigned to the FNP program. The FNP faculty salary is also $100,000 plus 25% fringe benefit for a total of $125,000. The FNP program has 25 credits per year for 2 years for a total of 50 credits. Examining the ROI of the PNP program over a three year period would reflect one year of development time for the PNP and two years for the first cohort to complete the program plus the addition of a second cohort in year 3 with income for their first year. The FNP program would immediately add 10 students and over a three year period would include two full years of tuition income plus the year 3 admissions for one year. The costs of the NP faculty would be the same over the three years. Assuming no change in salary or tuition rates, in comparing the two options you would find:

Pediatric NP program with income after 3 years: No tuition in year 1; $240,000 in tuition year 2 (10 students × 24 credits × $1000); and $480,000 in year 3 (10 continuing students and 10 new students). The total income for 3 years would be $720,000. The cost for faculty would be 125,000 × 3 = 375,000. The ROI would be 720,000 − 375,000/375,000 = 0.92

FNP program expansion with income after three years: $250,000 tuition in year 1 (10 students × 25 credits × $1000); $500,000 in year 2 (10 continuing students and 10 new students); and $500,000 in year 3 (The 10 initial students have graduated, 10 continuing students and 10 new students). The total income over 3 years would be $1,250,000. Cost of the faculty for 3 years would $375,000. The ROI would be 1,250,000 − 375,000/375,000 = 2.3.

From this simplistic approach to deciding options for program development or expansion based on ROI, expanding the FNP has a better return because the program begins immediately and there are 2 more credits in the FNP program. The higher the ROI, the better is the investment. However, the difference in ROI may not be the most important criteria for this decision. The community need may be for pediatric NPs specifically which may be a reason to develop the PNP program.

SPACE AND TIME AS ESSENTIAL RESOURCES

Space and Facilities

As an organizational leader, you will often be in the position of requesting additional space for new initiatives or staff, consulting on the build out of space being renovated, or determining the location of staff and programs within your area of responsibility. You may also be asked to work on a new building design. While these responsibilities might seem like simple, low risk activities, decisions you make about space and facilities are often represented as the value you put on the people and initiatives. For example, if a staff or faculty member gets assigned a large office with a window, they might be perceived as more valued than another staff or faculty member who are assigned an office further from the main office without a window. While you may have had no intention to communicate that message, the size and character of individual's offices and the location often says a great deal about what and who the leader thinks are important. Bottom line, assignment of offices is often perceived as a very personal decision reflecting how a leader values an individual.

An example of the impact of space decisions is the common occurrence of hiring new people but not having any additional space. Clearly some change needs to happen, and the question will be who gets less space? Many organizations have created cubicles to expand the number of people with desks or adopted an open space configuration. However, a common complaint includes that smaller space does not accommodate the work that needs to be done. Being so close together, noise from other people may be distracting and there is limited privacy. There also may be limited space to schedule private meetings. Another common comment is that furniture that is in small spaces does not support the work being done nor provide easy meeting space. People also notice that often people who have offices spend less time in them compared to people in cubicles. This reflects the power gradient of different levels and types of responsibility. All of the above complaints can lead to significantly disgruntled staff or faculty who feel disrespected because of the way space decisions may have occurred.

There are several ways in which the pitfalls of space allocation can be minimized. First and foremost, stakeholders within an organization should be involved in defining principles around space planning that will be the foundation of your decision-making and stick by them. For example, will everyone have their own office, or will there be shared offices for all? Will people at a certain level of the organization have a private office and others will share? Will researchers share their labs, or will each scientist have their own dedicated space? Will a clinical educator have space on the unit to conduct educational meetings? Making some of these decisions prospectively will help to reduce the number of individual decisions that need to be made around space. Participation in decision-making is an important principle that reduces conflict in organizations. The ability to have a voice and feel like your needs and concerns are being considered will go far in helping members of the organization feel like they are valued. It will also give the leader an opportunity to share the reasons why there needs to be a space or facility change and the thought behind the options to consider. Being able to compromise on certain issues helps everyone feel like they have been heard and are valued members of the team.

It will also be important to find an individual within your organization who has expertise in space utilization and bring them into the conversation and decision-making. There are experts in the art and science of space planning who know how to get the most out of the often-limited space resources. This individual might also have a perspective that is different from the leaders and allow for better decision-making processes about use of space. A leader can expect complaints about assignments and arguments for better personal space. By having established principles about sharing, the response to complaints needs to be linked to the principles.

Decisions around space for programs and initiatives should always be based on the organization's strategic plan. The strategic plan may be best served with a new configuration of personal space. For instance, the open space design where everyone is in a low walled cubicle for some organizations may help people work together more effectively by enhancing communication. For other organizations, having privacy available for members may work best because of confidentiality issues. Space is a critical organizational resource and should be allocated fairly and with an eye to the initiatives defined in the strategic plan.

It should be noted that in non-clinical delivery units and academic institutions, many leaders have established criteria for employees to work at home. This movement has been accelerated by the COVID-19 pandemic and has forced many organizations to develop extensive plans for employees to work at home. Working at home often provides the employee more work time and less commute time, as well as reduces the space needs of the organization. One of the outcomes of the pandemic is that more people working from home. With many educational programs being online, the need for faculty to be physically at the college or university is greatly reduced and therefore decreases office space needed. Telehealth is also opening the opportunity for some nurses to work at home. This clearly is not an option for clinical nurses who have to be on-site to deliver care.

Finally, anticipating potential conflict over space and facility decisions will help to minimize the conflict. Emotional response to space changes is to be expected. Address the issues that concern people and use the principles defined for space allocation, the strategic plan, and the space and facilities expert (when possible) to help with this challenge.

Time

Most would agree that time is a precious resource in any organization, and the one in shortest supply. Time management is a challenge for all members of an organization. It is critical for the leader to be aware of ways to create efficiencies and build effectiveness in work for themselves and their staff. Helping each member of the organization take responsibility for their roles and responsibilities prevents any one member from feeling they are overburdened with a larger share of the duties than other members.

As a leader, your plans and objectives for each day can be derailed by unexpected issues that arise. Sometimes the situation requires your attention while other times, the situation can be handled by others in the organization. It is important for a leader to be able to distinguish which issues they should be addressing, and which they can delegate to others. As a leader looks at their role and how they spend their time, a useful question is: "Is this something that I, uniquely, as leader of this organization, should be doing?" If the answer is yes, then the leader should take responsibility to address the issue. If the answer is no, the next question is: "If not me, then who can take this on?" By examining the role in this way, the leader addresses the issues and tasks that they uniquely must do, it empowers others to participate in work that may be new to them and therefore are learning experiences. If the leader takes on too much responsibility, their essential work does not get done and the organization will get stalled waiting for the leader to make decisions or address important issues. The leader creates the bottleneck in the effective running of the organization because of poor time management and delegation.

For example, in the academic setting, a school of nursing dean might spend a lot of time reviewing the details of course syllabi for the undergraduate BSN program. However, this responsibility is within the purview of the associate dean for undergraduate programs. Reviewing syllabi takes away time from activities, such as fundraising or recruiting new faculty, since these are major expectations of a dean of a school of nursing. Aligning work to the leader's responsibility is critical in effectively and efficiently managing time and work. This will have a direct impact on the organization's success.

A leader also needs to be aware of opportunities to provide time for their staff or faculty to reenergize themselves and extend their knowledge through continued learning thereby increasing the organization's effectiveness. In the academic setting, this is often accomplished through participation in continuing education programs or a sabbatical for faculty. In many academic organizations, faculty have the opportunity to take a semester- or year-long sabbatical leave for the purpose of personal renewal and focused work on a project that broadens or extends their scholarship. In the clinical setting, these opportunities may not be as prevalent or institutionalized, yet the need for professional growth or concentrated time for enhancing knowledge is just as important. The leader will need to find creative ways to invest in the professional development of staff or faculty. This not only enhances the capacity of each person, it communicates the organization's commitment to the individual for professional development to help them achieve their personal and professional goals.

Providing professional development has several benefits, including a more capable workforce and greater loyalty to the organization. However, it comes with a cost. The cost is both in the loss of work of the person engaging in professional development activities as well as the cost of replacing the person who may be at a conference or involved in another type of professional development activity. Supplemental pay for a short period of time or reorganizing responsibilities to allow for coverage are important ways to recognize those people who have to take up the slack when one of their colleagues is away. In times of budget crises, professional development funds often get cut and it is important to look for opportunities to have new sources of income. One way to expand the impact of professional development activities is for staff members to share their experience and the outcomes and thereby other empower staff to infuse new ideas and information into the organization.

SUMMARY

It is critical for nurse leaders to be budget savvy and know the financial underpinnings of the organization. Budgets reflect and support the priorities of the organization and therefore, need to be closely linked to the strategic plan and goals. Leadership decisions should be based on evidence as much as possible. Data is one of the critical inputs to being an effective leader and managing resources. In addition to the operational budgets, there is an array of opportunities for leaders to gain access to additional funds through grants, contracts, and gifts. Acquiring additional funds can be extremely challenging so careful consideration of time and effort is important when embarking on this process These types of funds can provide support for "proof of concept" ideas in both educational and clinical settings. Accessing and managing resources is challenging in today's environment with constant change in payment, expectations of providers, and new treatments and technology. Every leader at some point, will have resource constraints and must manage within those constraints.

In addition, leaders also need to be knowledgeable about making the case for resources, whether for internal or external resources. Making the case of resources is a critical responsibility of leaders. With the fast pace of change, additional resources are very helpful to meet a current need or try a new approach to education or patient care. There may be times that garnering additional resources is necessary because of concerns about the quality and safety of services, reputation, ability to compete with other institutions, accreditation/certification requirements, or future payment issues. However, usually to be persuasive in attaining resources, a ROI must be demonstrated. There may be various timelines for the return to take place depending on the needs of the organization. Making the argument for resources requires a clear vision of the return on the investment.

CRITICAL THINKING QUESTIONS

At the beginning of the chapter an academic and clinical vignette were presented. Please review the vignettes to address the following the questions. The questions are specific to the vignettes.

Academic Vignette Questions

1. As director of the advanced practice registered nurse programs how will you approach cutting your budget? What options do you see to address the budget issue and have the necessary faculty time and talent?
2. What impact will the budget cuts have on accomplishing the mission of the organization to prepare APRNs to meet the needs of vulnerable populations?
3. How will you use "ROI" to create an argument to have the funds needed to support hiring faculty?

Clinical Vignette Questions

1. How will you approach the budgeting process in terms of understanding the budgets of each of your units and the overall organizational budget?
2. How might the request for budget cuts compromise the attainment of the organizational mission?
3. What options do you have in reducing the budget and maintaining sufficient staff funding to ensure safe patient care?
4. How will you use ROI to create the argument for additional funds to support increased numbers of staff?

REFERENCES

Balanced Scorecard Institute. (2020). Strategic planning basics: *What is strategic plan-*

ning? Balanced Scorecard Institute.https://balancedscorecard.org/strategic-planning-basics/

CFI. (2021). *Types of budgets: Four common ways to creating a budget*. CFI Education Inc. https://corporatefinanceinstitute.com/resources/knowledge/accounting/types-of-budgets-budgeting-methods/

McCleary, E., Christensen, V., Peterson, K., Humphrey, L. & Hefland, M. (2014). Evidence brief: The auality of care provided by advanced practice nurses. In *VA Evidence Sysnthesis Program Evidence Briefs* (*Internet*). Department of Veterans Affairs. https://www.ncbi.nlm.nih.gov/books/NBK384613/

Surdez, S. (2018, March 1). *What are KPIs*. Illumine. https://www.illumine8.com/what-are-kpis-key-performance-indicators-best-practices

Yox, S. B., & Stanik-Hutt, J. (2016, July 12). *APRNs vs physicians: Outcomes, quality, and effectiveness of care according to the evidence*. Medscape. https://www.medscape.com/viewarticle/8657

CHAPTER 9

Human Capital Resources

ACADEMIC VIGNETTE

Dr. John Jones has been in the associate dean for academic affairs position for three months, coming from another institution that had created a coaching culture. During Dr. Jones's recruitment, there were expressions of wanting to build a culture of coaching and mentoring. His orientation to the school did not include any information about coaching. The school of nursing has undergraduate and graduate education including DNP and PhD programs. This current institution is also research-intensive, and the school of nursing has several faculty with major research projects. Two nurse-run clinics are also valued projects of the school. Thirty-five percent of the faculty are tenured professors. Dr. Jones has had the opportunity to assess the state of readiness for culture change and he was surprised that there is little understanding of what that means with some of the faculty saying that, "a coaching culture is nonsense." He has heard from new faculty that the senior faculty have not been helpful to them in developing a research area to pursue or in understanding the requirements for promotion and tenure. Although the dean of the school has expressed commitment to the establishment of a coaching culture, the dean's attention has been focused on urgent financial issues caused by the University's budget reduction. The dean has asked Dr. Jones to lead the effort to create a coaching/mentoring culture.

CLINICAL VIGNETTE

Debbie Smith is the vice president for nursing services and has been in the position for one year. Nursing turnover in the hospital has been significantly higher than the national average. Ms. Smith has worked with HR to review the hiring and orientation programs of the hospital but they are very traditional in their approach. They develop the job description for the exact needs of the unit today without any consideration of future needs. The orientation program consists of putting the new hire in front of a series of three ring binders and telling them to read the material. There is little discussion of how the institution will invest in the employee over the course of their tenure and opportunities for professional development including the opportunity for coaching.

Ms. Smith is charged with reducing turnover in her units and wants to create a recruitment and retention model that could have a positive impact on nursing turnover. She sees this as a model that will begin with the advertising for the position, through hiring and orientation and continue through the tenure of the individual with the organization. She meets resistance from her senior leaders who don't see the issue with the high turnover. They say, "If people don't want to be here, it's good that they just leave." In addition, her HR department is reluctant to change their models of recruiting and onboarding talent. Ms. Smith has been introducing the idea of a revised model of recruitment and retention to the CEO and other high-level leaders in the organization and there is a commitment to exploring this to move the organization to a higher performing hospital.

INTRODUCTION

In the last ten years, there has been so much change in organizations related to workforce planning and the workplace itself. Much of this change is due to the constantly changing health care landscape, everyday disruptions in work, and a strong desire by a new generation of workers for work-life balance. Engagement of employees, positive workplace culture, and, most recently, anti-racist workplace policy change, working from home, and workforce reductions have all been top priorities for organizations. Long-term workforce planning models are common, integrating generational differences and preferences. Organizational recruitment, retention, and engagement models must adjust constantly to the ever-changing external environment including most prominently, the national and global economy and emergent and urgent societal needs.

In the past, many organization's workforce planning consisted of a traditional recruitment model where the objective was to fill vacancies without a clear picture of the long-term needs of the organization. Organizations would place advertisements in various venues in hopes for a robust pool of applicants from which to choose their employees. Once hired, employees were onboarded with often unorganized approaches to orientation, leading to various levels of organizational success. The result was a workforce that met today's organizational needs but was unprepared for the needs of the future, resulting in unsatisfactory retention rates for the best employees.

Jim Collins (2001), in his classic book Good to Great talked about the importance of getting the right people for an organization. He uses the analogy of a bus. Having the right people in the right seats on the bus results in the ability for an organization to define a preferred future. If a leader hires people for distinct roles that currently exist, when the direction of the organization has to change, the employees may no longer be equipped with the right skill set to accommodate that change. According to Collins, the key to a great organization is hiring the right people who have the capacity to grow with the organization.

Talent Acquisition

A more contemporary approach to recruiting and retention is called talent acquisition. Recruitment refers to the process of filling a vacancy as the need arises. In the traditional recruitment model, when one person leaves, you fill the position with another person from within or outside the organization. Talent acquisition is a broader hiring strategy. The talent acquisition model (Figure 9.1) in HR is the process of identifying, recruiting, and retaining the right people for your organization based on today's needs and the organization's potential future. The model is represented as a funnel where you cast a wide net in the early stages of the process and continue to reduce the size of the pool as you get closer to making an offer to a candidate. Unlike the traditional model of hiring that separates recruitment and retention, the talent acquisition model sees both phases as part of the same process. In this model, retaining employees is as important as the recruitment process and each member of the team has a responsibility in both recruitment and retention.

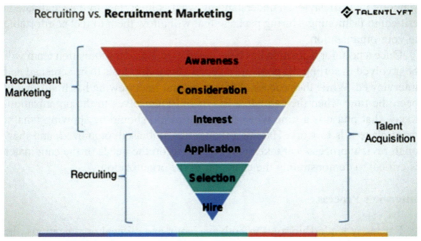

FIGURE 9.1 Talentlyft: Talent Acquisition Model—Used with permission.

Unlike the traditional recruitment process, the talent acquisition model begins before there are job openings at the organization with a careful review of the strategic plan and the organizational goals. For example, if an academic organization identifies a goal within the strategic plan that indicates that they want to increase the number of faculty of color, then the talent acquisition team might begin reviewing the literature to find the faculty of color who are publishing in a specific discipline. They might review listings of NIH awards or disciplinary honors to determine which faculty of color are included. Working with the current faculty, the organizations might reach out to invite a subset of candidates to campus to provide a lecture or have a symposium with students. In this way, the potential faculty of color begin to develop a relationship with the campus and faculty that can be nurtured over time (awareness). When a faculty position in an area becomes available, there is a list of potential candidates who already know and have a relationship with the organization (consideration). In this way, the leader is building the talent pipeline into the organization that will position it for the future.

Moving from consideration to interest to application is often a challenge in our highly competitive work environments. Most of the people being recruited in healthcare and academia have multiple opportunities and are making choices based on several organizational factors such as salary, benefits, space, responsibilities, culture of the organization, and colleagues. Helping the candidate define how the organizational values align with the personal values of the individual shows the candidate how they can contribute to the organization's future. Candidates are also including personal factors such as work-life balance, housing prices, availability of jobs for a spouse or partner, school systems, commuting time, and access to public transportation as important variables in the decision-making process for a position. People want a position that supports their lifestyle, so understanding what is important to the candidate is critical to fashioning a hiring package that will allow them to feel comfortable in your organization.

Once a pool for a position has been developed, a talent acquisition team will be involved in sorting the pool and selecting the individuals to be screened and interviewed. While the process of screening and interviewing has traditionally been the time when the candidate has to sell themselves to the organization, today, that phase is a time when the organization should be showing what a great place it is to work. Having a thoughtful, unbiased, organized, and thorough review process that takes into consideration the needs of the candidates is critical to demonstrating the character of the organization.

Interview Process

For many leadership roles in both academic and clinical organizations, the interview process usually includes a search committee that is a group of individuals who are involved in the hiring process to screen the applicants and make recommendations about hiring. The process varies from organization to organization. In some organizations, the HR manager will screen all applicants and just send the qualified applicants to the search committee or to a particular manager. In others, the search committee reviews all of the applicants. However the process unfolds, the key to a successful search is consistency and clarity of process. Often the search committee will develop a set of questions based on the key job functions that will be used for each interview conducted. Each candidate will be allotted the same time and the structure of the interview will not vary significantly from candidate to candidate. Evaluating each candidate using similar criteria helps to create an even playing field for all candidates.

Even with a consistent and clear approach to screening and interviewing, we all come to the search process as a product of our lived experiences. For some, that means having a life characterized by white privilege, and for others it might mean being raised in a multicultural low-income family or having experienced discrimination based on a particular identity. All human beings have prejudices and biases, some they are aware of and some of which they are not aware.

Implicit bias is when individuals have attitudes toward people or associate stereotypes with them without realizing they have those attitudes. Confirmation bias is seen when an individual interprets the information they see as a confirmation of their values and views. In this situation, any information that is not consistent with those values and views is ignored. While bias is present in all interactions, it is often not realized (it is unconscious) by the individual holding the bias. Michael Brainard (2016) describes unconscious bias as, "a form of social categorization, whereby we routinely and rapidly sort people into groups. In fact, we are hard-wired to prefer people who look like us, sound like us, and share our interests."

Many organizations are providing training in implicit bias for all leaders and faculty and specifically search committee members as a first step in the search process. The most commonly used program was developed in the late nineties by three Harvard University researchers. "Project Implicit" is a non-profit organization and international collaboration between researchers who are interested in implicit social cognition, thoughts and feelings outside of conscious awareness and control. The goal of the organization is to educate the public about hidden biases and to provide a 'virtual laboratory' for collecting data" (Greenwald and Nosek, 2011).

Another approach that organizations use to reduce the influence of individual bias includes adding an equity advocate to a search committee. Generally, someone who is outside the disciplinary specialty, the role of the equity advocate is to serve as a consultant to the search committee by raising awareness of implicit and confirmation bias in the review and selection process. An equity advocate might ask questions of the committee that helps members identify their implicit or confirmation biases. The advocate can explore assumptions, norms, and practices that might hinder full consideration of each candidate's credentials, and facilitate what might be difficult conversations for the committee about race or identities that may come up in the search process.

In addition to having an equity advocate as part of a search committee, many organizations require bias training for search committee members. This training is often available online and it is the responsibility of the chair of the search committee or the equity advocate to confirm that all members have taken the training. In the debriefing with the search committee members following the training, is important to address any question or concerns they might have. The goal of both the training and including the equity advocate in the search process is to promote and advance the diversity and social justice mission of the organization, making sure that the search process is fair and equitable with a minimal impact from implicit and unconscious biases.

Interview questions that infringe on protected privacy information can be the basis of a discrimination complaint during the hiring process. Examples of these questions include age, race, ethnicity, arrest or conviction record, financial information such as having a credit card or ever filing for bankruptcy, marital status, or information about children. It is useful to have an HR representative meet with all members of the search committee prior to interviewing any candidates to avoid any of these situations. HR can be very useful in reviewing with the search committee questions they can ask and ones they cannot ask.

Once the interview process is complete, the search committee will make a recommendation to the leader, or the person responsible for hiring, a specified number of candidates they propose for hire. Some leaders ask for the search committee to provide a non-ranked list of candidates while others might request a list of the three top candidates, ranked in order of priority. Once the leader makes the decision on who they want to hire, the leader will develop a recruiting package that will include salary and benefits but also might include start-up funds, sign-on bonuses, equipment, moving allowances, and space requests.

Job Offer

Making and negotiating a job offer is an inexact science. The leader will often create a recruitment package that includes benefits that they think would be attractive to the candidate. The applicant may want other resources or more of the resources than were offered. It is imperative that you have a maximum number of resources in mind, beyond which you will not exceed. Often this is determined by the salaries and sign-on packages of other members of the organization. It is not unusual for the process to be iterative, with each party presenting their offers and counteroffers several times. When the leader and the applicant come to an agreement on all the details of the position, it is important that the leader begin to create a welcoming environment that will help the applicant feel like they are part of the organization. Once an offer is accepted, the leader will work with their HR department to prepare and send an official offer letter. The processes of onboarding and retaining are the next steps.

In some situations, usually large clinical settings, the hiring may be done through the HR department. In many of the large healthcare organizations, sometimes hundreds of nurses may be recruited at one time or over a short period of time. Given the time demands of the recruitment and hiring process, the nursing staff may not be able to manage the recruitment and hiring process. However, even in these cases, there is usually an opportunity for the nurses being recruited, especially at the entry level, to meet the nurses they may be working with and tour the facility. The recruitment of nurses who have just completed their academic program and are entering the workforce are often the most important source of nurses to meet the needs of an institution. This is currently the case with many nurses retiring and varied roles in healthcare systems available outside of hospital nursing.

Retention and Engagement-Creating Practice Supportive Environments

Every 30 days, about 3.5 million people in the US voluntarily leave their jobs and it costs between 50% and 200% of their annual income to replace them (Maurer, 2018). The monetary cost is only a piece of the impact organizations feel when top talent leaves. There is also a loss of institutional knowledge, decrease in productivity and a reduction in organizational morale with employee turnover. Retention begins as soon as the applicant accepts the position, making them feel like they are a welcomed and valued member of the organization. An organized and structured onboarding process increases the likelihood that an employee will remain with the organization. The first 45 days on the job are critical (Llarena, 2013). If an employee does not feel like they fit into the organization or they are unsure about their future, they are likely to begin looking for another position. From the time the applicant accepts the position, the onboarding process begins. If there is a long lead time before the applicant begins work, making sure there is regular communication, engagement, and connections from members of the unit or organization will be important.

When the employee arrives on the first day, having a workspace that is prepared, and a plan for the next few days that includes some welcoming activities, gives the new employee a sense of being valued by the organization. During the first week, the job responsibilities and work life should be clear to the new employee. This will help the new employee have a sense that they can successfully integrate into and be a contributing member of the organization.

While not every employee will decide to have a long-term relationship with the organization, there are several things a leader can do to reduce employee turnover following a successful onboarding experience. Most employees want to work for an organization that is interested in them and their professional development. Professional development is often cited by nurses as one of the most important areas affecting job satisfaction (Coleman and Desai, 2019; Hariyati and Safril, 2018; Price and Reichert, 2017). A leader needs to budget the resources that will allow employees to engage in professional development which is essential to fostering job satisfaction.

Another significant aspect of job satisfaction is related to the effectiveness of the individual's manager. Fifty percent of employees who leave their job do so to get away from a bad boss (Garland, 2016). Effective leaders connect with their team members on a personal level, are effective communicators, and are active listeners. Being respectful of the employee's time by leading efficient meetings, setting clear expectations and goals, and assigning meaningful work all demonstrates how much the employee is valued. Also important is recognizing excellent performance and celebrating accomplishments. Promoting the performance of the team is an important strategy to build engagement and increase job satisfaction.

When there are more jobs than nurses, organizations try to position themselves to be competitive. Being competitive for hospitals and health systems often means having a culture that helps new nurses and nurses new to the organization feel that they are valued and supported. Organizations may also pay sign-on bonuses and provide other benefits to attract the best nurses in a tight labor market. Leaders must stay vigilant to projections of supply and demand for nurses. Many states have health workforce units that track supply and demand. At the federal level, the Health Resources and Services Administration provides information about supply and demand by state (U.S. Department of Health and Human Services, Health Resources and Services Administration, 2017). Attention to workforce trends will provide the data to allow leaders to stay ahead of the curve in recruitment and retention activities.

Consider: **Think back to when you were recruited and hired for your most recent position. Did your employer appear genuinely interested in you? Did you have a meaningful orientation program? Is your employer invested in your development as a professional?**

BUILDING A COACHING CULTURE

Leader as a Coach

Creating a practice environment that is attractive to new staff and retains current staff is vital to an engaged workforce. A culture of coaching and mentorship has been noted to increase worker satisfaction, engagement, and retention of talent (Human Capital Institute [HCI], 2014; International Federation of Coaching [IFC], 2014). IFC (2014) and HCI (2018) have also noted that coaching is a very effective means of managing change in an organization. A culture that values employee engagement co-creates a culture in partnership with employees. Such a practice environment is supportive, affords the opportunity for continued development and contributes to a just approach to quality issues. Developing a coaching culture is based on a mindset of how to best develop staff and get the work done. The mindset is different from traditional management styles in that it recognizes the importance of engaging staff in decision-making and problem-solving, with the leader committed to helping them develop. Within an organizational context, coaching and mentoring is good for staff and for the health of the organization. All leaders, whether the chief nurse or a team leader, have a responsibility to develop not only their team of direct reports but also to encourage others in leadership positions to develop their teams. The benefits of a coaching culture are benefits to the organization.

Coaching of leaders has become a more accepted method of developing leadership capacity. Everyone in the organization should benefit from coaching because everyone is a leader whether they are leading a clinical team or leading a patient through a difficult health issue. Developing teams through coaching creates more effective teams. In addition to a more effective workforce, coaching is likely to reduce turnover. There are many examples of coaching cultures that have drastically reduced turnover, especially in organizations that employ millennials who are expected to be 39% of the workforce by 2025 (Lettick, 2019). Reduced turnover translates into reduced cost of recruitment that has been estimated to be between $30,000–$45,000 per nursing staff recruit (Nursing Solutions, Inc. [NSI], 2018).

Developing a culture of coaching is tangible evidence of an organization investing in its staff and not just looking for productivity. It is a giving situation for the leader. There are benefits to leaders who coach/mentor in terms of seeing people achieve their goals and be successful in their career development. It also provides the opportunity to role model coaching behaviors and techniques to team members who can then employ them with their teams. It is a useful way of establishing the capability of individuals within the organization as part of succession planning. Succession planning needs to occur many years before a planned departure.

What Does a Coaching Culture Look Like?

If you were making a site visit for accreditation purposes to a coaching organization—whether academic or clinical—and had the opportunity to watch and listen to a variety of staff, you would see people helping each other, having honest conversations to help each staff member grow in their abilities, with team members being clear about the goals of team, and staff saying they are valued by the leadership of the organization. In addition, you would hear leaders empowering staff to solve problems. In a coaching culture, people feel that the work of the organization is everyone's work and each person contributes something important. While no organization is perfect and there are conflicts, disagreements, and frustrations between leaders and followers, a coaching culture can help address these issues in a way to help everyone learn and grow.

Executive coaching has been present in many companies to help leaders be more effective in their roles. A coaching culture includes everyone as a coach and a "coachee." The Chief Nurse might serve as a coach for the nurse managers and the nurse manager may serve as a coach for the staff nurses. The Hudson Institute of Coaching (2020) notes that a coaching culture is one in which:

- Teams operate with clear goals and roles
- Giving and receiving feedback is in the service of being at one's best
- Focusing on opportunities is done to help members of one's team grow
- Developing others when it matters most is important
- Asking and empowering is more the mode of communication than telling and fixing

A coaching/mentoring culture is an approach to maximize the effectiveness of an organization in achieving its goals. Coaching builds the capacity of individuals which translates into more effective functioning of staff in the organization.

How Do You Build and Evaluate a Coaching Culture?

Building a culture of coaching usually requires time. Any change of culture takes a commitment to a long-term, multi-pronged process. An organization may consider having one or all of different levels of coaching: external coaches who meet specific criteria established by the organization usually to work with leaders of the organization; internal staff to address leadership more broadly; and leaders doing the coaching. The steps to building a coaching environment include:

- *Leadership commitment to create the coaching/mentoring culture*: Top level leaders need to engage in learning how to be a coach leader in order to be role models and disseminate the model throughout the organization. The entire organizational leadership team might engage in experiential learning and visit an organization that has developed a coaching culture. Developing a coaching culture would be integrated into the strategic planning process for the entire organization. Working with outside experts would be useful. Leaders would begin to role model the behaviors associated with coaching and mentoring.

- *Engagement of all staff in learning about a coaching culture*: The nursing leadership team will identify those in the organization at the supervisory and director levels that can begin to seed the coaching/mentoring culture throughout the organization. Learning sessions and experiences need to be planned for all levels of staff. Learning will be ongoing and integrated into all meetings, continuing education, and professional development activities.
- *Embedding coaching/mentoring into the HR policies*: Integrate the expectation of coaching and mentoring in job descriptions, evaluation processes, and expectations at team meetings.
- *Make success visible*: Be clear and transparent about the performance measures that will be tracked related to the culture change. Include examples of successful coaching and mentoring in communications to staff at all levels. Start meetings with examples of coaching and mentoring.
- *Continually supporting the coaching/mentoring culture*: It is essential to continually support the culture even after there is evidence that the culture has changed to one of coaching and mentoring to improve the organization's ability to attain goals.

Evaluation of the success of the culture change includes assessment at the individual, team, and organization levels. Individuals would have their performance evaluation include behaviors related to coaching and mentoring. At the team level, assessing the culture of coaching and mentoring would include measures of feedback among team members, ability to problem solve and behaviors showing respect among team members. At the organizational level, evaluation criteria include achievement of organizational goals and patient or student outcomes. Table 9.1 provides examples of evaluation criteria relevant to the different levels to be assessed.

Implementation and evaluation of a coaching culture takes an effort of the entire organization. This effort has to be led and sustained by all of the high-level leaders. Nurses, all additional staff, and patients are the beneficiaries of coaching environments resulting in better outcomes, higher retention, and more effective recruitment of nurses.

Coaching and Mentoring

Coaching and mentoring have traditionally been distinguishable approaches to help people in their careers as well as personal lives. The traditional type of mentoring is helping another to follow a professional path that in many ways mirrors that of the mentor. For example, a senior person in a higher-level position may help a junior person move forward in their career. The senior/junior mentoring relationship provides information about how to be successful in specific areas, as well as making connections and helping a younger person network in a way that furthers their career. Examples of mentoring include a

TABLE 9.1. Examples of Evaluation Criteria.

Level of Organization	Examples of Evaluation Criteria
Individual	• Observed coaching or mentoring • Approaches feedback as constructive • Evidence that actions help professional development of others • Self-assessment and assessment by others of the above criteria
Team	• Goals are understood by each team member • Team adequately moves forward or accomplishes their goals • Team interactions consistent with a coaching culture • Team assessment reflects above criteria
Organization	• Organization meets its goals • Positive financial metrics • Patient/student outcomes • Metrics important to the work of the organization are positive • Staff feel safe to raise questions and recognize errors

faculty mentor providing guidance to a new mentee on how to achieve tenure in an academic setting, or a chief nurse providing guidance to a nursing director on how to become a chief nurse. Mentoring is often a life-long commitment with relationships that can be close and enduring.

Mentoring can evolve to where there is more of an equal relationship in which the mentor and mentee help each other to grow resulting in a relationship that is sustaining to both mentor and mentee. While the senior/junior mentorship model is common, there is also a mentorship model in which two people may be at the same level in an organization, but one holds information or has expertise that the other would benefit from having. This type of mentorship program is common among workers, one more experienced working with a newly hired person at a similar level, or when staff are cross trained to provide different functions. The relationship is not necessarily based on a senior-junior experience, both might be at the same level but have different experiences that are useful to each other and can be shared.

Coaching is helping another define their goals and help them move toward those goals. The relationship in coaching is usually shorter term than mentoring relationships but can extend from several coaching sessions to years of coaching. In a coaching relationship, the coach and coachee are working together unlike the mentoring relationship where there is usually an expert working with a novice. The goals of the coachee are the goals of the coach.

The science of coaching also includes the strategy of spot coaching. This approach can work well for busy leaders who cannot engage in a full coaching relationship. It is an approach to helping a person solve a problem in the moment. Spot coaching is intended to help the coachee be successful in meeting a defined challenge. A staff person may bring a problem to the leader, or the leader may see something that needs to be addressed immediately. Spot coaching involves identifying the issue and helping the staff member figure out the strategy of addressing the issue of who, what, when, and how, as well as establishing a plan to implement the solution. The conversation should be no more than 10 minutes and can be as short as two minutes. During spot coaching, it is important for the staff member to know that the coaching is not criticism, but a way to learn. This can be done by addressing the issue in a calm, non-judgmental way and unless there is a serious harm that is being or could be caused, engage the staff member in solving the problem for him or herself. There are times that it will take great restraint for a leader to not intervene to fix the problem and to approach an issue with a coaching mindset. The leader needs to ensure that there is the opportunity for the discussion necessary to help the coachee work through the problem.

Consider: **Think about a time when you were provided with spot coaching. How did it help you solve the problem you were faced with?**

Although coaching and mentoring are traditionally different ways of helping people advance, leaders frequently use a hybrid of coaching and mentoring. There are aspects of each that can be employed depending on the needs of the organization, the leader, and the individual. The focus of the goals for coaching and mentoring should be organizationally based; however, the lines between organizationally-related and personally-related goals are sometimes fuzzy. For instance, better time management crosses the lines of professional development and one's personal goals. In addition, while a coach helps focus on the individual's goals, those goals are often informed by the coach's experience and expertise. Within organizations, individuals may have several coaches/mentors depending on the need and interest of the staff member. A clinical faculty member may have a faculty coach for their academic goals and a clinical coach for their clinical responsibilities. A research clinician or faculty may have different mentors/coaches depending on the focus of their research that may change over time or with different aspects of a project.

Consider the following situation. Deja N. is a new nurse on the medical surgical unit of an 800-bed hospital. She chose to work at this hospital because of the residency program and the commitment to her learning she experienced in a student clinical rotation. She has just realized that she almost gave the wrong medication to a patient and reported it to her unit manager. How would the unit manager handle this in a coaching/mentoring culture as compared to a traditional management approach?

Knowing Oneself as a Leader Coach

Leaders can either be effective or ineffective coaches. Being a coach and leading others takes knowing yourself. Knowing yourself is essential to engage in being a coach which is one of the highest levels of personal interaction within an organizational context to help people develop. McLean (2012) has developed a useful model of "self as coach" as shown in Figure 9.2. While it was developed within a coaching context, it applies to a leader coach. This model includes six domains. These domains are essential to being an effective leader coach.

The first domain of range of feeling is presence. Presence means that you give focused attention to the person or group you are with. Wonfor (2016) states that presence is, "the cultivation of being with a heightened and expanded awareness; characterized by the felt experience of stillness, tirelessness and connectedness." This definition means giving full attention to the person being coached. For many leaders, it is extremely difficult to put all of the things that need to get done out of one's mind. We mentally carry our "to do" list. It is so easy to look at a message coming on a smartwatch or know that there is a

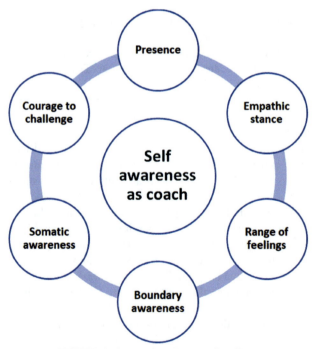

FIGURE 9.12 Domains of Range of Feelings.

complaint by a patient that needs attention. Leaders are often used to process-ing multiple inputs rapidly (multi-tasking is really quickly moving from one task to another) and setting those inputs aside is difficult. While being present sounds basic, often the basics are the most difficult to accomplish.

Perhaps a bigger challenge for leaders in being present is to help staff learn how to solve problems rather than telling them the solution to the problem. Moving too quickly to a problem solving mode inhibits being present. When a leader is already thinking about solutions, they have stopped listening. Lead-ers believe that it is their responsibility to know the answers. Telling people how to solve problems (while at times necessary) deprives them of learning how to solve problems. In addition, it is disempowering because that person may then tend to avoid solving a problem in the future and wait for others. It is temporarily faster and easier to tell someone what to do, but in the long run, leaders will continually have to be involved in the problem-solving that others should be doing.

A second element is empathy and requires a supportive and caring stance toward the person who is trying to make their way professionally. Empathy is the ability to understand and share the feelings of another. This does not mean the coach takes on the work of the coachee or allows the problem to go unresolved. It is important to emphasize that the work needs to be done by the coachee and not the coach.

Another important element of the model is the willingness to challenge the person. Coaching is about helping people move to a different place or level and can be done only by challenging them in their thinking and behaviors. For instance, people often blame others for creating difficulties and are reluctant to look at their role in creating a situation. Challenging them about their role in a problem can be very useful in helping to provide insight to changing behavior. Another situation where challenging is important is when someone is thinking about their limitations rather than their strengths and thus minimizing their potential for professional and personal growth. Challenging can be done in many ways and about many issues but it should always be done in a way that the coachee feels supported and safe.

The coach needs to be aware of the physical responses they have during interactions when working with a staff member. Everyone has some emotional response when working with another person. Somatic awareness provides very useful information in understanding feelings. The challenge is to acknowledge the physical signs that are associated with different feelings. Some people no-tice that they have a tightening feeling in their stomach when they get into uncomfortable conversations, others may run their fingers through their hair. If a leader, coach, or mentor is paying attention to their own feelings and man-ages those feelings, they will be more present and effective with the person they are coaching

It is also important to know your boundaries. It is, at times, easy to over identify with those that we are coaching, especially when there are commonly shared experiences. When coaching staff, it is important to maintain boundaries related especially to emotional involvement and taking on the work of the coachee. As nurses, we want to help and this commitment to help will disempower the person being coached and meet more of the coaches needs than that of the coachee. It is easy to get drawn into the coachee's world and their needs. If the person you are coaching is a direct report, it is particularly important that the boundaries are clear. If there is a concern about boundary setting, important questions to ask include:

- Am I taking on the work of my coachee?
- What are the factors that may be contributing to taking on my coachee's work?
- What emotional boundaries do I need to set to be both a compassionate coach yet empower, and challenge, when necessary, my coachee?

The final element in the model is being able to experience and manage a range of feelings. This is essential to letting the individual share their varied emotional responses and have the leader, coach, or mentor be comfortable with those responses and their own responses to the interaction. People may express anger, frustration, disappointment, joy, success, and every other emotion that exists. As a leader, being able to recognize and accept those feelings in another allows those feelings to be useful in moving the person toward their goals. The ability for a coachee to really move forward is based on getting to an emotional level of understanding of what might be keeping them from achieving their goal. Being comfortable with a range of feelings does not mean that it is acceptable for others to be disrespectful. The issue of boundaries is important in managing feelings of the other person. For instance, it is useful to be comfortable with a staff member crying because of a near miss of a medical error she made, but it is not acceptable for her to throw an object in frustration. Acknowledging another person's feelings is one of the most powerful interventions for coaches.

Coaching Process

The process of coaching has several decision points. The first decision is to determine who you will coach. A decision could be that you coach each of your direct reports, or your team as a group, or both. If you have individual meetings with each of your team members, you have the opportunity to do individual coaching as well as team coaching. There may also be promising young faculty or clinicians who are not direct reports that would benefit from the leader's coaching. If the culture values coaching and everyone is engaged, the role of the leader is to be a role model and to support the coaching culture.

Whether you are coaching an individual or team, establishing goals will drive the work in the coaching relationship. Within an organizational context, the goals may be the work goals of the staff, coachee, or a combination of goals established by both the coach and coachee. It is critical, at the beginning of the process, to identify how the coachee will attain the goals, as well as how they will know they achieved the goals. Revisiting the goals and making adjustments can be done on an agreed upon periodic basis.

Coaching provides the opportunity for the individual to find their own answers to achieve their goals (Reid-Ponte *et al.*, 2006). Useful coaching questions that can be used with an individual or team include (Rogers, 2012):

- What is the issue?
- What makes this an issue now?
- Who owns this issue?
- How important is it on a scale of 1–10?
- How much energy do you have for a solution on a scale of 1–10?
- What are the implications of doing nothing?
- What have you already tried?
- Imagine this problem has been solved: what would you see, hear, feel?
- What is standing in the way of that outcome?
- What is your own responsibility for what has been happening?
- What early signs are there that things might be getting better?
- Imagine you are at your most resourceful. What do you say to yourself about this issue?
- What are the options for action here?
- What criteria will you use to judge the options?
- Which option seems the best one against those criteria?
- What is the next step and when will you take it?

The point of coaching questions is to help define issues, clarify goals, identify barriers and strategies to attain the goals, and move forward with an evaluation component to assess attainment of goals. While the questions are very simple and straightforward, they are also powerful in that they get to the heart of a coaching process and enable an individual or team to move forward. Today, an important new question to add to this comprehensive list would be, "what are your identities" and "how do you think your own identities and those of others involved in the situation might be influencing you in your behaviors and thought processes?" One area of particular interest in this self-reflection work is the concept of intersectionality. This term was coined by scholar Kimberlee Crenshaw and colleagues, and is defined as how race, class, gender, and other individual characteristics "intersect" with one another and overlap. This phenomena often results in how individual's experience multiple sources of oppression (Cho *et al.*, 2013).

In addition to the coaching role, providing mentorship can be integrated into the coach as leader role. There are many activities that are characteristic of the mentor role but also can be incorporated into the role of the coach. Some include:

• Introductions to leaders in the field
• Nomination for relevant committee service
• Nomination for awards
• Inclusion on grants
• Recommendations for advancement
• Support of continuous learning—degree or non-degree
• Inclusion in meetings that will advance their understanding of the organization
• Providing support for attendance at professional meetings
• Feedback on articles and presentation
• Anticipation of challenges and exploring strategies that have worked

Consider the following situation. Ronna N. has been a nurse in a PICU for eight years working as a staff nurse, assistant unit manager, and then manager of the PICU. She has loved her work and has built an effective team. She is interested in eventually becoming a chief nurse. You are her direct supervisor. You are a strong advocate for supporting your direct reports and working with them on their goals. How will you structure a coaching relationship while maintaining the supervisory role boundary?

Consider: **Have you ever had to mentor a colleague or direct report? How have you structured that relationship?**

In coaching/mentoring an individual or team, the goal is to have a successful, productive, and meaningful relationship that helps the person be successful in accomplishing their work goals. There are relationships that just do not work, and either a different coach needs to step in or that person may not be the right person to stay on the team. However, relationships often last throughout the employment of each and also beyond. Many relationships last a lifetime. One of the best outcomes of the coaching relationship is to see individuals and teams grow and be successful. This leads to people being productive and satisfied with their jobs. Sometimes people have to leave an organization to attain their goals if there are limited opportunities within their current organization, and that is a reality. However, when staff feel like that have been strongly and positively influenced, when an opportunity comes open, they are likely to come back to an organization. Coaching is one of the very rewarding aspects of a leader's responsibilities. Seeing people grow and thrive is very heartening. Having people feel that they are making progress toward goals contributes to a strong and vibrant organization.

SUMMARY

One of the most important resources in an organization are its people. Bringing the right people in who can grow and change with the evolution of the organization will result in effective organizational outcomes and job satisfaction of its employees. Coaching and mentoring are critical elements of improving the effectiveness of the organization. A coaching culture results in improved teamwork and individual success.

CRITICAL THINKING QUESTIONS

At the beginning of the chapter an academic and clinical vignette were presented. Please review the vignettes to address the following the questions. The questions are specific to the vignettes.

Academic Vignette

1. How are you going to respond to the dean's request that you lead the effort to build a coaching/mentoring culture?
2. What do you feel you will need to be successful?
3. You have decided to take the lead on the coaching/mentoring culture. What will be your first steps? Next steps?
4. How are you going to work with the senior faculty? Junior faculty?
5. How will you know when the culture has changed?
6. How do you think the coaching/mentoring culture affect recruitment and retention of faculty and staff?

Clinical Vignette

1. What would you recommend as the first step in transforming the process for recruiting and retaining nurses in this hospital?
2. What would be the critical elements of a transformed recruitment and retention process, recognizing the resistance from HR to make any change?
3. How do you envision working with the senior leader in the organization? What is your plan for working with the direct supervisors?
4. How can you leverage the support of the CEO in this process?
5. How will you evaluate progress in changing the culture?

REFERENCES

Brainard, M. (2016). Strategy Leadership Pitfalls and Insights Into Unconscious Bias Brainardstrategy.com.

Cho, S., Crenshaw, K., McCall, L., (2013). Toward a field of intersectionality studies: Theory, applications and praxis. *Signs: Journals of Women in Culture and Society. 38* (4) 785–810

Coleman, Y.A., & Desai, R. (2019). The effects of a clinical ladder program on professional development and job satisfaction of acute care nurses. *Clinical Journal of Nursing Care and Practice, 3*, 44–48. https://doi.org/10.29328/journal.cjncp.1001016

Collins, J. C. (2001). *Good to great: Why some companies make the leap . . . and others don't.* Harper Business.

Garland, P., (2016). Why people quit their jobs. Harvard Business Review https://hbr.org/2016/09/why-people-quit-their-jobs

Greenwald, T., M., Nosek, B., (2011). Project Implicit Bias https://implicit.harvard.edu/implicit/aboutus.html

Hariyati, R. T. S., & Safril, S. (2018). The relationship between nurses' job satisfaction and continuing professional development. *Enfermeria Clinica, 28*(Suppl 1), 144–148. https://doi.org/10.1016/S1130-8621(18)30055-X

Hudson Institute of Coaching. (2020). *A coaching culture matters & here's why.* Hudson Instituteof Coaching. https://hudsoninstitute.com/a-coaching-culture-matters/

Human Capital Institute. (2014, October 1). *Building a coaching culture.* Human Capital Institute. https://www.hci.org/system/files/research//files/field_content_file/2014%2520ICF_0.pdf

Human Capital Institute. (2018, September 26). *Building a coaching culture for change management.* Human Capital Institute. https://www.hci.org/research/building-coaching- culture-change-management

International Federation of Coaching (2014) What is Coaching? https://experience-coaching.com/

Lettick, A (2019) No, Millennials will not be 75% of the workforce in 2025 (or ever!). Linkedin https://www.linkedin.com/pulse/millennials-75-workforce-2025-ever-anita-lettink

Llarena, M. (2013). How not to lose new employees in the first 45 days. Forbes. https://www.forbes.com/sites/85broads/2013/07/19/how-not-to-lose-your-new-employees-in-their-first-45-days/?sh=4fe7738d3be3

Maurer, R. (2018). Why are workers quitting their jobs in record numbers? SHRM. https://www.shrm.org/resourcesandtools/hr-topics/talent-acquisition/pages/workers- are-quitting-jobs-record-numbers.aspx

McLean, P. (2012). *A completely revised handbook of coaching: A developmental approach*, 2nd Ed. Jossey-Bass.

Nursing Solutions Inc (2018) 2018 National Healthcare Retention and RN Staffing Report. Nursing Solutions Inc. https://pdf4pro.com/view/2018-national-health-care-retention-amp-rn-staffing-1292b3.html

Price, S., & Reichert C. (2017). The importance of continuing professional development to career satisfaction and patient care: Meeting the needs of novice to mid- to late-career nurses throughout their career span. *Administrative Sciences, 7*(2), 17. https://doi.org/10.3390/admsci7020017

Reid-Ponte, P. Gross, A., Galante, A., Glaser G., (2006). Using an executive coach to increase leadership effectiveness. *Journal of Nursing Administration Vol. 36* (6), pp. 319–324.

Rogers, J. (2012). *Coaching skills: A handbook.* Open University Press.

U.S. Department of Health and Human Services, Health Resources and Services Administration, National Center for Health Workforce Analysis. (2017, July 21). *National and regional supply and demand projections of the nursing workforce*: 2014-2030. Bureau of Health Workforce. https://bhw.hrsa.gov/sites/default/files/bhw/nchwa/projections/NCHWA_HRSA_Nursing Report.pdf

Wonfor, D, (2016) Working with Presence: A transformational learning experience for coaches. Linkedin. https://www.linkedin.com/pulse/working-presence-transformational- learning-coaches-damion-wonfor?trk=public_profile_article_view

CHAPTER 10

Organizational Decision-Making

ACADEMIC VIGNETTE

The college of nursing's deans and faculty of a fairly large university in the Southwest region of the US were faced with an important decision in 2017. Their graduate nursing program prepared advanced practice nurses in five specialty areas. One of the programs was a Certified Registered Nurse Anesthetist (CRNA) program. A recent proclamation by the national organization that governs the certification of all CRNAs mandated that a DNP degree would be necessary to attain in order for graduates of a CRNA program to sit for the CRNA exam. The college of nursing had not yet implemented a DNP program in any specialty area so the deans and faculty needed to decide. At least four options were available as discussed below.

1. Close the MSN CRNA program but continue to provide MSN programs for the four other APRN specialties.
2. Design and implement a DNP CRNA program but maintain the other MSN APRN programs.
3. Design and implement an APRN DNP program for all specialties while simultaneously eliminating the MSN APRN programs all together.
4. Design and implement the APRN DNP program for APRNs but continue to provide the option of MSN only for the four specialty programs not currently mandating the DNP as a terminal degree.

CLINICAL VIGNETTE

A hospital in the Midwest ended the 2019 fiscal year with a three-million-dollar annual operating deficit and the nursing department in the hospital was charged with eliminating $1.2 million from their 25 million-dollar operating budget. The chief nurse and the nurse executive team began brainstorming about how to implement this cost reduction without involving direct care resources. One idea that emerged in the brainstorming exercise was the consideration of eliminating the role of the clinical nurse specialist (CNS) and/or to reduce the number of personnel in this job category. The nurse care coordinator role was one that had been very successfully piloted on two services. The idea on the table was to eliminate the CNS role function altogether and replace that role with unit-based educators and nurse care coordinators, both groups were less expensive than the CNS and more importantly, the two new role groups were thought to meet the needs of patients and staff more directly. The nursing staff in this organization is represented by a bargaining unit.

INTRODUCTION

Individual employees and groups of employees at all levels and roles within all organizations make decisions every day. Decision-making in organizations can be complicated and messy with decisions requiring leaders to be knowledgeable about services provided, human nature, budgets and finance, social interactions, power dynamics, and politics. Leaders often have to make high stakes decisions in high pressure environments. Decisions likely affect many people and have implications for the future success of the organizations. The bottom line is that leaders make many important decisions everyday ranging from very impactful decisions to minor decisions.

Types of Decision-making

There are many different lists of characteristics associated with what is a good decision. The following are generally associated with good organizational decisions: there are clear reasons for the decisions based on good information, the decision aligns with the organization's values, options are carefully considered, experts are consulted as necessary, and the decision can be reasonably implemented (Parsons, 2016; Dholakia, 2017). It is great if leaders could always take the time to carefully consider options and make the best decision. However, decisions are often made in crisis mode. Quick decisions may need to be made with imperfect knowledge with a lot at stake. For instance, during the COVID-19 pandemic crises, decisions regarding the spread of the coronavirus impacted organizational function. Clinical institutions had to make decisions about how to best manage the pandemic and academic institutions had to make decisions about how to handle closure of institutions and continue to offer education.

Even though the ideal decision is based on thoughtful consideration, Kahneman (2011), a Nobel prize winner for his work on thinking, decision-making, and bias, has adopted the idea that there are two systems of thinking: System 1 and System 2. He describes the systems as follows: System 1 operates automatically and quickly, with little or no effort and no sense of voluntary control; System 2 allocates attention to the effortful, mental activities that demand it, including complex computations. The operations of System 2 are often associated with the subjective experience of agency, choice, and concentration. (Kahneman, 2011, pp. 20–21).

The everyday life of leaders whether in an academic setting or clinical organization are filled with System 1 and System 2 thinking. As noted above, System 1 thinking is much more common and based on a lifetime of experiences that are unconsciously applied to decision-making. Within either setting, a leader decides to look at email as it comes in on their smart watch, or to know to go to the next meeting now. The vast majority of daily decisions fall into the System 1 thinking that requires little to no data or thoughtful analysis. It is simply looking at the clock and knowing it is time to leave for the meeting. However, when major decisions are required, a leader may need to move into System 2 thinking and actively analyze data related to the situation, get as much input as possible, and engage in systematic analysis of the issue and come to a conclusion. The conclusion may be to set up a process to make recommendations about an issue such as in the above vignettes. Decisions that require System 2 thinking are usually more complicated and may fall outside of the experience of a leader. Leaders do not always have the opportunity to talk with others about decisions because a decision may be urgent or confidential, but getting input from others may help make better decisions when there is limited experience or evidence.

Decision-Making Process

Decision-making consists of several steps. Decisions by individuals and groups that would follow System 2 thinking is systematic. It begins with identifying the decision that needs to be made, including the goal of the decision. This step is followed by gathering information relevant to the decision. The information is assessed and alternatives or options for decision-making are identified. Evidence related to each alternative is considered and an alternative is selected. Once a decision is made, the outcome is evaluated. The evaluation is based on criteria that are pre-established based on the goal. While this may seem like a very simple, stepwise approach to decision-making, it is often (though not with System 1 thinking) very messy. There are significant questions that need to be addressed especially for large organizations in terms of who is responsible, how will the decision-making proceed, and who and how will the decision be implemented. When there are multiple units and committees that have intersecting responsibility for a decision, the decision-making can be challenging. Later in this chapter is a discussion of a framework for the context of decision-making in organizations.

Cascade of Decision

We often think of a decision as a unitary event; however, every decision can lead to a consequence and often results in multiple consequences. These consequences do not all happen simultaneously and are likely to be influenced by multiple other decisions. The intersection of multiple decisions can either move an organization forward or stymy achievement of goals. One way of thinking about a cascade of decisions is to think about the impact of a primary decision and the intended consequences with the decisions that then follow. In the cascade of decisions, there are usually the intended and the unintended consequences. Leaders are fortunate when decisions have limited unintended consequences.

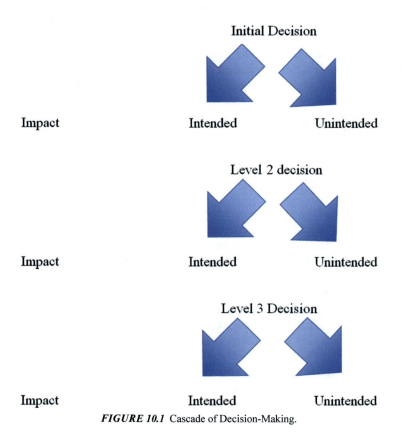

Initial Decision

Impact   Intended   Unintended

Level 2 decision

Impact   Intended   Unintended

Level 3 Decision

Impact   Intended   Unintended

FIGURE 10.1 Cascade of Decision-Making.

Decision-making is often like a chess board in which you need to think at least 2–3 moves ahead. The critical questions include: "what are the intended impacts, and how will we identify and address the unintended impact?" Each unintended impact will require additional decisions, which is why decision-making is dynamic and multi-leveled. That is why decisions are very rarely one and done. It is also important to note that each decision level interacts with the previous decision and may create a need to change the previous decision.

Emotions, Fatigue, and Decision-Making

A leader likes to think that their decisions are rational, objective, and based on evidence. However, the reality is much different. Every decision has an emotional component. There are many factors that affect decisions including how a person is feeling when they decide, the context, who is involved in the decision, and other factors. There is a growing literature on, and therefore greater recognition of, the relationship between emotions and decision-making. It is not as simple as happy people make better decisions than angry people, or vice versa. Exploring the role of emotions is very complicated because of the many factors that go into emotional responses including how a person is feeling, the context of decision-making, the quality of interpersonal relationship, and factors such as certainty related to a decision (Lerner and Keltner, 2001).

There are many studies that comprise our understanding of emotions; this chapter is not intended to be a comprehensive exploration of this topic, but to point out the importance of acknowledging the emotional underpinnings of decisions. Studies of the emotions of anger and fear have shown some interesting findings. Anger is an activating emotion and may lead to quicker action, more willingness to take risks, and a greater reliance on stereotypic thinking (Keltner, D. *et al.*, 1993). Studies to date have suggested that sadness can be useful in generating more systematic decision-making. On the other hand, too much sadness can create a state of indecision based on excessive thinking about the pros and cons of a situation (Keltner, D. *et al.*, 2019). The perception of control, whether internal or external, are important factors in decision-making when someone is fearful or sad. Fearful individuals see future events as more uncertain and that they have limited control, while angry individuals tend to view future events with more certainty and with a greater sense of control (Lerner and Keltner, 2001; Tiedens and Linton, 2001). These differences produce different inputs into decision-making.

Lerner *et al.* (2015), in a review of the literature relating emotions and decision-making, found themes that included a view that decisions have an integral emotion. In other words, we have feelings about the decision itself. An example of an integral emotion is having feelings about needing to cut back personnel costs by changing the staff mix, or having to change an educational program that is recognized as a model of effective learning. In addition to integral emotions, decisions hold incidental emotions that carry over from one situation to another, even though that emotion is not related to the current situation. Interesting research on how to manage incidental or integral emotions has found that people with high emotional intelligence can mitigate the impact of these emotions on decision-making (Yip and Cote, 2013).

Another theme identified by Lerner et al. (2015) was that emotions play a role in interpersonal decision-making. How someone feels about another person will influence the approach and ultimate decision. If someone is not trusted, a decision will be made that takes this emotion into account. If the perception of an interaction is that one party is angry, this will trigger a response by the other. What can we do to minimize decisions that may be compromised by emotional factors? Lerner et al. (2015) identified two major strategies to manage emotions in order to make more rational-based decisions. First, minimizing the magnitude of the emotional response through time delay, reappraisal, or induction of a counteracting emotional state. Second, insulating the judgment or decision process from the emotion by crowding out emotion, increasing awareness of misattribution, or modifying the choice architecture (Lerner et al., 2015, p. 811).

Pausing before responding when a leader is angry, overwhelmed, or fearful is a well-known adaptive response. Writing the angry communication, waiting until the next day, and re-evaluating the communication has saved all of us from creating situations that compromise thoughtful decisions. Friday afternoon messages can be especially perilous. Pausing gives time to reassess a situation and to possibly reframe our understanding. For instance, a chief nurse may feel very angry when told by the CEO that she needed to reduce the number of nursing staff so that new, very expensive diagnostic equipment could be purchased. This question came at a time when nurses were already complaining of having a too high nurse-to-patient ratio. An initial reaction might be to send an email to the CEO refusing to do this and threatening to resign. Waiting until the next day to respond will, in all likelihood, change the response. In addition, as the CNO was reflecting on the financial issues of the institution, she re-appraised the request and understood that the institution needed this equipment to stay competitive. By pausing and re-appraising, she offered some ways to cut costs that would be equitable across the institution and not compromise patient care. If she had sent the original email, the resignation may have been accepted. This example includes both strategies of managing one's emotions. While both strategies are noted to help, reappraisal has the strongest effect on moving out of an emotional decision (Gross, 2002).

Consider: **What decision in your current role would be difficult for you to make and why? How can these decision-making approaches help you frame the decision for effective decision-making?**

Fatigue

Decision fatigue has been noted as having an effect on decision-making. This is defined as deteriorating decisions after a long day of decision-making. Because of the fatigue, poor decisions may be made that compromise the success of an organization. Some leaders, such as Steve Jobs, have been known to eliminate the need to make decisions by wearing the same style of clothes every day, black pants and black turtleneck shirt. Decision fatigue is in play after a day of making many decisions, many of them requiring considerable mental effort and having an emotional response.

A relevant and interesting study of Israeli judges found that prisoners fared least well if their case came before the judge before a break (Danzinger, S., *et al.*, 2011). Studies of account analysts support this in tracking the quality of their decisions throughout the day. As analysts become tired their assessments are lower in quality. The data in nursing also supports that the quality of decisions is decreased with fatigue, as there are more errors when nurses are fatigued. This has become a well-recognized concern with the American Nurses Association, SIGMA, and the American Academy of Nursing having position statements related to fatigue (Stimpfel and Aiken, 2013; ANA, 2014; Drake and Steege, 2016; Caruso *et al.,* 2017).

Decision fatigue can be a factor when leaders engage in the following (See Figure 10.2).

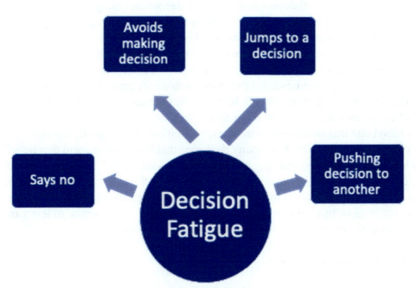

FIGURE 10.2 Decision Fatigue Factors.

- *Avoidance of Decisions.* When exhausted we often avoid deciding and make statements such as, "I can't make this decision now," or just saying, "later." However, the decision is unlikely to go away, and it will either need to be addressed sooner or the issue requiring a decision will snowball and become a more complicated decision later. It is better to take a break, meditate, take a walk, or do whatever will provide the energy and focus to make a decision that works.
- *Pushing the Decision to Another Person.* Often when we are tired, we look to others to pick up the responsibility that is really ours. This may be reasonable on occasion but if done too much, others will see a leader as not leading.
- *Jumping to a Decision.* Leaders may decide just to get the decision done without carefully considering the implications.
- *The Answer is No.* When tired leaders may not be able to think about taking on one more activity, idea, or plan, they are more apt to say no. Many followers purposely avoid meetings with leaders just before lunch or late in the day if they want to get a positive reception to an idea or plan.

Many decisions are plagued by incomplete information and conflicting evidence, leading to ambiguity. Coupled with ambiguity is the need to often decide within a time constraint. In these types of situations, leaders may say their decision was a gut level decision. When people talk about gut level decisions, they are really talking about relying on their previous experience and applying it to the current situation as best they can. There has been considerable research into gut level decisions or intuitive decisions. Going with our gut does not guarantee the best outcome. It may be the best decision given the circumstance, but can also result in an unwanted outcome.

In addition to an intuitive decision being based on previous experience, it may also be based on beliefs and values. Beliefs can be a double-edged sword in that our beliefs are based on experiences that may provide inaccurate information about something. People believed that the earth was flat, and we also believed that our DNA limited our ability to change. Now, we know the world is round and that changes in genetic expression create change. Given that there is likely limited evidence for many decisions that leaders make and that beliefs play a role in decision-making, it is important to understand that beliefs are difficult to change. Beliefs may not be accurate or useful to a particular situation. It is important for leaders to reflect on the basis of their decisions that are based on gut level or intuition rather than evidence, in order to continue to learn and incorporate new experiences into their arsenal of experiences.

Bias and Decision-Making

A phenomenon that is common in humans and therefore within any group is the presence of various forms of bias (Kahneman, 2011). Often, we are not aware of a bias. Being unaware of a bias is called unconscious bias, and it influences our decision-making. It influences how we categorize people, objects, thoughts, and ideas. Unconscious bias often comes into play around how we see others based on race, color, weight, how they dress, and many other characteristics. There are hundreds of different types of biases that have been identified but common forms of bias are: status quo, anchor, framing, and confirmation bias.

- Status quo bias includes a tendency to want to keep things the same. Keeping things the same provides some sense of safety in knowing what is, and being more uncomfortable with the unknown. Studies by Kahneman (2011) indicated that people had more regret about bad outcomes from new actions taken than from bad outcomes from inaction.
- Anchor bias involves relying too heavily on a first piece of information that influences all subsequent information. An example is the recent corona virus outbreak with some hearing first the information about it going to be like the flu, and ignoring or discounting the evidence of spread and mortality as more information was available. Related to the above cases, an anchor bias could be that the CNS is more effective than lower cost nursing roles in spite of evidence to the contrary.
- Framing bias occurs when information is presented in a way that influences a decision in one direction or another. This could apply to the academic scenario in framing the decision as either creating a DNP program or discontinuing the CRNA program, and not exploring other possibilities such as partnering with another school.
- Confirmation bias is at play when people favor information that supports a preconceived idea or belief. People will also interpret ambiguous messages and data in a way that confirms their beliefs. They will also more heavily weigh information that confirms beliefs rather than information that challenges those beliefs. For instance, during a leader's 360 assessment, areas that others have found to be needing attention are identified. If the leader believes she is strong in these areas, the 360 information may be ignored or discounted. In the academic vignette, any information that might question the decision to require the DNP for the CRNA program would be given more credence than other statements.

Individuals and groups make decisions every day in organizations. If there are questions such as, "whose decision is it, anyway?" time is wasted, efforts may be redundant, conflicts arise and organizational outcomes ultimately suffer.

Organizational Decision-Making Context

Within organizations, decision-making occurs at the strategic and operational levels. Both types of decision are ideally evidence based, that is driven by timely, relevant information and the process of decision-making is based on an organization approach to decision-making.

Highly effective organizations design and routinely use accountability structures and processes to advance mission driven decisions and related outcomes. Accountability drives effective decisions creating a "decision-making model." The primary aim of defining and using such a model is to clarify accountability of individuals and groups in their decision-making role, provide resources and support for effective decision-making, and ultimately effective implementation of decisions. Organizations are dynamic and ever changing, particularly in terms of employees at all organizational levels coming and going. It is critical for organizations to use a decision-making model.

Decision-Making Approach: Setting the Stage for Good Decisions

The best organizational decisions are made by individuals or groups of people who ask the following questions to lay the foundation and agree on a context for an effective decision-making process. These questions are:

1. What is the problem/challenge/issue that is generating the need for a decision?
2. What are the assumptions that are framing the need for a decision?
3. What are the *principles* that will guide the decision-making-process and outcome of the decisions?
4. Who is/are the decision maker(s)? Is it a committee, an individual, or a dyad? If the decision maker is a committee, does the committee function effectively? Are there known behavioral biases among members of the group? Who, beyond the individual or committee, is ultimately accountable for the decision, who is responsible, who needs to be consulted, and who needs to be informed?
5. Who is responsible for implementing the decision and how will the decision be communicated to that individual, group, and organization-wide?
6. How will the organization know the outcome of the decision was accomplished, and by when? What performance measures will be used to monitor and control the results of the decision?

These questions form the basis of a decision-making model that guides individuals and groups who make decisions on a regular or irregular basis. In addition to this foundational, context setting approach, there are three additional components of a decision-making model.

First, organizations should ideally formulate a "decision inventory," which is a comprehensive list of the key decisions that must be made by organizational leaders, by individuals and by groups, at both the operational and strategic levels (McDowell and Mallon, 2011). An annual review of key decisions is good practice. Second, to realize the full potential of individuals and groups to make effective decisions, a set of organizational procedures and resources such as committee charters, well defined role descriptions, standing agenda templates, dedicated time, tracking tools, and more should be made available. Finally, intermittent review and assessment of the organizational structure (roles/ functions of individuals and groups) is necessary to clarify decision-making accountability and authority or "decision rights" of specific roles and groups, both standing (committees) and short term (task force). This review process should occur annually as well.

Clarity of the Decision to Be Made

The reason for an organizational approach to decision-making is that decisions significantly impact the organization. It is important to make sure that the decision that needs to be made is clear. Often the decision is well defined and obvious. In the academic example the main decision was to move the MSN level CRNA program to the DNP or close the program. However, not all questions that require a decision are that clear. For instance, in the clinical example, replacing the CNS with other roles is a decision defined within specific boundaries. However, a more basic question requiring a decision is, "what is the highest value overall staffing model?" Defining the decision to be made is similar to finding the root cause of a problem and it may take considerable thinking to figure this out. Clarity could be achieved by using a brainstorming mode or the five whys used in the quality improvement processes (Ohno, T., 1988). In addition to defining the basic decision to make, it is important to keep in mind that every decision has many other decisions that follow, but the major or first decision is critical to addressing questions that must be answered. Defining the decision is the basis for all of the next steps of the process.

Assumptions that Guide the Decision

Defining assumptions is a critical first step. Individuals and groups should spend 15–30 minutes brainstorming and then developing consensus about a list of assumptions that form the basis of the decision-making process and outcome. An assumption is a thing that is accepted as true or as certain to happen, without proof; a fact or statement taken for granted as true. In the first scenario, the faculty and dean may make the following assumptions as they begin the process of decision-making: our decision will affect our enrollment, the president and provost of the university will want input into our decision, the composition of our faculty may have to change.

In the second scenario, the CNO and executive team may make the following assumptions as they begin the process of decision-making: Care Coordinators can easily be recruited; eliminating a role group will cause individual and organizational angst; the labor union will likely have major concerns about any change that results in reduction in force of a role group.

Principles That Guide a Decision

A principle is a fundamental truth or proposition that serves as the foundation for a system of belief or behavior or for a chain of reasoning. Principles that may drive the decision-making process and outcome in the academic vignette: the AACN's DNP Essentials will frame our new program and curriculum; the state board of higher education and the state board of nursing that will need to approve the development of a new degree program will be consulted and kept informed on progress on a routine basis; the faculty will be fully engaged in every step of the decision-making process and will ultimately approve all changes.

In the practice vignette, the following principles may guide the decision-making process and outcomes: cost, quality, and employee satisfaction will form the basis of our decisions and implementation plans; evidence based best practices about leading organizational change will guide our decision and the changes that require implementation; the bargaining unit will be fully engaged in the implementation plan.

Decision Makers

It is critical for organizational leaders to be very clear about who or what group owns a decision or a set of decisions. This is commonly referred to as "decision rights" (McDowell and Mallon, 2011). Decision rights relate to the structure of the organization and role of specific groups, but are not necessarily hierarchical in the classic sense. More organizations broaden decision-making authority to individuals and groups closest to where a decision meets the operations. Organizations in which professionals are the main employee groups drive decisions to interdisciplinary committees and co-leaders of functional areas. Advisory groups are often used to assure a wide net of inclusivity, and ultimately buy-in, for a particular decision or a set of related decisions.

In such organizations, role descriptions and committee charters describe the decision-making authority of individuals, pairs or triads, and committees. This important clarification serves to diminish overlapping or redundant decisions by various decision-making bodies. It also helps to clarify the domain(s) of accountability and authority of similar roles or role groups across departments or disciplines. The clarity will also aid in reducing conflict among different groups of decision makers.

When committees have the authority to make key organizational decisions, leaders should routinely assess the committee's composition, productivity, and overall effectiveness. This assessment should include a self-assessment by committee members of their effectiveness on the committee, as well as the effectiveness of the committee as a whole. This assessment can be done every year or two.

Consider: Are you and others in your organization aware of who or what committee is accountable for key decisions?

Paying attention to the role description of individuals and groups is paramount. To initiate the process of clarifying roles and responsibilities related to key organizational decision-making, a responsibility assignment matrix (RACI) (McDowell and Mallon, 2011) may be used. RACI stands for responsible, accountable, consulted, and informed and is described as:

- *Responsible*: This person or committee does the work to complete the task. Every decision needs at least one responsible person or committee.
- *Accountable*: This person delegates work and is the last one to review the decision before it is communicated more broadly and implemented. In some scenarios, the responsible person or committee may also serve as the accountable one.
- *Consulted*: Every deliverable is strengthened by review and consultation from more than one person or committee. Consulted parties are typically the people who provide input based on either how it will impact their future work or their domain of expertise on the deliverable itself.
- *Informed*: People or committees that simply need to be kept in the loop on progress of a decision-making process or final decision rather than involved the details of the decision-making process at hand.

Together the RACI elements provide a complete model for who is doing what. Although this matrix is sometimes designed for a specific project, the matrix is also conducive to clarifying the responsibilities of each individual and group that will have a role in making the decision happen. Clarity about who is ultimately accountable, what their job functions are, what level of autonomy they have, when collaboration and consultation is needed, and who to keep informed and when. Table 10.1 provides an example of how information can be organized. In the table we are using the RACI headings however, the names of individuals and groups can be used.

The process requires clarity about who assumes what roles related to decision rights. Individuals and groups need to communicate with one another in a

TABLE 10.1. Using the RACI format in Decision Making.

Decision	Responsible	Accountable	Consulted	Informed
Move forward with CRNA DNP program				
Decision 2				
Decision 3				
Decision 4				

structured and formal way to begin the process. This may seem like a straight-forward task, but it is frequently complicated in large organizations because of the many groups that often have purview over decisions. Committees and cross functional team leaders often have shared accountability for key decisions. For this reason and more, it is especially important to undertake the work of creating RACI matrices for clarity of the decision-making process.

At the leadership level of the organization the process begins by creating a decision-making inventory that is made up of a comprehensive list of the key decisions that must be made by an organization including the leaders, teams, business units or function. This work is a large undertaking, but once completed, it is a list that can be revisited and updated annually. The decision questions should be based on the goals and strategies of the strategic plan. The timing of the decision-making will be driven by the strategic plan timetable. In addition, annual operating plans also yield a set of decisions that require a shorter time frame for action. Both organizational activities may drive the composition of the decision inventory.

After creating the decision questions, the next step is to create a collaborative effort involving key stakeholders in a business unit, functional unit or cross functional units, and committees to determine roles in the decision-making process as noted in the table above.

In the academic vignette, the administrative deans and faculty chairs would ideally refer to college and university bylaws, committee charters and role descriptions before embarking on the decision to create a DNP level CRNA program. They would also initially clarify what changes are within the purview of the college of nursing or department level and which are made at the university level. The first question on the decision list would likely be: whose decision is it to move forward with the DNP? Who makes this decision: The provost? The dean? The chair? The faculty? For this example, a series of approvals is likely needed. Decision-making may start with the dean of the school to move forward with a proposal, that would then go to a committee to create, then to the full faculty for approval and then to the provost and possibly the Board of Trustees for the institution. RACI will be a way of organizing who will be responsible for each aspect.

In the clinical vignette, the CNO and her team would want to answer the question, "Since the care coordinator role has implications for the medical departments, is this decision one for both the CNO and CMO?" Another question that would require careful consideration is, "How does the bargaining unit contract potentially impact our decisions?" It may be known that the CNO tends to frame information in a way that limits creativity and brainstorming by people and groups. In a situation like this, it is incumbent that the leadership team working with the CNO have some frank conversations about preparing information and material for decision makers, and for decision-making groups to be as informed as possible.

Implementing the Decision

Deciding and implementing a decision are related but two separate processes. Often, work groups, committees, and individuals conduct the process of coming to a good decision and most often the carrying out of the decision is transitioned to an operating team or individual to take the necessary steps to fully implement the decision. An action plan is often created to assure that the outcome of the decision-making process is carefully planned and executed. The action plan consists of a timeline, a communication plan, and a set of steps necessary to assure completion.

In the academic vignette, a decision will be made to either proceed or not with a DNP program. If the decision is to proceed, a designated business owner of the new DNP program would likely be necessary to identify. It may be an associate dean, department chair, or perhaps a dyad consisting of an administrator and faculty member. It might entail posting and hiring into a new role, perhaps a director of the DNP program. In the clinical services vignette, assuming the idea on the table is agreed upon (eliminate one role and replace with two roles) by the decision makers, a reduction in workforce plan as well as an operating plan would need to be developed and communicated with HR assistance, finance, and appropriate managers of the cost centers/units/services affected by the decision.

Evaluation of the Decision

Evaluation of the decision should be based on what the decision was attempting to address and the criteria that were established, a priori, for a good outcome. There are many measures of achievement in academic and clinical organizations. Most of the measures are required to be reported by accrediting and certifying agencies, payers for service, professional organizations as part of recognition programs, and others. However, the required measures may or may not be related to the decision that needs to be made. The measure of the success of the decision needs to be specific to the decision. For some decisions the measure may be very straightforward, such as whether something was done. For instance, in the academic vignette either the DNP CRNA program was developed, or it was not. In the clinical vignette the measure may be to substitute other roles to replace the CNS staff. However, there are many sub-measures of the decision that could also be important.

In the academic vignette, measures that would already be collected would include the number of applicants and matriculation, student evaluations of the courses and overall program, and the tuition income compared to the costs of the program. There could also be measures associated with recruitment of faculty to teach in the program and how faculty perceive the importance of the program. In the clinical area, measures could include the perception of staff on the change in staffing pattern as well as measures that reflect impact on patient care, such as measures that are required to report such as falls, infection rates, readmission rates, and others. An important measure in this case would be the measure related to financial impact, which would include any financial impact related to the patient care measures. The results of the measures related to the decision should be transparent to all of the stakeholders and decision makers.

How Is Decision-making Different from Problem Solving?

Decision-making is action oriented and problem solving is process-oriented, and some authors consider both as components of the broader conceptual framework of conflict resolution (Weitzman and Weitzman 2000). Both decision-making and problem solving have to do with making choices and taking actions. Problem solving tends to be more process oriented and often involves trial and error or small tests of change (when individuals or teams test out ideas based on evidence). Decision-making also involves a process-oriented approach but tends to be a more specific set of mental activities in which judgment or discernment takes place as the primary action or outcome.

In a meta-analysis by Thornton and Dumke (2005), the terms problem solving and decision-making are integrated. A problem occurs routinely, the problem solver is required to generate alternative solutions or strategies to solve the problem, and then they are required to make a decision that results in a desired resolution of the problem.

SUMMARY

The problem solving and decision-making process is a complex one. While we frequently make decisions quickly based on past experiences, given the complex and high stakes decisions facing leaders today, a systematic, thoughtful approach is necessary. Recognition of bias that comes into the decision, as well as the intended and unintended consequences of decisions, are important to consider. Leaders of organizations will benefit from applying a framework to decision-making. Staying focused on the decision, applying a useful process, and ensuring adequate evaluation are keys to effective decision-making to address complex problems, issues, and challenges.

CRITICAL THINKING QUESTIONS

At the beginning of the chapter an academic and clinical vignette were presented. Please review the vignettes to address the following questions. The questions are specific to the vignettes.

Academic Vignette Questions

1. What factors should be considered in making these decisions?
2. What steps could the teams use to decide what to do?
3. What would constitute a positive outcome for the organization?
4. How would you communicate the changes?

Clinical Vignette Questions

1. What are the variables that should be considered in making the decision to eliminate the CNS role?
2. How does the bargaining unit factor into the decision-making?
3. Are there some decisions that take precedence over other decisions and why?
4. How would the chief nurse determine if her decision resulted in a successful outcome?

REFERENCES

American Nurses Association. (2014, December 2). *ANA position statement on nursing fatigue*. Patient Safety Solutions. https://www.patientsafetysolutions.com/docs/December_2_2014_ANA_Position_Statement_on_Nurse_Fatigue.htm

Caruso, C. C., Baldwin, C. M., Berger, A., Chasens, E. R., Landis, C., Redeker, N. S., Scott, L. D., Trinkoff, A. (2017). Position statement: Reducing fatigue associated with sleep deficiency and work hours in nurses. *Nurse Outlook, 65*(6), 766–768. https://doi.org/10.1016/j.outlook.2017.10.011

Danziger, S., Levav, J., & Avnaim-Pesso, L. (2011). Extraneous factors in judicial decisions. *PNAS, 108*(17), 6889-6892. https://doi.org/10.1073/pnas.1018033108

Dholakia, U. (2017, July 9). *What is a "good" decision?* Psychology Today. https://

www.psychologytoday.com/us/blog/the-science-behind-behavior/201707/what-is-good-decision

Drake, D. A., & Steege, L. M. (2016, March 17). *Dimensions of hospital nurse fatigue: Improving clinical outcomes with translational research.* Sigma Repository. https://sigma.nursingrepository.org/bitstream/handle/10755/601767/2_Drake_D_p72469_1.pdf?sequence=1&isAllowed=y

Gross, J. J. (2002). Emotion regulation: Affective, cognitive, and social consequences. *Psychophysiology, 39*(3), 281–291. https://doi.org/10.1017/s0048577201393198

Kahneman, D. (2011) *Thinking Fast and Slow.* Farrar, Straus and Giroux

Keltner, D., Ellsworth, P. C., & Edwards, K. (1993). Beyond simple pessimism: Effects of sadness and anger on social perception. *Journal of Personality and Social Psychology, 64*(5), 740–752. https://doi.org/10.1037//0022-3514.64.5.740

Keltner, D., Oatley, K., Jenkins, J. M. (2019). *Understanding emotions.* Hoboken, NJ Wiley & Sons.

Lerner, J. S., Keltner, D. (2001). Fear, anger, and risk. *Journal of Personality and Social Psychology, 81*(1), 146–159. https://doi.org/10.1037//0022-3514.81.1.146

Lerner, J., Li, Y., Valdesorro, P., Kassam, K. (2015). Emotion and decision making. *Annual Review of Psychology, 66,* 799–823. https://doi.org/10.1146/annurev-psych-010213-115043

McDowell, S. W. J., & Mallon, T. R. (2011) *It's your decision.* Deloitte Insights https://www2.deloitte.com/content/dam/insights/us/articles/6360_getting-decision-rights-right/DI_Getting-decision-rights-rights

Ohno, T. (1988), Workplace Management, Productivity Press, ISBN 0-915299-19-4

Parsons, J. (2016, December 21). *Seven characteristics of a good decision.* University of Nebraska: Agricultural Economics. https://agecon.unl.edu/cornhusker-economics/2016/seven-characteristics-good-decision

Stimpfel, A. W., & Aiken, L. H. (2013). Hospital staff nurses' shift length associated with safety and quality of care. *Journal of Nursing Care Quality, 28*(2), 122–129. https://doi.org/10.1097/NCQ.0b013e3182725f09

Thornton, W. J. L., & Dumke, H. A. (2005). Age differences in everyday problem solving and decision-making effectiveness: A meta-analytic review. *Psychology and Aging, 20*(1), 85–99. https://doi.org/10.1037/0882-7974.20.1.85

Tiedens, L. Z., & Linton, S. (2001). Judgment under emotional certainty and uncertainty: The effects of specific emotions on information processing. *Journal of Personality and Social Psychology, 81*(6), 973–988. https://doi.org/10.1037/0022-3514.81.6.973

Yip, J. A., & Côté, S. (2013). The emotionally intelligent decision maker: Emotion-understanding ability reduces the effect of incidental anxiety on risk taking. *Psychological Science, 24*(1), 48–55. https://doi.org/10.1177/0956797612450031

Weitzman, E. A., & Weitzman, P. F. (2000). Problem solving and decision making in conflict resolution. In M. Deutsch & P. T. Coleman (Eds.), *The handbook of conflict resolution: Theory and practice* (pp. 185–209). Jossey-Bass/Wiley

CHAPTER 11

Leading Quality and Safety

ACADEMIC VIGNETTE

As the chair of the department of psychiatric nursing and behavioral health you are responsible for the psychiatric and behavioral health nurse practitioner program as well the psychiatric and behavioral health content in the pre-licensure program. You have five faculty members in your department who are engaged in teaching. Three of these faculty members received excellent ratings from students on their teaching from both the NP and pre-licensure students. Two faculty members, newly hired two years ago, received average ratings their first year and poor ratings this year. The most problematic areas for the two faculty members included measures of timely feedback on assignments, consistency between objectives and course content, motivating students to learn, and treating students with respect. In addition, the results of the last NCLEX pass rate showed that those students who did not pass scored low on the psychosocial integrity content of the exam and the two new faculty members were the primary faculty for the pre-licensure students.

You have worked with the two faculty members over the past year to improve their teaching and had them attend faculty development workshops to enhance their course content and teaching approaches. However, even after the year of supporting their further development, they continued to receive ratings lower than in the previous year. The three faculty members who have consistently received high ratings for their teaching have voiced concerns that the two poorly rated faculty members are not team players and are not carrying their fair share of work. You have substantial concern about keeping the two faculty members and talk with the senior associate dean (whom you have kept informed about your concerns) to begin a process of termination, to be followed by recruitment of two new faculty members. In contrast, the senior associate dean has determined that there should be another effort to help them improve their teaching. As the leader of the department, what are you going to do to maintain the quality of the teaching?

CLINICAL VIGNETTE

Wayne Memorial Health System serves people in the Southeast region of the country. Heather Smith, the CNO has been receiving feedback from the nursing and patient care services (NPCS) leadership team that the nursing staff across the system were expressing dissatisfaction with staffing shortages in clinics and in many of the inpatient units. Simultaneously, she was seeing patient satisfaction rates fall, particularly in the areas of nursing responsiveness. Pressure ulcer prevalence in the ICUs across the system had increased above national benchmarks.

This information confirmed what she was already seeing from data she regularly monitored including: RN and PCA hours per patient day; HCAHPS patient satisfaction, pressure ulcer prevalence, and other measures. She was concerned that the indicators she was following may be the tip of the iceberg in terms of overall quality and safety. Her index of concern became heightened when some measures showed a decrease in error reporting, knowing this could be a sign of more quality and safety issues, not less, because of failure to report errors.

She decided to pull together the shared governance nursing council, which included members of the NPCS leadership team and chairs of all the professional practice model committees who were clinical nurses and advanced practice nurses, to a 2-hour work session to begin to map out plans and priorities to address the issues of concern about insufficient staff and patient experience. She also invited members of the patient and family advisory council to participate in this workshop as well as participate in any future work. She also engaged the chief medical officer and the chief operating officer, who were part of a triad of leaders she served with, to join her in leading the session. Engaging her co-leaders was a strategic decision to get them on board with her efforts.

In preparation for this meeting, she asked the quality department to create control charts related to staffing and patient experience of care. The CNO understands that addressing the quality issues will likely require additional resources and that some of the work that will need to be done is to link quality to increased resources. This would be hard work and would continue indefinitely. She and others would determine a structure (task forces, committees, individual Quality Improvment (QI) team leaders, and more) to assure accountability for results. A communication plan would be needed to keep all members of NPCS and the other participants in the effort, including the CEO, informed and engaged. She would report this work in the quality/safety update to the board of trustees at every meeting. She felt energized about the work and knew that in both the short and long run patient outcomes, workforce outcomes and organizational outcomes would improve.

INTRODUCTION

The US health delivery system continues to harm patients at alarming rates. Prior to the COVID-19 pandemic, estimates indicated that medical error was the third leading cause of death in the US with between 250,000 and 400,000 people dying per year from error (Makary and Daniel, 2016). Nurse leaders in clinical and educational positions have the opportunity to improve the quality of care provided throughout our care delivery, and quality of education delivered in our educational programs. Clinical nurse leaders are responsible for the care that all nurses provide directly to patients. Academic leaders are responsible for the quality of the programs offered, and ensure that students have the knowledge and skills to fully engage in patient safety and QI activities. American Association of Colleges of Nursing (AACN) revised *Essentials for Practice* highlights this commitment (AACN, 2020).

Nurses are positioned to lead and engage in quality and safety initiatives. First, nursing is the largest health workforce providing and influencing care at all levels and in all settings. The magnitude of the workforce is directly related to the level of improvement that can be achieved. As more nurses are knowledgeable and engaged in quality and safety issues, the better the healthcare delivery system will be. Second, nurses have been rated the most trusted profession for nearly twenty years in a row, with 85% of Americans regarding nurses as high or very high in honesty and ethical standards Nurses Ranked Most Trusted Profession 19 Years in a Row (Nurse.Org, 2021). https://nurse.org/articles/nursing-ranked-most-honest-profession/ retrieved December 14, 2021. The level of trust Americans have in nurses carries the responsibility to provide the best care possible, and consistently work to improve care.

Third, nurses are committed to continually expanding, disseminating, applying, and continually evaluating new knowledge in order to best serve our patients. Evidence-based practice is the standard of practice. Evidence is employed in both our direct care skills and processes as well as our caring, compassion, and empathy in building therapeutic relationships to improve quality and safety. Both clinical and academic leaders serve the objective of nurses providing the best care possible to patients. Through academic partnerships, each brings research and clinical care expertise together to address critical quality issues. Clinical leaders will best serve their patients through active, evidence-based QI efforts, and academic leaders will serve patients by preparing students to participate and lead improvements in care.

It is clear that there are serious issues that compromise patient safety and the quality of care delivered by nurses. Nurse leaders working with leaders of other disciplines together have the authority and accountability to create a culture of quality and safety, and to adequately prepare and reinforce competencies and commitment to these efforts. Improving quality and safety requires everyone working as a team leveling out power gradients among the professions, addressing systems that contribute to the harm of patients or near misses, decreasing unnecessary waste, and improving the value of care processes. Nursing alone can only take improvement so far, having all the health professions, as well as patients and families, working together will create transformational change to keep patients safe and receiving the highest quality care.

Quality and Safety Concepts

While the role of leaders in improving patient safety and healthcare quality is to provide vision, strategy, and engagement of followers, leaders must also embrace the fact that measures of quality provide the information necessary to know the quality of care provided. Measures of quality are essential to assess and improve the work we do. The Quality and Safety Education for Nurses (QSEN) project defined competencies and knowledge, skills, and attitudes that should be integrated into all educational programs and clinical practices (Cronenwett et al., 2007). The competencies identified built on the Institute of Medicine (IOM) competencies that all health professionals should have and included teamwork and collaboration, informatics, evidence-based practice, QI, and patient-centered care (IOM, 2003, p.4). The QSEN faculty added the competency of safety because it is conceptually different from QI. QI and safety are defined by QSEN as (Cronenwett et al., 2007, p. 123):

- *Quality improvement* (QI): Use data to monitor the outcomes of care processes, and use improvement methods to design and test changes to continuously improve the quality and safety of healthcare systems.
- *Safety*: Minimizes risk of harm to patients and providers through both system effectiveness and individual performance.

Taken together, these definitions integrate the concepts of data use in order to prevent harm and to continually improve care processes and systems effectiveness. Both definitions recognize both individual accountability and systems failures, as well as the necessity of data in knowing the state of quality and safety. In addition to the QSEN definitions, there are several other definitions of note that apply to both the clinical as well as educational realms. The IOM defines quality and safety as: ". . . quality of care is the degree to which health services for individuals and populations increase the likelihood of desired health outcomes and are consistent with current professional knowledge"

(IOM, 1990, p.4). Further, the IOM indicates that, "patient safety is the prevention of harm to patients."

The World Health Organization (WHO, 2020) defines quality and safety as: "... the extent to which health care services provided to individuals and patient populations improve desired health outcomes." Patient safety is the absence of preventable harm to a patient and reduction of risk of unnecessary harm associated with healthcare to an acceptable minimum.

While the QSEN, IOM, and WHO definitions are the most referred to as a guide to the meaning of healthcare quality and patient safety, you as a leader need to be clear about your definition of quality and safety. Your definition may differ from those noted above to incorporate elements of mission, vision and values. However, several aspects should be incorporated, including the importance of data, individual and systems accountability, effectiveness, and preventing harm. The definition that embodies the above elements within the context of the organization needs to be communicated and strongly woven into the fabric of the organization.

Scientific Inquiry and the Relationship to QI

The nursing profession has advanced a broad set of terms that includes QI and other related systematic approaches to scientifically based inquiry, improvement, translation of evidence, and implementation of evidence-based standards of care. Practice inquiry, scientific inquiry, scholarly inquiry, clinical inquiry, and related terms (such as clinical scholar, scholarly practice, and evidence-based practice) are terms that many healthcare disciplines and professions use to prepare their clinicians and providers to base their practice on available scientific information and to ask important, relevant questions about advancing knowledge and improving care. While there are specific differences in the use of the above terms, there is also considerable overlap.

These terms, often used interchangeably, refer to the application of systematic approaches for asking pertinent questions based on a commitment to plan, deliver, and evaluate evidence-based care.

Quality Improvement

QI is the application of techniques and instruments to improve the structure, process and outcome measure of a product or service. QI is about developing new, locally useful knowledge, most often accomplished through small tests of change (plan-do-study-act [PDSA] cycles) using Rapid Cycle Change Methods.

Such practice-based, contextually confined improvement efforts are not intended to be generalizable beyond the setting and population involved. These initiatives and the evaluation methods used in them are considered formative in nature where improvements, also often called interventions, are experimented with and often adapted while running small-scale tests of change. Some interventions or improvements following these tests of change when considered successful are adopted, sustained, and disseminated more widely beyond the initial unit or context in which they occurred. A note about the word "interventions" is warranted here.

Interventions are purposefully implemented change strategies that may be simple or complex. This term is often used in a systematic inquiry area called "intervention research" and in the public health program planning and health services research area in which community "interventions" are planned, evaluated, disseminated and implemented. The term "intervention" is also used in implementation science or dissemination and implementation science (D-I Research). Finally, at times the word intervention is used in QI and improvement science.

Improvement Science

The term improvement science, while related to the practice of QI, is based on a more rigorous research methodology than QI. QI activities include a focus on a well-defined, single problem in one microsystem that is not generalizable. Improvement science is based on a more summative evaluation that takes place, often across multiple sites, using quasi-experimental evaluations such as time series, equivalent time series, multiple baseline, and factorial experiments. Improvement science is used to design generalizable interventions and innovations that aim to improve the health services structures, processes, and outcomes. The units of analysis can be patients, or the people served, typically in the form of outcomes, practices, and health system level improvements. This type of research is less about reducing complexities in the design of the study, as found in randomized control trials, and more about robust experimentation that incorporates system complexity directly (Toulany *et al.,* 2013).

Implementation Science

Implementation science consists of a body of knowledge directed at how to establish proven effective interventions in everyday practice. (Bauer and Kirchner, 2020). Implementation is defined as the transition period following adoption of a change or the decision to use a new QI idea or practice when intended users put that new idea or practice into use.

The leading international journal in the field of implementation science, the British Medical Journal of Implementation Science (2021), defines implementation as, "the methods to promote the systematic uptake of clinical research findings and other evidence-based practices into routine practice and hence improve the quality and effectiveness of health care."

Implementation science is a knowledge base aimed at making more effective change through the use of practical tools and guidance. Part of preparing for an improvement initiative is to assess whether the unit or place where changes will occur is ready and able to implement and sustain the improvement. Implementation science also offers something called an "implementation outcome stages map", which highlights what parts of the implementation have occurred and which parts have not. This tool also provides a method for cost effective alternatives to assure full implementation.

The focus of implementation research efforts, as well as the application of implementation methods and tools, include the contextual factors as explanatory variables in the conduct of implementation research and in the application of the methods and approaches in practice. There are implementation tools that could be useful for QI teams to use in the four phases of a QI initiative as noted later in this chapter.

The improvement and implementation of scientific communities overlap in many ways. For instance, the Six Sigma/DMAIC (design, measure, analyze, improve, and control) model "Control Phase" includes the important step of creating new standard operating procedures (SOPs) and new structures (roles and functions) to assure fidelity to the original change idea. This step is a critical component to sustaining and disseminating the change within the microsystem. This is one example of many in which practice inquiry scientific disciplines merge, overlap, and reinforce each other.

Evidence Based Practice and Translation Science

Improvement and implementation science overlap in many ways. The classic discovery process of turning observations in the laboratory, clinic, and community into interventions that improve the health of individuals and the public, from diagnostics and therapeutics to medical procedures and behavioral changes, is the most inclusive definition. It is often thought of as taking research findings and applying them to the bedside in clinical settings, or to the process of teaching in academic institutions. This translation process is related to the work of identifying evidence-based practices, standards, and interventions that have been identified through research. The research is often contextually accomplished, and considers the microsystem, the people served, and the providers to determine the highest and most comprehensive level of evidence to drive what we do in clinical care to achieve safe, timely, equitable, efficient, effective, and people focused care by translating new evidence into practice.

Creating robust and rigorous QI research to provide more generalizable information about best practices and improving outcomes of care. Putting scientific inquiry approaches into practice no matter what lexicon is used is paramount for assuring high performance healthcare delivery.

QI Models and Methods

There are four prominent models used today in healthcare including the IHI model, Toyota Lean Model (TLM), Six Sigma DMAIC Model, and the FOCUS-PDSA Model. The IHI model is built on the work of the Associates in Process Improvement that largely adopts the work of Edward Deming. The model asks three questions. What are we trying to accomplish? How will we know that a change is an improvement? What changes can we make that will result in improvement (IHI, 2021)? After addressing the questions, a PDSA cycle for small, rapid-cycle tests of change is completed. This model is the basis for all QI work of IHI.

The TLM grew out of the Toyota production system developed by Toyota founder Sakiichi Toyoda beginning in the 1930s, and further developed by his son Kiichiro Toyoda along with Tiichi Ohno (Toyota, 2021). The Toyota production system was committed to the elimination of waste. It incorporates two important concepts. The first is Jidoka, meaning when there is a problem noted, a machine must come to a stop to prevent any additional defective parts being produced. The second is just in time production making what is needed, when it is needed, and in the amount that is needed, thus creating an efficient system. The book *The Machine That Changed the World* (1990, 2007) by James P. Womack, Daniel Roos, and Daniel T. Jones provides a thorough description of the history and impact of the Toyota production system that is used worldwide.

Six Sigma is frequently combined with DMAIC. Six Sigma was introduced at Motorola by Bill Smith in 1986 and provides tools and methods to reduce variation in production and therefore defects. DMAIC is the approach to solving problems that occur in production and provides the roadmap to reducing defects.

FOCUS PDCA provides an approach to QI that includes the following steps: (1) Find an opportunity for improvement; (2) Organize a team; (3) Clarify processes; (4) Understand the process and root causes of the problem; and (5) Select and improve. After completing these steps, a PDSA is completed.

There are common steps across all of the above models, and they are:

1. Problem definition and preparation
2. Improvement design and planning
3. Implementation and evaluation
4. Sustainment and spread

Making change happen is an essential component of all models. To successfully make changes that will lead to better patient outcomes, better system performance, and better learning organizations, QI teams need to apply knowledge, methods, tools, and approaches that have evolved over time in the QI field and within improvement science.

> *Consider*: What model of QI has been adopted in your organization? Is quality and safety embedded in your organizational culture?

As noted, each of the four most commonly referred to and used QI models share common characteristics or steps, which are described here.

Step One: Problem Definition and Preparation

During the first step of a QI initiative, a problem is identified. The problem identification can come from a number of different sources including reportable data, observations of staff, complaints of patients or students, the organization's team of leaders, or the organization's QI team. Once a problem is identified, a QI team is charged with doing a QI project. The team that addresses the problem needs to include people who are directly affected by the problem as well as those who are knowledgeable about the problem. The responsibility for forming the team may fall to the chief nurse, dean, or person responsible for quality in the organization.

The problem identified may be very clear to everyone, such as too many falls with injuries, or it may be less well defined, such as poor morale among staff. After naming a problem, there is additional work that needs to be done to further clarify the problem. Additional information needed to address falls includes answering questions such as: Is there a specific unit that is contributing to the number of falls? Are falls happening at a specific time of day? What are the circumstances of the fall? Were patients trying to get to the bathroom? Were the staff unresponsive in a timely way to a call light? On the educational side, what programs contribute to the most student complaints? What are the most often cited student complaints? Data need to be collected in a systematic manner and analyzed to provide a targeted approach to identifying the problem and doing PDSA to address the problem.

This step often involves the identification of the problem by understanding the trend of the data. Is a particular area of concern getting better, worse or staying the same? In some cases, statistical process control (SPC) is used to evaluate current performance particularly as it relates to the common cause variation (variation that is expected and measurable within a system) and special cause variation (variation that is not expected, is unusual, not quantifiable and not previously observed) that occurs in a process. There are several tools to see variation including statistical control charts, histograms, scatter plots, and regression analysis. It is very useful to have statistical support to create the visuals of events in order to easily track them. For instance, the statistical control chart shown in Figure 11.1 provides data related to the average number

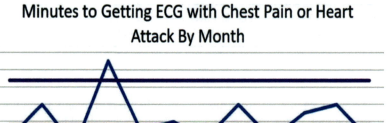

FIGURE 11.1 Example of Statistical Control Chart.

of minutes before getting an ECG in the emergency room. The upper line represents the upper control defined statistically based on the mean. If the mean number of minutes goes above the upper control limit, there is a problem to be concerned about. The lower line is the lower control limit and going below this line shows better than average performance. The control lines are based on statistical averages and standard deviations. IHI (2021) has numerous templates for these tools in the QI Essentials Toolkit.

The first step also involves the application of diagnostic methods to explore the cause of the problem and to generate change ideas. These methods may include root cause analysis, cause and effect analysis using a fishbone diagram (shown in Figure 11.2), SIPOC (Supply, Input, Process, Output, and Customer) analysis, and more. Understanding current performance allows a QI team to generate an aim statement for the improvement project, and begin to hypothesize reasons for the issue or problem and ideas for change that would result in improvement. The fishbone diagram shown in Figure 11.2 incorporated the problem identified, the major areas likely contributing to the problem (people, environment, process, and equipment), and more detail about each of the areas contributing to the problem.

Step Two: Improvement Design and Planning

The second common step in the process of QI is to clarify the aim of the project, the measures to be used to evaluate the outcome, and who is going to do what and when. In this step, QI teams invite people to become engaged in the initiative. The team will work best when staff who are most affected by the problem, and most knowledgeable about the problem, are included. Team members need to be committed to change, to perform in a different way, or to learn something new in order to improve a process or outcome. This step often includes brainstorming sessions, work sessions, and training. Later, when trials of change begin, performance feedback, presentations of analyzed data for review, and input regarding current performance are reviewed.

In addition, an assessment of other contextual factors such as team skills, microsystem motivation, leadership and organizational culture, and strategic priorities of the healthcare system. As part of the design work, the data to be collected and analyzed need to be defined. The design and planning phase should clearly identify who is going to do what, by when. The design of the project should be basic in terms of being able to implement the intervention and test it in a short period of time. While many QI projects may be considered research, the point of doing QI interventions is to have a quick turnaround of information about what might work to improve care within a focused context. IHI has worksheets available to help create the design of the project and track the work being done (IHI, 2021).

Step Three: Implementation and Evaluation

This step includes the use of short, iterative tests of change to garner better understanding of the impact of the intervention. This is the PDSA step. All QI models involve the actual implementation of a change idea and the concomitant collecting, analyzing, and reviewing data related to the planned intervention. In this phase of improvement work, feedback about the change in a process, structure, or outcome to those who are responsible for performing

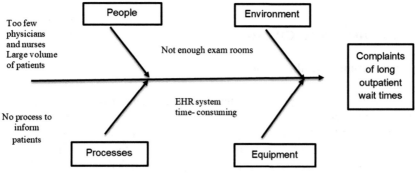

FIGURE 11.2 Example of a Fishbone Diagram.

differently is obtained to gain a better understanding of the impact of change on the process and the people involved in doing it.

It is during this phase that a QI team may decide to abandon a change idea, due to the intervention not being successful in producing the expected outcome. The failure of the intervention could be due to flaws either in the planning or in the intervention itself. A small change in the intervention or the process of change could produce a different result and is considered. During this phase, the documentation about the new process is communicated, improved, and clarified to begin the process of communicating a change. The implementation and evaluation processes are iterative, in that efforts need to remain focused on the problem being addressed in order to institutionalize changes in the future.

Step Four: Sustainment and Spread

The fourth step used consistently within QI models is the process for decision-making to adopt, sustain, and spread the change; to drop the change idea; or select a new change idea and begin again. Sustaining a change is complicated and includes re-enforcing the habits and routines of staff that have contributed to the promising results. It also includes sustaining the changes by changing policies and procedures and ensuring that there is adequate training about the change. Resistance to change requires anticipation, communication, and reinforcement for adoption in order to address the issues staff are concerned about.

Implementing and managing change is complex, is often phased in and takes rigorous discipline and attention over time. The acknowledgment of the contextual factors, as well as human factors such as behavior change, that inherently make change difficult and challenging is at the core of implementation science. Applying the knowledge, tools, and methods from the field of implementation science that can assist QI teams in improving the likelihood of successfully implementing, sustaining and disseminating change.

QI READINESS TO CHANGE

Organizational Readiness and Context

Tools that assist improvement teams or implementation research teams to do their work are related to whether a unit or organization is ready and able to implement and sustain the change. The conditions and influences inside and external to a unit/microsystem might help or hinder the implementation and sustained operations. For instance, the Organizational Readiness to Change Assessment Tool (ORCA) (Helfrich et al., 2009) and the Ready-Set-Change

Tool (Timmings *et al.,* 2016) or Will it Work Here Innovation Assessment Tool (Brach *et al.,* 2008) are examples of assessments that help QI teams and Implementation researchers know the readiness level of the people who need to embrace the change.

Change Capability

Another category of tools that could be useful to QI teams are the many tools and resources compiled by IHI, such as the Improvement Capability Assessment that assesses whether the skills of the people making the change are present within the context in which the change will happen (IHI, 2021). Another method to determine capability of the team to engage in QI is determining "intervention fit" (Aarons *et al.,* 2014), which can be used by QI teams to choose from a list of potential solutions or interventions based on the evaluation of the best fit to the context and readiness of the people (implementers).

The People Side of Change

QI teams may also undertake a planning phase in order to create the expectations, capacity, and environment for all members to implement a QI initiative. Engaging all staff in QI efforts may take changes in staff behavior, and there is a consensus list from expert implementation scientists of 93 intervention techniques (Powell *et al.,* 2017) and a similar list of behavior change techniques available for QI teams to consider for use (Michie *et al.,* 2013). Some examples of these techniques and concepts include: beliefs about capabilities, beliefs about consequences, environmental context and resources, attitude toward behavior, motivation, and social learning/limitations (Michie *et al.,* 2013).

Analytics

Analytics are critical to QI efforts. Every QI project should have metrics associated with a before and after approach, in order to know whether or not the intended outcome of the change was a result of the intervention(s). Analytics may include SPC, time series analysis, and other statistical tools and tests to give QI teams the information needed to assess the impact of the intervention on intended outcomes.

Documentation

Changes associated with a QI intervention need to be carefully documented. A framework for describing an intervention or change uses criteria such as: fidelity, dosage, program differentiation, personnel, or community factors. These factors can assist QI teams in knowing whether a change is feasible and replicable beyond one microsystem.

Sustainability

A related set of tools that focus on sustained implementation include evidence-based intervention strategies such as the realistic appropriation for resources to sustain change. Another is the need for continued organizational support of the change. The concept of "sustainment climate" is useful to QI teams when thinking about and planning for sustaining the change (Greenlaugh *et al.*, 2017). The tools from implementation science that address fidelity, adaptation-assessment, and documentation of the change are considered most useful.

Consider: What is the greatest challenge in your organization or an organization you worked in related to QI efforts that consider the readiness for change?

FRAMEWORKS FOR QUALITY IMPROVEMENT

Clinical Frameworks

In addition to the definitions above, the IOM identified characteristics of healthcare quality. These characteristics describe care as: safe, timely, equitable, efficient, effective, and patient-centered known as STEEEP. The definitions of each are (IOM, 2001, p. 5–6):

- *Safe*: Avoiding harm to patients from the care that is intended to help them.
- *Timely*: Reducing waits and sometimes harmful delays for both those who receive and those who give care.
- *Effective*: Providing services based on scientific knowledge to all who could benefit and refraining from providing services to those not likely to benefit (avoiding underuse and misuse, respectively).
- *Efficient:* Avoiding waste including waste of equipment, supplies, ideas, and energy.
- *Equitable*: Providing care that does not vary in quality because of personal characteristics such as gender, ethnicity, geographic location, and socioeconomic status.
- *Patient-centered*: Providing care that is respectful of and responsive to individual patient preferences, needs, and values and ensuring that patient values guide all clinical decisions.

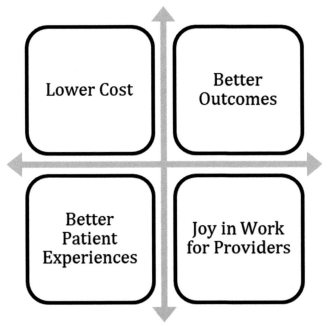

FIGURE 11.3 Quadruple Healthcare Aim.

Consider: **Is your organization committed to improving joy in work and a healthy work environment? How do you lead joy in work efforts?**

A national framework for healthcare quality began as the triple aim and evolved to the quadruple aim, as noted in Figure 11.3. The triple aim included reducing the cost of care and therefore making it affordable to all, improving the experience of care, and improving the health of populations. The fourth aim added recognizes the importance of providers and maintaining or attaining joy in work.

Educational Perspective

Nursing education has approached quality nursing education by identifying characteristics and standards for programs and validating the incorporation of standards through an accreditation process. The NLN (2016) has identified five standards that characterize nursing education quality including: (1) Culture of Excellence—Program Outcomes; (2) Culture of Integrity and Accountability—Mission, Governance, and Resources; (3) Culture of

Excellence and Caring—Faculty; (4) Culture of Excellence and Caring—Students; and (5) Culture of Learning and Diversity—Curriculum and Evaluation Processes.

The CCNE has defined four areas of importance to quality and effective nursing education: mission and governance, institutional commitment and resources, curriculum and teaching/learning practices, and assessment and achievement of program outcomes. The AACN (2020) draft essentials on core competencies for professions nursing education includes quality and safety as one of the domains for educational programs.

QUALITY AND SAFETY MEASURES

Measures of quality and safety are foundational to improving the efficacy, quality and cost of care and keeping patients safe. Quality measures are also critical to ensure that students experience high quality educational programs that prepare them to provide evidence-based care driven by continuous commitment to QI. Measurement allows the organization to see progress toward goals and provides direction for the organization. It is critical that the measurements taken can be used to influence the success of the organization. All too often data are collected that have no bearing on the decisions to improve systems or processes. These data should not be collected. Data that are focused on the results of strategic initiatives and inform decisions about how to improve the organization are data that communicate to the organization what the leader feels is important.

Measures are defined as a standard unit used to express the size, amount, or degree of something. Measurement is the action of measuring (Oxford Dictionary, 2020). The terms metric, indicator, and measures are used synonymously in healthcare QI efforts. We cannot know how good our care is if we do not have measures of care. It is not enough to rely on intending to provide outstanding care, measures will tell us if we are indeed providing outstanding care. For a long time, healthcare providers believed that the care provided was good. However, when we started to measure care structures, processes, and outcomes, we discovered we were falling far short of what we thought.

While some leaders may be experts in quality and safety, others may have basic knowledge related to quality processes and measures. Indicators that provide measures of quality have multiple uses including for internal QI, public information to help people make decisions about providers based on quality, and for payment. There is significant overlap of measures used for the three purposes. An example is the reporting of patient experience measures used for public reporting also having consequences for payment by third parties. An organization may want to know more about the patient experience of care and have their own complementary measures that go beyond the required patient experience survey. Another example is the HCAHPS (Hospital Consumer Assessment of Healthcare Providers and Systems) survey which is the first national, standardized, and publicly reported patient perception of hospital care. However, an organization may, and most do, want to know more about the patient experience of care and have their own complementary measures that go beyond the required patient experience survey.

It is important for leaders to avoid getting into the weeds with measures and measurement issues and to rely on individuals who are experts, whether in the organization or outside as contractors/consultants. Leaders are not the ones to do the data collection and analysis; leaders determine the measures that are important and required (this may be done through leading a team effort), as well as create the support system to accomplish the work of interpreting, applying findings to changing process of care and improving systems, and evaluating the outcome. Knowing the right questions to ask, specifically around common cause and special cause variation is important. Leaders should understand what SPC is, how run charts and control charts work, and how to interpret the meaning of descriptive and enumerative statistical tests.

Leaders need to understand what constitutes a useful measure. The National Quality Forum (NQF) reviews proposed measures and either endorses or does not endorse the measure based on a number of criteria including (NQF, 2021):

- *Importance*: Extent to which the specific measure focus is evidence-based, important to making significant gains in healthcare quality, and improving health outcomes for a specific high-priority (high-impact) aspect of healthcare where there is variation in, or overall less-than-optimal, performance.
- *Reliable and valid*: Extent to which the measure, as specified, produces consistent (reliable) and credible (valid) results about the quality of care when implemented.
- *Feasibility*: Extent to which the specifications, require data that are readily available or could be captured without undue burden and can be implemented for performance measurement.
- *Usability*: Extent to which potential audiences (e.g., consumers, purchasers, providers, and policymakers) are using or could use performance results for both accountability and performance improvement to achieve the goal of high quality, efficient healthcare for individuals or populations.
- *Comparison to related or competing measures*: If a measure meets the above criteria and there are endorsed or new related measures (either the same measure focus or the same target population) or competing measures (both the same measure focus and the same target population), the measures are compared to address harmonization and selection of the best measure.

In addition to the NQF criteria, Rose (1995) in a seminal article described a model for quality measurement and data collection that includes eight steps:

1. Define performance categories that answers the question: What do we do?
2. Define the operational definitions of the performance goal or target.
3. Define performance indicator(s) related to each performance goal.
4. Define what is actually measured—the measurement data sources.
5. Define the parameters of the measure—context, constraints, and boundaries.
6. Define the means of the measurement—a how-to action statement.
7. Define the notional metrics—how the concept of how the information is compiled will be applied to measuring organizational performance.
8. Define the specific metric—an operational definition and a functional description of the metric. How the data are described, collected, and used. What data mean and how they affect organizational performance. This step shows what actions might be taken as a result of the measurement. This enables subsequent improvement activity.

The criteria of useful measures should be a guide to leaders in determining the measures to use that will have the greatest impact on the most serious problems affecting patient care.

Types of Measures

Nurse leaders are responsible for quality and safety at several levels. These levels include consumers, processes and people in an organization, the organization's systems, and finally the organization as a whole, as shown in Figure 11.4. Examples of measures for each level are:

- *Consumer*: Patient satisfaction, functional health status
- *Process and people*: Access, wait time, staff satisfaction or employee engagement
- *Organizational systems*: Cost, workforce supply/demand, volume
- *Organization as a whole*: Measures of competitiveness, diversity of patient population, social determinants of health.

There are several different types of measures that can be applied at each level of the work of the organization. Donabedian's work in the 1960s has provided a lasting framework for considering quality measures (Donabedian and Rosenfeld, 1962). The structure, process, outcome framework recognizes the type of measure. In addition, there has been growing attention to composite measures. Composite measures are defined by NQF as, "a combination of two or more individual measures in a single measure that results in a single score." The benefit of a composite measure is that it can summarize

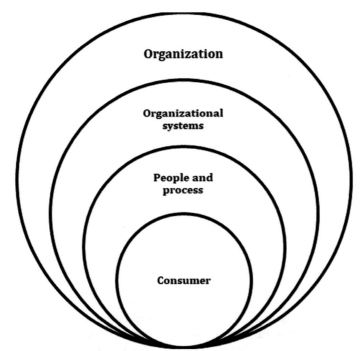

FIGURE 11.4 Scope of Quality Measures.

overall quality by combining several measures. A composite measure needs to have a high reliability, validity, and usability.

Within the outcome measures (and in some cases considered separately) are consumer satisfaction measures. Within clinical care, this would be patient and family centered satisfaction, and within an educational program it would be student, faculty, and staff satisfaction. There are many measures that have to be reported by clinical and educational organizations and will be considered separately below.

Clinical Organizational Measures

There are many healthcare quality measures. Numerous organizations have worked to create measures of care. Measures reflect specific settings, specific health conditions and specific populations. They can be structure, process or outcome measures. Well known measures include the Health Effectiveness and Data Information system (HEDIS) developed by the National Committee for Quality Assurance (NCQA) (NCQA, 2021). HEDIS measures were developed to evaluate health plans and a number of the HEDIS measures. Other measures were developed by CMS, AHRQ, accrediting organizations such as The Joint Commission, and professional organizations. Measures that have been proposed are reviewed by NQF for endorsement as noted above.

The Centers for Medicare and Medicaid Services (CMS) Measures Inventory Tool lists over 700 measures that includes the measure title, description of the measure, whether it is NQF endorsed, and the program/s that use the measures (CMS, 2022a). The tool also provides the opportunity to compare measures. Information available when comparing measures includes a description of the measure, the description of the numerator and denominator, the rationale for the measure and the developer and steward as well as other information. This tool is robust and the measures can be searched in a variety of ways and compared to other measures related to a similar issue so that the best measures for a given situation within an organization can be selected for use.

Measures that reflect nursing care are embedded in the broader set of quality measures. Historically, NQF had endorsed nursing specific measures that included measures of the rate of falls, restraint use, catheter related urinary tract infections, pressure ulcer prevalence, central line infection rate and smoking cessation. The rationale for not having discipline specific measures is that results of measures are difficult to attribute to a single profession.

CMS require reporting of quality measures both for public reporting as well as payment. A useful Website for consumer information about the quality of care of a variety of healthcare settings is https://www.medicare.gov/care-compare/#search (CMS, 2022b).

This information includes outcomes data as well as patient survey data. A five-star rating is used as an effort to make the results easy for users to understand. One star is the worst and five the best. There has been concern voiced by providers about the accuracy and validity of the data reported, as well as concerns about how the star ratings are calculated. However, public reporting of measures is now firmly embedded in CMS and will continue to evolve. In addition to the settings noted in Table 11.1, there are comparison websites for hospice care, inpatient rehabilitation services, long-term care hospitals and dialysis facilities, and physicians. The physician site does include advanced practice nurses but is limited to name, address, and whether or not Medicare is accepted. CMS is currently planning to integrate the comparison sites into one tool that will simplify consumer use.

Using measures to improve care requires benchmarking. The comparison sites provide data in terms of percent of patients or events for at least two additional institutions, as well as state and national averages for each of the items in the category of measures reported. Benchmarking is comparing performance with the performance of others and usually best practices. While benchmarking can be external, benchmarks can also be internal and can exceed or create steps in comparison to best practice. For instance, a hospital may report that 76% of patients responded that their nurses "Always" communicated well on

TABLE 11.1. *Summary of Selected CMS Required Reporting of Quality Measures for the Public. (CMS (2022c) Quality measures for each setting can be found at https://www.medicare.gov/care-compare/)*

Setting	Description
Hospital	Data include general information, patient experience, timely and effective care, complications & deaths, unplanned hospital visits, psychiatric unit services and payment and value of care.
Nursing Home	Ratings of nursing homes include star rating for: • Overall Rating • Health Inspection Results • Staffing Levels • Quality Measure Data (of resident care and uses minimum data set assessments of individual residents and the measures differ for short stay and long stay residents) • Facility safety inspection
Home Health Quality Reporting Program (HH HRP)	Patient quality of care measures (OASIS) and patient survey (HHCAHPS) reported in Home Health Compare OASIS based outcome measures Types of measures collected: • Improvement measures • Measures of potentially avoidable events • Utilization of care measures • Cost/Resource measures

the patient experience survey. This compares to 71% for another hospital, 81% for the state, and 86% for the nation. In this case the best practice could be defined as the national average of 86%, and the hospital could set an initial short-term internal benchmark of 79%, with the longer-term goal of 86% as the best practice.

In addition to Medicare measures, Medicaid also has measures of quality that include the Adult Core Set and the Child Core Set (CMS, 2020b). The core measures are updated annually and can be found by searching Medicaid Adult and Child Core Measures. Measures from each of these sets have been integrated into an additional Core Set of Maternal and Perinatal Measures for Medicaid and CHIP. Reporting of data is voluntary for the states, and states are encouraged to report on both the Medicaid as well as CHIP. The median number of measures reported by states as well as the number of states reporting has continually increased since the beginning of the program in 2010. Reports on these measures are required by the Affordable Care Act annually.

The Magnet hospital program incorporates measurement reporting and benchmarking for participating hospitals. This program has five components that incorporate forces of magnetism including: transformational leadership, structural empowerment, exemplary professional practice, new knowledge, innovations and improvement and empirical quality results. There are specific measures reported for each area, especially related to the empirical quality results that include clinical outcomes related to nursing, workforce outcomes, patient and consumer outcomes, and organizational outcomes.

Link of Clinical Quality Measures to Payment: Value-Based Payment

It is important for nurse leaders to understand the payment models for whatever setting in which they work. The linkage of payment to quality will continue to be a strong force in healthcare, with CMS coupling quality performance to payment for hospitals, nursing homes, outpatient care, and other services. The linkage of payment to quality provides an incentive to improve care. The aim is to promote high quality and low cost in order to create greater value in our health system. CMS considers how individual hospitals compare to other similar hospitals and how much they improve their own performance compared to a baseline. The Hospital Value Based Purchasing (HBP) Program reduces select payment to hospitals (currently 2% defined by law) and uses those funds to provide incentive payments to those hospitals that meet specific criteria for performing well. Hospital performance includes four areas: Clinical outcomes, person and community engagement, safety, and efficiency and cost reduction. Each of these areas carries a 25% weighting that creates a Total Performance Score (TPS). Each participating hospital gets an annual report on the TPS and the incentive payment that will be added to each fee-for-service discharge.

The skilled nursing home value-based payment model is built on a single quality score for hospital readmissions. The measure used is the 30-Day All Cause Readmission Measure. Scoring of the measure distinguishes planned from unplanned readmissions. The program applies to Medicare Part A payment authorized in the 2014 Protecting Access to Medicare Act, and was initiated in 2018. Medicare withholds 2% of payment for Part A and is required to use 60% of the funds for incentive payments for Medicare Part A fee-for-service claims paid under the SNF Prospective Payment System (PPS). All facilities (15,000+) that participate in the PPS must participate.

The Medicare Access and CHIP Reauthorization Act (MACRA) of 2015 established the Quality Incentive Payment Program is intended to reward clinicians for high value care and to streamline the multiple different programs into the Merit-based Incentive Payment System (MIPS) program for Medicare Part B payments. In addition, it provided the opportunity for bonus payments through the Alternative Payment Models (APM). APRNs and other types of providers can participate in the MIPS if they meet specific requirements as do physicians. MIPS payment requires the reporting of quality measures that fall into four categories and will contribute to the final score. The categories and percent contribution to the final score are: quality (45%), cost (15%), interoperability and information exchange (25%), and improvement activities (15%). Practices can select the required number of measures to report in each category. Numerous measures from multiple data sets have been approved for reporting with the measure requirement changing on an annual basis. Currently the optimal amount of additional payment is 9% for meeting a specific score threshold and –9% is the penalty for poor performance on reported measures. Updates to MIPS are done annually and can be found through a search of MIPS Update.

Consider: **How can a clinical nurse leader use the value-based payment to access the resources to support high quality nursing care?**

APMs provide the opportunity for added incentive payments. While APMs are mandated in MACRA for Medicare physician payment, private insurers and Medicaid are also moving away from fee-for-service models and toward APMs to lower cost and increase quality. The most common types of APMs include capitated plans for practices to care for a large population, bundled payments for populations with specific conditions such as heart failure or cellulitis, and patient-centered medical homes. Each of the APMs requires the reporting of measures and those practices and institutions that can lower cost and maintain or increase quality will get incentive payments. However, the practices take the risk that they will lose income if they do not meet the cost and quality metrics.

Measures of Educational Quality

Nursing education programs have many measures of quality. There are standards and measures that apply to the educational organizations through accreditation processes and standards and measures, usually through national examinations and licensure that address the quality and safety of nurses. Often the measures used to make judgments about the quality of nursing education are not tested to the same extent as clinical measures in terms of reliability and validity. The penalty for poor quality education is reputation, ability to attract students, and possible closure of the program. In addition to accreditation and licensure that are professionally generated efforts to protect the public, ranking educational programs based on data submitted to the organizations doing the ranking, such as US News and World Report, has become an important measure of quality. Programs work to be ranked in the top institutions.

Education quality is informed through several processes including accreditation, licensure of graduates, and certification processes. In order to be approved as an accrediting agency, certification by the U.S. Department of Education (USDoE) is required. In addition, the Commission on Higher Education Accreditation (CHEA), a non-governmental organization focused on non-governmental regulation of institutional quality, also reviews and approves of accrediting organizations. Many accrediting organizations meet the standards of and are recognized by both the USDoE and CHEA. It is important to note that CHEA is independent of USDoE.

The landscape of accreditation at the institutional level has changed dramatically. Up until 2020, the accreditation process, particularly for non-profit institutions, was within the purview of one of seven regional accreditors such as the New England Commission on Higher Education and the Middle States Commission on Higher Education. Each regional accrediting agency accredits institutions only within their geographic region. The seven regional accrediting bodies comprised the Council of Regional Accrediting Commissions. However, with the emergence of for-profit online programs, national accredited bodies emerged more strongly. The landscape for institutional accreditation changed in 2020 with new rules issued by the USDoE that removed the geographic focus of regional accreditors allowing them to cross boundaries and putting them on the same footing as the national accreditors. This will create greater competition among all of the accrediting agencies, with a likely outcome being confusion for institutions in choosing which accrediting agency with which to work. All of the institutional accreditors have standards that each institution must use. While the standards are not specific to nursing, as a constituent unit of the college or university, nursing schools are required to meet the standard identified by the regional accrediting body. These standards reflect critical elements of academic life such as financial resources, diversity and inclusion work, governance and learning outcomes.

In addition to the institutional accrediting bodies, there are nursing specific accrediting organizations. The purpose of nursing accreditation is to provide a set of standards that will drive excellence in nursing education and improve the overall quality and integrity of nursing programs. Standards speak to the structure, process, and outcome measures of nursing education with a strong emphasis on evaluating the outcomes of the educational program.

The CCNE, an autonomous arm of the AACN, primarily accredits bachelor and graduate nursing programs and the Commission for Nursing Education Accreditation (CNEA) is a subsidiary of the the NLN and accredits all levels of programs. Accreditors use the standards that are set by the professional organizations of the AACN and the NLN. AACN standards for educational programs are "essentials" that define essential content areas for entry level, masters and

DNP nursing programs. The new Essentials document is competency-based with domains for both entry level and advanced observable abilities that integrate multiple components such as knowledge, skills, values, and attitudes that are measurable (AACN, 2020). Their document, *Standards for Accreditation* (2018) includes criteria for assessing each standard, elaborations to explain the criteria, and examples of evidence to support meeting the criteria. CCNE standards are closely linked to the 'essentials' documents. (CCNE, 2018 Standards for Accreditation of Baccalaureate and Graduate Nursing Programs).

The NLN's *Hallmarks of Excellence* provides guidance on the characteristics that constitute quality education (NLN, 2020). The hallmarks include engaged students, diverse faculty, and continuous improvement to name a few.

Both CCNE and CNEA accredited DNP programs but neither accredited PhD programs in nursing. This is consistent with other PhD programs within the university and excluded because PhD programs in all disciplines are tightly integrated into the university PhD structure and evaluation of these programs is overseen by the university's graduate school.

Accreditors of nursing education focus on programs meeting defined standards. The standards include areas such as having sufficient resources for students in terms of faculty and support services, governance, providing facilities and equipment that support learning, having faculty who are qualified to teach the courses assigned, and having a QI/evaluation plan in place. The accrediting bodies require that nursing programs have an active quality evaluation process and demonstrate that findings are acted on when needed. Examples of measures reported include: application, admission and matriculation numbers, student demographic data, availability of clinical sites, quality of clinical experiences, hours of clinical contact, course and program evaluation data, student to faculty ratio, cost per student, time to graduation, pass rates on national exams, student complaints, and others.

The responsibility of boards of nursing is to safeguard the public through two processes: educational program review and licensing of nurses. In addition to accrediting bodies, boards of nursing review new and established educational programs. While this is redundant of accreditation efforts, a board of nursing usually works to coordinate efforts with accrediting organizations. Board criteria for evaluating nursing programs are usually worded differently from accreditation standards but consider similar aspects of nursing program quality. The National Council of State Boards of Nursing Education Committee (2016) found that the major issues that programs have on review included:

- Faculty shortage/lack of qualified faculty
- Clinical site shortages
- Concerns about quality of pre-licensure education programs, signaled by low NCLEX pass rates, student attrition, etc.

- Lack of robust outcome measures for nursing education programs (besides first-time NCLEX pass rates)
- Rapidly changing expectations for nursing practice

A second process that boards of nursing use to ensure quality of nurses is to test the knowledge of nurses. The NCLEX exam is a national exam that tests the knowledge of entry level nurses in four categories: safe and effective care environment, health promotion and maintenance, psychosocial integrity, and physiological integrity.

An often-used measure of the quality of a program is the percent of students that pass their licensing or certification exam on their first attempt. State boards of nursing establish benchmarks for program performance. For instance, in Virginia, if an entry level program falls below an 80% pass rate of their students for two years in a row, they may be put on probation. If there is no improvement, the program will be noted as not approved by the state board. State boards also review and work with nurses who have been reported for unsafe practice. Licensing is intended to protect the public through an examination process as well as required continuing education in many states. Entry level nurses are required to pass the NCLEX to be licensed.

In order to align the regulatory aspects of nursing licensing, accreditation, certification and standards of professional organizations, representatives of all stakeholders came together and put forward an Advanced Practice Nurse

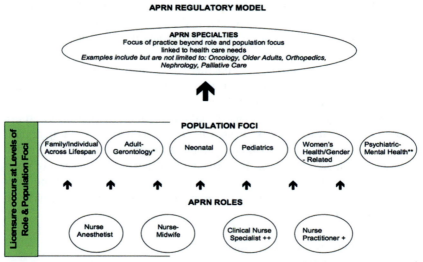

FIGURE 11.5 APRN Regulatory Model. Consensus Model for APRN Regulation: Licensure, Accreditation, Certification & Education," ncsbn.org, National Council of State Boards of Nursing. https://www.ncsbn.org/Consensus_Model_for_APRN_Regulation_July_2008.pdf

Regulatory Model also known as the Consensus Model (NCSBN, 2008) https://www.ncsbn.org/aprn-consensus.htm At the time of writing this book 18 states had fully implemented the model with at least 29 states are on their way to implementation (NCSBN, 2021). This model defines the scope of regulation of state boards of nursing and the role of specialty organizations in providing specialty practice certification. In the figure below, the four APRN roles have expertise in providing care to one or more of the population foci. In this model licensure by the state board of nursing occurs at the role and population foci levels. Specialty recognition is through certification not overseen by state boards of nursing. To be licensed by a state board of nursing, an APRN has to pass a national exam that tests knowledge related to their role. Exams are given by national certifying agencies such as the American Midwifery Certification Board, the National Board of Certification and Recertification for Nurse Anesthetists (NBCRNA), and for nurse practitioners the American Academy of Nurse Practitioners Certification Board (AANPCB), and the ANCC Certification Program. After the graduate has passed the certification exam and confirmed completion of the program to the board of nursing, the board reviews the application to approve practice.

Consider: **What is the basis for selecting the quality measures in your organization and how is the information about how well the organization is doing get communicated to stakeholders? In academic institutions, are all faculty and staff aware of the findings? How are the measures used to improve the quality of educational programs and student experiences? In clinical settings, who is informed about the measure results, and how are they used to improve care?**

Nurses, both entry level and APRNs, can be certified in a specialty that does not require board approval. Specialty certification can be in areas such as oncology, pediatric care, critical care, diabetes management, etc. Specialty certification is often offered through a professional organization that supports the specialty.

CALL FOR LEADERS TO ENGAGE IN COMMUNITY LEVEL QUALITY IMPROVEMENT

Don Berwick, who has done much work to move our health system to provide better care, has recently noted that there is now a "glut" of QI measures. He suggests that the focus of QI should be on streamlining the required measures by identifying those measures that will make a difference in patient

TABLE 11.3. *Quality and Safety Resources for Clinical Leaders.*

Resource Sponsor	Description	Access
AHRQ	Weekly Updates: Source of up-to-date information from the patient safety literature, news, tools, and events. Past versions of Weekly Updates are archived on the PSNet website Web M&M Cases and Commentaries: Consist of expert analysis of medical errors reported anonymously by our readers. Commentaries are written exclusively by patient safety experts and published monthly. • Spotlight Cases: include interactive learning modules with available free CME. Perspectives on Safety: Features expert viewpoints on current themes in patient safety, including interviews and written essays published monthly. • Annual Perspectives highlight vital and emerging patient safety topics and are released yearly. Primers: Guides for key topics in patient safety through context, epidemiology, and content. Training Catalog Database updated monthly, of patient safety training programs, events, and meetings. Email updates.	https://www.ahrq.gov/cpi/about/otherweb-sites/psnet.ahrq.gov/index.html
CMS	Provides updated information on quality reporting programs and initiatives.	https://www.cms.gov/Medicare/Quality-Initiatives-Patient-Assessment-Instruments/MMS/Quality-Programs

(continued)

TABLE 11.3 (continued). *Quality and Safety Resources for Clinical Leaders.*

Resource Sponsor	Description	Access
IHI	Starting at the home page will provide many opportunities for resources including publications, tools, conferences and more.	http://www.ihi.org/
AHA	Provides trends, updated information to broad topics with information about disparities, emergency readiness, measurement and other topics	https://www.aha.org/advocacy/quality-and-patient-safety
TJC	Information about activities, high reliability organizations, communications, current articles and more.	https://www.jointcommission.org/resources/patient-safety-topics/patient-safety/
DHHS	Email updates, training resources and conferences, tools and more	https://health.gov/our-work/health-care-quality/trainings-resources/resources
Patient Safety and Quality Health Care	Provides podcasts and daily updates on their website related to a wide range of issues including cybersecurity, clinician burnout, events, and more.	https://www.psqh.com/
Collaborative Healthcare Patient Safety Organization	List numerous organizations worldwide that are resources to leaders	https://www.chpso.org/organizations-focused-patient-safety

care (Berwick, 2017). Berwick also noted the importance of committing to the moral determinants of health. He strongly asserts that healthcare leaders in addressing the social determinants of health need moral determinants for the will to act. Berwick is taking the quality movement beyond the institutional boundaries into areas that greatly affect health and require moral determination such as human rights, universal coverage, climate change, and criminal justice reform (Berwick, 2019). Berwick's challenge will take all leaders beyond their immediate organizational responsibility.

In addition to knowing the quality of care or education at the organizational level, leaders will best serve their constituents by understanding the context of the patients they serve. Community based information about the health of communities is now available. For instance, social determinants of health have been integrated into the Healthiest Communities assessment done by US News and the Aetna Foundation that include data related to community vitality, equity, economy, education, environment, food and nutrition, population health, housing, public safety, and infrastructure (US News and World Report Aetna Foundation, 2021). In addition, the RWJ Foundation sponsored project on County Health Ranking includes a broad look at the health of each county in the US incorporating data about health behavior, clinical care, social and economic factors, and physical environment (University of Wisconsin Population Health Institute and Robert Wood Johnson Foundation, 2020). The challenge to leaders is to act on the information related to social determinants of health in a way that serves the people cared for within the organization.

Quality and Safety Resources for the Clinical Leader

Clinical resources listed below include major organizations that focus on healthcare quality and safety. The resources listed generally provide information about measurement, tools, and newsletters to help clinicians be consistently updated. Our advice is to choose two sources that best match your leadership responsibilities with which to remain current since there is overlap among the resources listed. It will be useful to review the resources related to academic leadership to be knowledgeable about quality and safety issues of nurses you will be recruiting and hiring as well as forging academic-clinical partnerships focused on quality and safety.

SUMMARY

This chapter recognizes that nurses being the largest health profession and the most trusted have a responsibility and capability to lead quality and safety efforts. Quality can be broadly defined as using data and systematic interventions to produce desired patient outcomes and safety is the minimization of harm. Quality improvement (QI) interventions are increasingly based on improvement and implementation science. There are several approaches to QI including the TPS, Lean, and Six Sigma as well as hybrids of these approaches. Healthcare frameworks for quality and safety include the quadruple aim as well as the IOM STEEEP. CMS has a useful inventory of measures that provides meaningful descriptive information about each measure. There are also numerous measures applied to academic institutions including measures related to educational standards, accreditation, and national rankings. Rich resources available for both academic and clinical leaders are noted to help expand efforts in quality and safety.

CRITICAL THINKING QUESTIONS

At the beginning of the chapter an academic and clinical vignette were presented. Please review the vignettes to address the following questions. The questions are specific to the vignettes.

Academic Vignette

1. How might the chair of the mental and behavioral health department manage the conversation with the associate dean to get her support for removal of the two faculty who were not performing?
2. What QI framework might work best for the chair in thinking about how to continue to work with the underperforming faculty?
3. How might the chair involve the three experienced faculty in improving the teaching performance of their colleagues?
4. What metrics would be most useful in assessing the ongoing efforts to improve the teaching of the faculty?

Clinical Vignette

1. What might be three goals of the CNO in efforts to improve the quality of care in the health system?
2. What quality framework would be most useful in the CNO efforts and why?
3. How might the issue of getting additional resources be addressed by the CNO? What arguments related to quality might be most useful?
4. How might the CNO inspire all nursing staff to be active participants in quality and safety efforts?

5. Review the CMS Measures Inventory to assess whether there are measures, in addition to what is required by CMS, that would provide useful information about the patient experience for the CNO.

REFERENCES

Aarons, G. A., Ehrhart, M. G., Farahnak, L. R., & Sklar, M. (2014). The role of leadership in creating a strategic climate for evidence-based practice implementation and sustainment in systems and organizations. *Frontiers in Public Health Services and Systems Research, 3*(4). https://doi.org/10.13023/FPHSSR.0304.03

American Association of Colleges of Nursing. (2008, July 7). Consensus model for APRN regulation: Licensure, accreditation, certification & education. American Association of Colleges of Nursing. https://www.aacnnursing.org/Portals/42/AcademicNursing/pdf/APRNReport.pdf

American Association of Colleges of Nursing. (2020, November 5). *Draft: The essentials: Core competencies for professional nursing education.* American Association of Colleges of Nursing. https://www.aacnnursing.org/Portals/42/Downloads/Essentials/Essentials-Draft-Document-10-20.pdf

Bauer, M.S. & Kirchner J., (2020) Implementation science: What is it and why should I care? P*sychiatry Research* https://doi.org/10.1016/j.psychres.2019.04.025

Berwick, D. M. (1989). Continuous improvement as an ideal in health care. *New England Journal of Medicine, 320*(1), 53–56. https://doi.org/10.1056/NEJM198901053200110

Berwick, D. (2017, May 24). *5 missteps on the patient safety journey.* Becker's Review Clinical Leadership and Infection Control. https://www.beckershospitalreview.com/quality/dr-don-berwick-5-big-missteps-on-the-patient-safety-journey.html

Berwick, B. (2019). *Quality, mercy and the moral determinants of health.* Institute for Healthcare Improvement. http://www.ihi.org/resources/Pages/AudioandVideo/Don-Berwick-Forum-Keynotes.aspx

Brach, C., Lenfestey, N., Roussel, A., Amoozegar, J., & Sorensen, A. (2008). *Will it work here? A decisionmaker's guide to adopting innovations.* RTI International under Contract No. 233-02-0090. Agency for Healthcare Research and Quality (AHRQ) Publication No. 08-0051. https://innovations.ahrq.gov/guide/guideTOC

BMJ Implementation Science. (2021) https://implementationscience.biomedcentral.com/about retrieved December 14.

CCNE (2018) CCNE Standards and Professional Nursing Guidelines https://www.aacnnursing.org/ccne-accreditation/resource-documents/ccne-standards-professional-nursing-guidelines

Centers for Medicare and Medicaid Services. (2022a) *Measures Inventory Tool.* Centers for Medicare & Medicaid Services. https://cmit.cms.gov/CMIT_public/ListMeasures

Centers for Medicare and Medicaid Services. (2022b). Find and compare hospitals, nursing homes and other providers near you. https://www.medicare.gov/care-compare/

Centers for Medicare and Medicaid Services. (2021). *Nursing homes including rehab services*. Medicare. https://www.medicare.gov/nursinghomecompare/search.html

Commission on Collegiate Nursing Education. (2018). *Standards for accreditation of baccalaureate and graduate nursing programs*. Commission on Collegiate Nursing Education. https://www.aacnnursing.org/Portals/42/CCNE/PDF/Standards-Final-2018.pdf

Cronenwett, L., Sherwood, G., Barnsteiner, J., Disch, J., Johnson, J., Mitchell, P., Sullivan, D. T., & Warren J. (2007). Quality and safety education for nurses. *Nursing Outlook, 55*(3),122-31. https://doi.org/10.1016/j.outlook.2007.02.006

Donabedian A., & Rosenfield L.S., (1962) Some factors influencing prenatal care Nursing Research: Volume 11, Issue 2, p. 113.

Gaines, Kathleen. "Nurses Ranked Most Trusted Profession 19 Years in a Row." Nurse. Org, Nursing News, Education and Community Stories, 19 Jan. 2021, ttps://nurse.org/articles/nursing-ranked-most-honest-profession/.

Greenlaugh, T., Wherton, J., Papoutsi, C., Lynch, J., Hughes, G., A'Court, C., Hinder, S., Fahy, N., Procter, R., & Shaw, S. (2017). Beyond adoption: A new framework for theorizing and evaluating nonadaptation, abandonment, and challenges to the scale-up, spread, and sustainability of health and care technologies. *Journal of Medical Internet Research, 19*(11), e367. https://doi.org/10.2196/jmir.8775

(Health IT.Gov., 2021) https://www.healthit.gov/faq/how-do-i-use-rapid-cycle-improvement-strategy#:~:text=The%20Basics,standard%20eight%20to%20twelve%20months.

Helfrich, C. D., Li, Y. F., Sharp, N. D., & Sales, A. E. (2009). Organizational readiness to change assessment (ORCA): Development of an instrument based on the Promoting Action on Research in Health Services (PARIHS) framework. *Implementation Science, 4*(38). https://doi.org/10.1186/1748-5908-4-38

Institute for Healthcare Improvement. (2021). *Science of improvement: How to improve*. Institute for Healthcare Improvement. http://www.ihi.org/resources/Pages/HowtoImprove/ScienceofImprovementHowtoImprove.aspx

Institute for Healthcare Improvement. (2021). *Quality improvement essentials toolkit*. Institute for Healthcare Improvement. http://www.ihi.org/resources/Pages/Tools/Quality-Improvement-Essentials-Toolkit.aspx

Institute of Medicine. (1990). *Medicare: A strategy for quality assurance*, 1. The National Academies Press. https://doi.org/10.17226/1547.

Institute of Medicine, Committee on Quality of Health Care in America. (2001). *Crossing the quality chasm: A new health system for the 21st century*. National Academies Press.

Institute of Medicine. (2003). *Committee on the health professions Education Summit*, Greiner A.C., Knebel, E, editors. National Academies Press (US).

Makary, M. A., & Daniel, M. (2016). Medical error-the third leading cause of death in the US. *BMJ, 3*(353), i2139. https://doi.org/10.1136/bmj.i2139

Michie, S., Richardson, M., Johnston, M., Abraham, C., Francis, J., Hardeman, W., Eccles, M. P., Cane, J., Wood, C. E. (2013). The behavior change technique taxonomy (v1) of 93 hierarchically clustered techniques: Building an international consensus for the reporting of behavior change interventions. *Annals of Behavioral Medicine, 46*(1), 81–95. https://doi.org/10.1007/s12160-013-9486-6

Modernizing Medicine. (n.d.). *What you need to know about MIPs changes in 2020.* https://www.modmed.com/blog/mips-changes/

National Committee for Quality Assurance. (2021) *HEDIS and performance measurement. National Committee for Quality Assurance.* https://www.ncqa.org/hedis/

National Council of State Boards of Nursing. (2021) *Consensus model implementation status.* National Council of State Boards of Nursing. https://www.ncsbn.org/5397.htm

National Council of State Boards of Nursing (2008) *Consensus Model for APRN Regulation: Licensure, Accreditation, Certification & Education.*

National Council of States Boards of Nursing Inc. (NCSBN 2008) https://www.ncsbn.org/aprn-consensus.htm

National League for Nursing Commission on Nursing Education Accreditation. (2016). *Accreditation standards for nursing education programs.* http://www.nln.org/docs/default-source/accreditation-services/cnea-standards-final-february-201613f2bf5c-78366c709642ff00005f0421.pdf?sfvrsn=12

National League for Nursing. (2020). *Hallmarks of excellence.* National League for Nursing. http://www.nln.org/professional-development-programs/teaching-resources/hallmarks-of-excellence

National Quality Forum. (2021). Measure evaluation criteria. National Quality Forum. http://www.qualityforum.org/Measuring_Performance/Submitting_Standards/Measure_Evaluation_Criteria.aspx

Nurse.Org, (2021). https://nurse.org/articles/nursing-ranked-most-honest-profession/ retrieved December 14, 2021.

Øvretveit, J., Garofalo, L., & Mittman, B. (2017). Scaling up improvements more quickly and effectively. *International Journal for Quality in Health Care, 29*(8), 1014–1019. https://doi.org/10.1093/intqhc/mzx147

Oxford Dictionary. (2020). *Measure.* Lexico. https://www.lexico.com/en/definition/measure

Powell, B. J., Beidas, R. S., Lewis, C. C., Aarons, G. A., McMillen, J. C., Proctor, E. K., & Mandell, D. S. (2017). Methods to improve the selection and tailoring of implementation strategies. *The Journal of Behavioral Health Services & Research, 44*(2), 177–194. https://doi.org/10.1007/s11414-015-9475-6

Rose, K. (1995) A Performance Measurement Model *Quality Progress*, vol. 28 issue 2

Reinhart, R. J. (2020, January 6). *Nurses continue to rate highest in honesty, ethics.* Gallup News. https://news.gallup.com/poll/274673/nurses-continue-rate-highest-honesty-ethics.aspx

Timmings, C., Khan, S., Moore, J. E., Marquez, C., Pyka, K., & Straus, S. E. (2016). Ready, set, change! Development and usability testing of an online readiness for change decision support tool for healthcare organizations. *BMC Medical Informatics and Decision Making, 16*, 24. https://doi.org/10.1186/s12911-016-0262-y

Toulany, A., McQuillan, R., Thull-Freedman, J. D., & Margolis, P. A. (2013). Quasi-experimental designs for quality improvement research. *Implementation Science,* *8*(Suppl. 1). https://doi.org/10.1186/1748-5908-8-S1-S3

The Toyota Production System (2021) https://global.toyota/en/company/vision-and-philosophy/production-system/

University of Wisconsin Population Health Institute & Robert Wood Johnson Foundation. (2020). *2020 County Health Rankings: State Reports.* County Health Rankings & Roadmaps. https://www.countyhealthrankings.org/

U.S. News & World Report. (2021). *Healthiest Communities.* U.S. News & World Report. https://www.usnews.com/news/healthiest-communities

Womack, J. P., Jones, D. T., & Roos, D. (1990, 2007). *The machine that changed the world.* Simon & Schuster.

World Health Organization. (2020). Quality of Care. https://www.who.int/maternal_child_adolescent/topics/quality-of-care/en/#:~:text=Quality%20of

CHAPTER 12

Communication and Organizational Leadership

ACADEMIC VIGNETTE

You are the assistant dean for community outreach and academic-practice partnerships. During the COVID-19 pandemic you have worked with community partners to set up testing sites throughout the city. The testing sites are in communities of vulnerable populations that have a high risk of being infected with COVID-19 and you have secured a $2 million dollar grant to help pay for setting up the sites and people to provide the testing. You report directly to the dean of the school with a dotted line to the vice president of community relationships for the university. The dean and VP have a strained relationship centering on the division of indirect funds from a research grant. You also need to communicate with community leaders, faculty colleagues, and students to engage them in helping at the testing sites. You are clear that to get all of the pieces in place to implement the testing site, your communication plan needs to be in place. You also know that how you manage the conversations with the dean and VP will be critical in gaining the support of both and moving the work forward. You are thinking that the communication challenges are similar to crisis intervention communication. You know that effective communication is absolutely essential to successfully mounting the testing sites.

CLINICAL VIGNETTE

You are the chief nurse for a large life care organization that has a 120-bed nursing home, 500 units for assisted living and 500 units for independent living residents. All of the residents of the community are over 65. You have 800 care providers that include personal care aids, RNs, and LPNs. You have received a

235

weather alert that a hurricane has formed and is likely to hit your area in four days. You have responded to hurricane threats in the past, so your team is ready to go into crisis response mode and follow the plan. However, you are aware that the response plan must include communication to various stakeholders living and working in the community, to critical community resources, and family members of the residents. Calls from worried family members are beginning to flood the switchboard. The CEO of the organization is new and has no previous experience with hurricane response procedures. You are concerned about how to help her be effective in managing the organization's response, yet you don't want to have to spend time bringing the CEO up to speed on the emergency response plan. Although the logistics of managing this situation are daunting, the nursing staff members have previous experience with a hurricane response plan. You are now in the process of developing your communications plan recognizing the complexities and the possibilities of ineffective communication.

INTRODUCTION

Communication is the heart of leadership because it is foundational to establishing trusting, effective relationships, and positive relationships are what gets things done. Communication is a dynamic and interactive process between two or more people. A leader communicates every day to many people and each communication is important. The importance of communication cannot be overstated. While leaders communicate everyday using different mediums of communication (verbal, non-verbal, in writing and through synchronous and asynchronous virtual modalities), we may take for granted that we know how to communicate and fail to appreciate the complexity of conveying a message. Often, we use patterns of communication that are ways we communicated with family and friends, and in those situations, they may have been useful. But, patterns and modes of communicating need to be carefully examined before using them in the role of a leader. For instance, we may have a way of communicating that lacks authority or is too authoritarian. We may tend to avoid difficult conversations or be uncomfortable with communications that challenge an idea or another person. On the other hand, we may have no problems addressing challenging situations or people. No one is a perfect communicator. Communicating effectively requires a willingness to engage in self-reflection, seeking and accepting feedback from others and continuous learning.

CONSIDERATIONS FOR EFFECTIVE COMMUNICATION

There are many aspects to effective communication. We begin to learn how to communicate at birth. We become progressively competent in learning the meaning of words and nuances of language. We learn about what words to use in public, with family, and with friends. Certain styles of language and communication are acceptable in church or in school, and we learn to understand what communication works in a variety of situations. Learning to communicate is a very complex process that ultimately for many people results in everyday communication being automatic.

As a leader, developing a communication style that works for you takes time and effort and the understanding that a style that works with one group of people or one person, may not with others. Leaders are expected to develop communication skills that are well-honed, and those who work with leaders notice when they are not.

Thinking Theoretically about Communication

Communication is a complex process, and this chapter will consider a variety of communication types, styles and contexts. We will begin with a brief review of the basics, which reminds us of why communication can be so hard to get right.

Communication starts with a sender and is directed toward a receiver(s). The sender may have a particular intent in mind but one of the most difficult lessons to learn is that the receiver may miss that intention, experiencing an entirely different impact. Intent and impact are distinct, and the better we are at communicating, including knowing our audiences and the cultural importance of language and power, the more likely our intent will match the impact.

Communication is highly personal and, as Figure 12.1 shows, both the sender and the receiver have experiences that will the understanding of the message by both the sender and receiver. Perception is everything in communication. After the received message is processed and a response goes from the original receiver back to the original sender, the perceptions of the original receiver give flavor to the message, which will be perceived by the original sender. It is easy to see how communications that are not closely monitored for impact, or are between two strangers, can be misaligned. Communications that go out to an organizational audience are particularly subject to misunderstanding if not intentionally monitored for impact. For these reasons and more, we will explore the ways we communicate within organizations and the contexts that will influence approaches to communication.

Be Clear About the Purpose

Being clear about the purpose of the communication may seem very basic, and it is. Many communications that really do not need a lot of time are quick and simply informational. However, messages that are important need to have

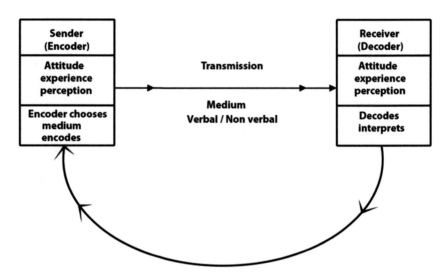

FIGURE 12.1 The Process of Communication.

a clear purpose. What do you want to accomplish with the message? How do you want the person/people to respond? Do you need the receiver of the message to do something? Do you want to motivate people or recognize a difficult situation? The purpose of the important communication should be clear, and the message should be consistent with the purpose. For instance, an associate dean for practice sent an email to his team that he thought they should begin a bi-monthly newsletter. His team was stretched in their teaching load with cutbacks in budgets due to the COVID-19 pandemic. When asked about the purpose of the newsletters, the dean responded that other schools had newsletters about their clinical activities. This was not a sufficient reason. There was no carefully thought-out purpose, and he did not identify a problem that a newsletter would solve. His request lacked sensitivity and good timing.

Quickly communicated requests or statements are often a response to a situation that is immediate with limited time to think about the purpose. Much of what we communicate reflects "fast thinking." Kahneman (2011) described the work he did with his colleague Amos Tversky in his book about "fast" and "slow" thinking. Most of our thinking is fast in that we react quickly without much or any conscious thought. If someone asks about the time of a meeting, the response may be automatic with no real need to analyze the question or dwell on the purpose of our response. However, leaders are faced with many issues that require slow thinking. Slow thinking is deliberate, analytic, and takes more time to process information. Many communications from a leader require the integration of complex information, and therefore slow thinking is critical when communicating important information.

Understand Every Communication has an Emotional Context

As leaders, we often believe we work within a context of objectivity. However, every communication is influenced by an emotional context for both the sender and receiver of a message. The emotional context varies from highly emotional, such as managing the communication around impacts related to the COVID-19 pandemic, compared to an announcement about the change of an entrance to the hospital cafeteria or an update on admissions statistics. Leaders need to be aware of the emotional context in all messages. Even the message about admission statistics may trigger a sense of accomplishment for some, concern about being furloughed for others and anxiety for still others. Important factors that affect the intensity of the emotional context include the amount and type of change indicated in the communication. Change nearly always generates some level of fear, anxiety or pleasure, and relief.

An example of a large emotionally contextual communication is messaging a change of ownership of an organization. People may not know if they will have a job, how the mission and vision will change, or how the workflow will change. Both the sender and the receiver may be significantly emotionally impacted. An example of a low emotional impact message in an academic setting may be the announcement of a change in the room for a meeting. Leaders will be well served to be aware of the emotional context of messages and create a plan to address the high impact emotional messages. The most important way of managing highly emotional communication is to recognize, with the recipients, that they may be worried about their future and perhaps angry if they had no warning that the communication was coming. Other strategies for managing the emotional impact is to have repeated opportunities for communication about an important issue including availability of the leader through additional meetings, personal contact, phone, email, or text. When leaders are uncomfortable with high emotion impact communication, there may be a tendency to avoid them or to try to put bad news in the best possible light. It is very useful to be honest about bad news and have a plan to address the emotional responses.

On Listening

The most important and sometimes most challenging aspect of communication is to listen. The Simon and Garfunkel song "The Sound of Silence" speaks of, "people hearing without listening." That is very descriptive of a lot of communication within an organization. Stephen R. Covey (1989), author of *The 7 Habits of Highly Effective People*, noted that people usually listen to respond

TABLE 12.1. Description and Implications of Covey's Continuum of Listening.

Type of Listening	Description	Implications for Leaders
Ignoring	Person is not paying attention while someone is talking either directly or in a group. They may be looking at their cell phone, constantly engaging with others, and avoiding eye contact.	People will feel disrespected and that what they have to say is unimportant. Most people can understand occasionally ignoring a communication, but a pattern of ignoring will compromise morale, inhibit useful and creative ideas, and limit critical information.
Pretending	This may be the most disrespectful because it is intentionally ignoring while trying to give the impression of listening. It is giving meaningless acknowledgments of listening such as occasional head shakes or "un ha". In this case there is a lack of presence and engagement with the speaker.	Some people can be fooled sometimes but a pattern of pretend listening will be noted. The implications are similar to those for "ignoring."
Selective listening	The listener hears what will support their beliefs, positions on issues and interests. There is a lack of interest in communications that present new ideas and creative ways of dealing with issues/problems/concerns.	Selective listening limits the understanding of important issues and responses that might be more effective but fall outside of the plan of the selective listener. This limits effective responses to change and creativity.
Attentive listening	The listener is present and engaged from their frame of reference of the communication. There is an effort to understand what is being communicated.	Attentive listening can encourage communication from others. They feel respected and recognized. The frame of reference for the communication is the from the listener's perspective.
Empathic listening	Empathic listening is listening until the other person feels understood. It is listening with ears, eyes, and heart.	The highest level of listening is not only having the other person feel understood, respected, and recognized, it is important in building intentional, productive relationships that are mutually satisfying.

rather than understand. This statement is profound and worth thorough consideration. Your job as leader often involves a lot of information giving as well as having answers. Leaders are assumed to have all the answers, all the information. When we listen without understanding we are missing an opportunity. We may be reinforcing assumptions that limit our ability to understand more fully, which limits our ability to develop more productive relationships and effective organizations. Listening is a critical leadership role and Covey described a continuum of listening that includes: (1) ignoring; (2) pretending; (3) selective listening; (4) attentive listening; and (5) empathic listening. Each of these are described in Table 12.1 and includes implications for leaders.

While leaders need to generate information, listening gives a leader a lot of information about an organization. Leaders who are more focused on giving information will miss the opportunity to deeply learn about concerns of staff, what is really going on in an organization, and what is important to external partners. When people know that a leader listens at least attentively, the leader generates the trust that is essential for effective leadership.

Use Effective Language

Being concise, concrete, and clear is so much easier said than done. The more concrete and specific the information shared, the more likely the language will be understood, as intended. Vague statements such as, "patients are complaining about the noise at night," would be better understood if communicated as, "we had complaints from Unit 5B about the noise every night between midnight and 3 a.m. occurring at the nurse's station." In an academic setting we might be told, "the course is not taught well," which contains less useful information than, "the student evaluations indicate that the content did not align with the course objectives." While making concrete statements that provide sufficient information may take more words, trying to use as few words as possible is important. Busy people have the time or interest to read more than a few paragraphs. Useful approaches for business communication include use of bullets, key points, diagrams, or figures. These are examples of communication that concisely convey a good deal of information. For instance, showing a bar chart of falls over a specific period of time will provide an easy and quick way to view information and understand the rate of falls and whether falls are increasing or decreasing over time. In addition, linking the message to something known by the target audience will aid in better understanding the message.

Recognize Tone

How often has someone interpreted an email message as telling people they have not been doing a good job, when the sender thought they were simply conveying a new policy? We often believe that the information in a message is the most important part of a message. While the content is very important, the tone of a message communicates the attitude of the sender. The intended tone and content will be perceived differently by different people. The tone may convey authority, friendliness or formality, concern or calm, anger or joy, and other emotional states. The words we use and how we put the words together convey more than the information in the message. Depending on the medium of conveying the message, different ways of constructing communication will convey different attitudes and feelings. The tone of communications from an organizational leader should be more formal than friendly. It should convey authority as well as caring about the audience. For instance, if there was a miscommunication about an issue, saying, "oops, I made a mistake," is too informal and a better approach would be to say, "I am sorry that the error in the message was sent and will, in the future, review all outgoing messages. I hope this did not inconvenience or disrespect anyone."

Tone will convey a negative or positive attitude. One approach to creating an inviting message is to begin by setting a positive context, or even offering appropriate praise, before describing a problem. When talking with a staff or faculty member about poor performance, an opening statement such as, "people have been complaining that you have not been doing your job and this cannot continue," will immediately cut off listening. A better approach, one that employs a tone of empathy, might begin with, "I have noticed that you are struggling in getting your job done. Here are three things that worked for me when I was in the role:" The latter example acknowledges the effort and joins the listener in a commitment to solve the problem.

Paul Garland outlines the research that shows, "First, managers are not reliable raters of other people's performance; second, that criticism inhibits the brain's ability to learn; and third, that excellence is idiosyncratic, can't be defined in advance and isn't the opposite of failure." Managers can't "correct a person's way to excellence." (Garland, 2019). Negative criticism and displays of anger, annoyance, or displeasure puts the recipient of the message on guard and defensive, and hardly in a place of potential learning and development. Putting a difficult message into a context of caring about the person as well as the job performance will help to jointly develop a plan with accountability measures. A negative tone will produce defensiveness and anger.

Tone can also be conveyed by pitch and loudness of one's communication. Both men and women tend to select leaders with a lower pitched voice. Women have been referred to as shrill when using a high-pitched voice, and women generally have a higher range in terms of pitch. In communicating verbally either through video (e.g., Zoom), or in-person, it is useful to be aware of the pitch. As a leader becomes more passionate about a topic, their voice may rise. An example is an associate dean who led meetings that could be contentious.

When she tried to make a point in a meeting and people kept asking questions and arguing about the topic, she would communicate by raising her voice, and would lose control of the meeting. She was subsequently coached to be aware that when she gets frustrated the pitch of her voice gets progressively higher and that does not help deliver her message, nor maintain people's attention or confidence. With practice and awareness, she was able to manage her voice and was more successful in managing her team meetings. It is very useful for a leader to be aware of how their emotions influence their tone in communication.

Consider: **Reflect on a time when you had been given the feedback that an email or in-person communication was felt by the receiver as dismissive, disrespectful, or terse. How did you feel when that was not your intent? How did you handle the situation?**

Communicate Important Messages More Than Once and in Different Ways

We often wonder why a policy has not been implemented after we either send a memo describing the new policy or talk about it once. When communication involves change, there will need to be multiple communications. We refer to this as over-communicating because it is a necessary approach for people to really hear the message. Communications can be delivered through different modes including in conversations, newsletters, meetings, webinars, emails, texts or video clips. Communicating in different ways through different media will also address issues of learning styles for staff. There is an array of backgrounds and different learning styles within an organization, and different types of communication are useful in recognizing those differences.

Know Your Stakeholder Audience

Leaders interact with many different constituencies. Every constituency has people with different backgrounds that create a challenge in constructing effective communications. Knowing the audience for the message and understanding the potential interpretations of the receiver is vital. In constructing a communication plan, the following may be useful questions to consider related to the stakeholder audience:

- Am I sending a message to an individual or group or both?
- Is that person or persons internal or external to the organization?
- Is the person or persons at the same level or role as I within the organizational hierarchy?

- What are the identities of the individuals in the group?
- What are some of the person or persons' interests or responsibilities?
- What does the person or persons need to know and what do they expect to know?

A leader communicates with many different people every day including one-on-one meetings and meetings of small and large groups. The communications can be through hard copy and electronic means including video, audio, text, email, or social media. Each person has their way of learning and hearing messages, so a leader needs to plan the structure of the communication to effectively work with a diverse population.

Internal and External Audiences

There are many internal and external audiences that leaders communicate with on a regular basis. Clinical leaders communicate internally with individuals within their unit as well as outside of their unit including their boss, leaders from other units, and individual staff. They also communicate with patients and family members when on their units. Academic and clinical leaders communicate with a variety of external stakeholders, ranging from governmental agencies, accreditors to consumers. The challenge is crafting messages and interacting personally in a way that best gets the intended message across, engages others in important conversations, and listens to what others say.

Number of People in the Stakeholder Audience

There are communication approaches to consider for in-person or zoom meetings based on the number of people in the communication. Regardless of the number of people you are meeting with, take a moment and deep breath before beginning the meeting so you can be present to the person or people with whom you are meeting. Table 12.2 provides suggestions to think about when communicating in person with small and large groups as well as individuals.

Consider: Who are the stakeholders to target in your everyday communications? How do you communicate with them? What is different about "the what" and "the how" you communicate with each stakeholder group?

Talk to People Directly

We all get used to using a specific type of communication such as email or text, even when we are in an office two doors down from the person to whom we are sending the email. There are reasons to put some communications in

TABLE 12.2. *Suggestions for In-Person or Zoom Meetings based on the Size of Audience (Internal and External).*

Large Group	Small Group	Individuals
Large groups in person or using Zoom (Town Hall meetings, presentations to external stakeholders/groups)	Small Groups in person or using Zoom (Committees, work teams, leadership group, external stakeholders)	Individuals in person or using Zoom (regular meetings with direct or indirect report, your supervisor, an external stakeholder)
Always recognize the mission and vision of your organization	Know the "hearing" preferences of group members and vary the communication such as in-person meetings, use of emails, texts.	Know the format, mode, and type of information that the individual prefers.
Address the "why" you are communicating, data that supports the "why" and the objective of the communication.	Frame the communication in a way that engages members of the group—begin the meeting with an issue that needs input from everyone and move from providing information to asking open ended questions.	Understand the decision-making position—is the person higher level, same level, or is it a direct or indirect report?
Tell a story that has emotional impact to gain the attention of the group and sets the intent of the communication to follow.	Ensure each person participates in the discussion.	Be clear what you want to achieve in the meeting.
Present main message providing context as appropriate	Organize agendas, having the most important items first rather than the easiest.	Listen to understand the person with whom you are meeting.
End with a positive statement about the importance of the message.		Be respectful to the person by being on time.
Repeat the main message several times in different ways.		Confirm the meeting a day before the meeting (done by an assistant or automatic confirmation).
Use words that are simple and commonly understood.		
Use visuals for visual learners.		
Leave time for questions and comments. If there are no immediate responses offer one, saying "you may be wondering..." to facilitate responding.		

writing (e.g., to have a paper trail) but getting up and talking to someone has many benefits, in addition to conveying specific information. Making rounds and being visible is an important way of communicating specific messages, as well as the message of valuing the people that work for you. While email and texts can fit into busy schedules, they must be accompanied by in-person (including Zoom) communication within the organization, as well as with external stakeholders through rounds, town hall meetings, or being present at committee meetings.

Recognize Non-verbal Communication

Non-verbal communication conveys important messages and tells a lot about each person in the dialogue. People who work closely with each other will recognize certain gestures that signify distress, displeasure, concern, relief, joy, fear, confusion, and other emotions. Even strangers can recognize emotions conveyed by non-verbal gestures. What a person wears provides important non-verbal information. For example, a dean that goes to a meeting wearing jeans and a college sweatshirt will be viewed and have their message received very differently than the dean who goes to that same meeting wearing a suit. Depending on the context of the gathering, either may be appropriate. Non-verbal behaviors can include subtle gestures, such as a fleeting facial gesture, running fingers through hair, jiggling a leg, being overly enthusiastic, crossing arms on the chest, and many more. Some non-verbal gestures and behaviors can be distracting, such as making silly faces or waving arms around like a propeller. Leaders can effectively enhance their communication by use of gestures to make points, provide clarity and emphasis, and show enthusiasm. Use of hand gestures as a way of making points can be effective, as well as standing to make a point. Table 12.3 provides examples of different types of non-verbal communication.

COMMUNICATING IN SPECIAL CIRCUMSTANCES

Communicating with Your Boss

There is often a complicated relationship between a leader and their boss. The range of relationships goes from being friends to being competitors and having a contentious relationship. The contentious relationships rarely last very long, and unless there are circumstances that go beyond the relationship, the boss will usually remain. The nature and ease of communicating with a boss depends on several variables: trust, level of commitment to a common goal, ability to communicate, and emotional intelligence of each person. There will be disagreements and trust will allow each person to safely state those

TABLE 12.3. *Examples of Non-verbal Communication..*

Type of Non-verbal Communication	Implications for Leaders
Appearance	Dressing to respect followers and stakeholders consistent with organizational culture and context of the situation includes hair, jewelry, make-up, and clothing choices. Remember that we are all individuals and what's right for one person may be different for another. Posture is part of your appearance and standing suggests confidence, slouching suggests avoidance, disengagement, or fear.
Touch	Leaders should not use touch with their employees unless they have expressed permission by the employee. With permission, the appropriate use of touch can be comforting and reassuring.
Facial expressions	Emotions are readily seen in facial expressions. There is general agreement about the interpretation of expressions reflecting joy, anger, confusion, etc. However, checking with the person about what they are feeling is important before assuming you understand. (Cherry 2019).
Eye contact	Different cultures interpret eye contact differently. Eye contact for some individuals and groups may indicate presence and respect. But it may not be the case for other individuals and groups. (Uono and Hietanen 2015).
Gestures	Emphasis can be added to verbal communications. Emphasis (point to people and things) can be added to describe what you are talking about (draw a circle), and describe emotions (hand pump to show enthusiasm) (Social Triggers, 2018). Don't overdo gestures as they could be distracting.
Space	Different cultures have different preferences about space between people. Consider the cultural preferences and situation. Social distancing during COVID-19 pandemic has influenced our preferences for space (Sorokowska, A. *et al.*, 2017).

disagreements. Trust is also knowing that your boss has your back. There are many stories of people whose boss did not support them in a tough situation. For instance, a chief nurse was told by the CEO that he strongly supported the development of a Designated Education Unit (DEU). At the CEO's leadership meeting, the chief finance officer and the chief medical officer voiced their opposition because of a diversion of resources to the unit. The CEO responded by suggesting perhaps it was not time to move in that direction, and that there would be a careful review process of the impact on costs and benefits. The CNO felt blindsided as she and the CEO had anticipated concerns and planned for responses. The CEO had not informed her of the resistance to the plan. This situation created distrust of the CEO that required follow up by both the CEO and CNO to determine clarity.

While alignment of the commitment to organizational mission, vision, and goals by the leader and boss is critical, it also provides a common language and context for understanding communications leading to a greater likelihood of limiting misunderstood communications. The ability to communicate, of course, has a massive impact on the quality of messaging. As noted above, the ability to listen may be the most important aspect of communication with a boss. Attentive and especially empathic listening gives the opportunity to more fully understand the content and the emotion of the communication. Emotional intelligence, the ability to recognize and manage one's own emotions in a positive way, as well as recognizing and managing the emotions of others, is a very important aspect of managing self and relationships (Goleman, 1995). Having self-awareness, self-management, social awareness, and social management provides the foundation of healthy communication between a leader and boss.

There are several important tips in communicating with your boss. These include:

- If you come to your boss with a problem, also bring options for a solution.
- Do not delegate work to your boss. The help you need is best framed as a request.
- Ask how your boss wants to communicate—regularly scheduled meetings, email updates, texts, or all of the above. Adapting to your boss's communication style will provide the routine of messaging.
- Do not let your boss be blindsided. Communicate all important information in a timely fashion that might come to him or her through some other person.
- Remember that your relationship with your boss is a two-way street, one that requires trust building by both. If something occurs that results in you not trusting your boss, you should make every effort to clarify the situation that resulted in the distrust. You should expect your boss to do the same with you.

Communication that feels easy and unstrained with a boss is often a sign of a very good working relationship. Knowing when, what, where and how to communicate is critical to an effective working relationship. Listening is key to any effective relationship. Both you and your boss should listen carefully to each other.

Engaging in Difficult Conversations

There are many definitions of a difficult conversation. One definition is anything we find difficult to talk about (Stone *et al.*, 1999). The difficulty lies in the emotional context of fearing the outcome of the conversation. The content of a conversation is often not the difficulty, but instead, it is the relationship with the person and the meaning of the conversation in terms of emotional investment. The situation is one in which there is a conflict of ideas, priorities, behaviors, and goals. The key word is the *conflictual* context.

There are many different reasons that a leader will have a difficult conversation. These conversations are usually one-on-one and frequently center around job performance, changes in positions, job termination, and addressing workplace conflicts. Effective, well thought-out communication is critical to convey a difficult message and manage the emotional responses. Difficult communications are highly emotionally charged, and that is why they are difficult. There may be leaders who welcome difficult conversations, but most leaders would prefer to not have them. Difficult conversations are emotionally uncomfortable because the response may be defensiveness from feeling threatened and will likely engender anger, fear, or sadness. While it is useful to plan for a difficult conversation, it is not always possible. Some conversations turn into difficult ones, and it is important to have the skills to manage them effectively in the moment.

Difficult conversations may center on disagreements about resources, priorities, processes, job performance, HR issues (e.g., unfair evaluation or getting a raise), and many others. How you handle the conversation may affect future employment and the ability to have a constructive and trusting working relationship. Suggestions for handling any difficult conversations are:

- Understand that difficult conversations are difficult because of the emotional context and high stakes
- Come to the conversation with optimism and the intent to be respectful
- Be clear about what you want for the outcome
- Know what you are willing to negotiate and what is not negotiable
- Know your plan if you get nothing you want from the conversation
- Be creative in looking for and creating middle ground
- Practice deep breathing to manage your emotions
- Avoid using threatening language such as, "I guess I will have to look for another job"
- If the emotional level gets high, take a break from the conversation. Suggest that you both are emotional about the issue and get a cup of coffee or just say, "let's take a breath and come back"

In addition to the suggestions above, there are several excellent books on having difficult conversations, including *Crucial Conversations: Tools for Talking When Stakes are High* (Patterson *et al.*, 2012) and *Fierce Conversations* (Scott, 2004).

Consider: **Reflect on a time that you had to have a difficult conversation with someone you reported to. How did you prepare for that conversation? Did the conversation go as you had planned? If not, what would you do differently?**

The Art of Saying No

Almost every day as a leader there will be instances where you have to artfully and skillfully say no to your boss, a colleague, a student, or a stakeholder. Sometimes it is because the proposed idea is inconsistent with the organization's direction and strategic plan, or it may be that the idea is not well thought out and fails to recognize its impact on essential dimensions of the organization. Many times, the idea is a good one, but the organization is unable to financially support moving in that direction. The resources are just not available. The way a leader says no to an idea or project is just as important as the decision itself because the individual(s) suggesting a project or idea often have a vested interest in seeing their project come to fruition. The challenge for a leader is to be able to say no in a professional manner while maintaining relationships, preserving the trust of the organization, and retaining a sense of fairness and mutual respect (Perlmutter, 2020).

There are strategies you can use to say no that are helpful in all communications. For example, recognizing the importance and value of each question, idea, or suggestion is a leadership tool that creates a sense of trust in the leader, that every voice has value, and that every idea is worthy of consideration. By creating that sense of trust within their organization, people are encouraged and are not afraid to think big and bring bold, transformative ideas to the conversation. Transparency is a critical communication attribute of the leader, especially when the response is going to be no. Being able to be clear and reasonable about why the decision is no is important. If the response to the request is vague or uncertain or even worse, untruthful, the person or people will become frustrated and trust in the leader will be eroded. A leader's most helpful communications strategy is the pause. By pausing, the leader gets the opportunity to think through the response and craft a message that is supportive of the organization and the members who suggested the idea. The message, "Let me think about this and get back to you," is one of the most powerful communication tools of a leader. That said, if you don't get back about the idea, you will have eroded significant trust.

One of the most important strategies in communicating the message of no is to provide the data that supports the decision. As a leader, you often have a broader view of the organization and access to data that members of the organization do not have. This is especially true around budgets and finances. A data-driven decision-making process is crucial (Perlmutter, 2020). When presenting the data, it's important to acknowledge the original idea and the work that went into formulating it.

Often members of the organization will come forward with a suggested change in process but without clearly defined desired outcomes. By reframing the conversation to defining the desired outcomes, the leader might be able to address the important issues that precipitated the suggestion without having to say no. In this way, the leader finds alternative pathways to support the suggestion, avoiding the need to say no, and hopefully improving the organization through the change (Perlmutter, 2020).

Being fair, equitable and not showing favoritism is an important process of decision-making as a leader. Most leaders have spent a great deal of time in a specific discipline or area of study before assuming a leadership role. If the leader shows preference to one person, one discipline or one area, dismissing suggestions or recommendations from others or financially supporting only their area of practice, the leader loses credibility. For example, a nurse leader in the role of vice president for patient care services has to be as open to suggestions and recommendations from the director of physical therapy and the director of environmental services, as they are from the directors of the nursing units. In academia, a dean who is prepared as a critical care nurse and researcher, must also be invested in the community health curriculum and other program areas. Equitable and data-driven decision-making must be visible and palpable for all employees to have trust that the leader will make decisions in the best interest of the entire organization.

Saying no is never easy, but it is an essential skill of a leader, especially in challenging fiscal times. The approach to communicating the decision is just as important as the decision itself. By focusing on the decision in the context of the organization's goals and strategies, the leader avoids making the decision a personal choice. However, paying attention to and managing the emotion of others when a leader does say no will build trust.

Use of Electronic Communications

Electronic communications have enabled efficiency and expansion of communication. It also brings challenges in terms of how leaders relate to others. The number of daily messages for a leader can be overwhelming. Many emails are simply informational, including being copied on emails to others. There are many tips to manage the volume of email. Some basic ways include:

- Designate specific times twice a day to go through emails and let people know this
- Do a quick review and delete junk emails
- Unsubscribe from emails with low value
- Create specific folders for different projects or issues
- Act on each email
    —Respond
    —Move to a folder related to that information
- Keep responses as short and concise as possible
- Get administrative help to do the above

When sending email, it is important to note the tone of the email as described earlier in the chapter. Without the benefit of physical cues such as facial expressions and gestures, there can be significant misunderstandings about an email or text message. A terse email can be interpreted as disrespectful or angry when the intent was to be concise. It is important to let people know your style of writing email, that you are working to keep them short and concise to save not only your time, but the time of the receivers of the messages.

Many organizations have a social media presence and use Twitter, Facebook, Instagram, Reddit, LinkedIn, and other social media platforms to promote their organization and specific unit within the organization. Social media from an organizational perspective is useful for marketing and can reach specific groups with a common interest such as alumni of an academic institution or patients with specific health issues. Information can be posted that is available to the public or can be created through private accounts limiting access to only those approved by the account holder. Even with private accounts, there have been examples of user information being shared, such as Facebook giving app developers user information.

Leaders need to be clear about the purpose and benefits of a social media account for the organization. Is the purpose to create support groups, provide information, market, or other? Maintaining a meaningful social media presence requires resources in terms of someone's time to maintain and update the site(s), creativity in what and how information is communicated, and constant evaluation of the impact, e.g., number of views, how long someone has stayed on the site, the feedback from comments, and the likes. If the site has limited impact, either it needs to be refocused or discontinued.

Many people have personal accounts on social media. While it is great to share family photos and share other personal information, it is unwise for a leader to post political positions, information about their organization, and leadership experiences. A leader should never post an email that can be interpreted as angry or hateful. Many people have had experiences with very negative consequences (such as being fired or not considered for a promotion) with employers seeing posts on social media that are inconsistent with the mission and values of the organization they work for. Most organizations have social media policies, and the leader should be fully aware and compliant with those policies.

Consider: How do you manage the emails you get every day? Do you prioritize them? Take the most difficult ones first? How might you better manage your email traffic? How do you help your staff manage their email? Have you established guidelines for times to send and not send email?

Brand Management Communication

Brand management communication is messaging that puts a brand in a positive light and communicates the value of the brand. A leader is responsible for promoting the organization's brand as well as their individual brand. Attention was brought to the importance of a personal leadership brand by Tom Peters (1997). There should be a strong relationship between the personal leadership brand and the organizational brand to be effective in communicating who you are, what you value, and your commitment to the organization as a leader. It also needs to be concise and understandable by a widely diverse audience. Every communication should reflect your personal brand as well as the brand of the organization. The commonalities of a personal brand and nursing education or clinical service could be the importance of science-based care, commitment to quality, and compassionate care. The brand would need to be distinguishing and consider the unique commitments such as creating partnerships, caring for vulnerable populations, commitment to addressing social determinants of health, creating high performing teams, and conducting turn arounds on poor performing care delivery. Some organizations have people use their strengths as a personal brand assessed by a tool such as VIA strengths (Peterson and Seligman, 2004) or Gallup's Clifton Strengths (Rath, 2007). The leader's description of their distinguishing characteristics is essential in the personal brand. Whatever your personal brand is, it must align with the mission and vision of your organization.

The Center for Creative Leadership (CCL) (2021) provides ideas about how to create a brand to advance both a leader's career as well as the work of the organization. CCL recommends thinking process not position. A title does not create a brand. How you work with others to achieve the mission and vision of the organization should be the basis of the brand. It is important to recognize that others have perceptions of what you get done and how you work. You need to be aware of what others think about how you work. At the same time, be aware of how you learn, communicate, make decisions, influence others, and get things done. Determine what aspects of these is the brand you want to be known for and what you would change in terms of how others understand you. Having others see you in the way you want to be seen takes focused efforts and a personal strategic plan.

It is useful to continually reflect on what your personal brand is and how that forwards the mission and work of your organization. As a leader within an organization, every communication reflects the brand of the organization. If the leader's brand is a mismatch with the brand and culture of the organization, the nursing unit or school will be at odds in goals, decision-making, and ultimately productivity. People will feel the difference in the mission and culture of the organization and that of their leader. An example is a mismatch of an organizational brand that values service to students or patients and the leadership brand is to streamline the organizational unit to be more profitable. This difference can create considerable dissonance that could lead staff to looking for other jobs. Alignment of leadership brand and organizational brand is important.

CREATING A COMMUNICATIONS PLAN

A communications plan will clarify the sharing of information to achieve a goal(s) and is useful to advance the strategic plan, as well as day to day operations and processes. A plan will also clarify the consistent messaging to individuals and teams such as meeting reminders, minutes of meetings, newsletters, etc. It is particularly important when any change of policy or process is planned. Creating a communications plan also provides an opportunity to engage key stakeholders.

The communications plan, for whatever purpose, should include key information including the topic, purpose/objectives, audience, content, timing, method, and person responsible. The process of developing the communications will provide the opportunity for meaningful interaction among leaders and their staff. If the communication plan requires resources beyond what may be integrated in annual budgets, the various costs related to communication will need to be integrated into a budget. Budgetary items can include consultants, advertisements in print and electronic media, communications personnel, and other costs. An example of some elements of a communications plan related to the roll out of a strategic plan is shown in Table 12.4.

CRISIS COMMUNICATION

A crisis is defined as any event that will or may lead to a dangerous or unstable situation affecting individuals, groups, a community, or a whole society (Wikipedia, 2021). In an organization, a crisis is any situation that is threatening or could threaten to harm people, harm property, significantly damage reputation, and/or negatively affect the bottom line (Bernstein, 2016). By definition, a crisis usually refers to an event with negative consequences that is serious and calls for the attention from leadership. Crises can arise from events out of our control such as hurricanes, earthquakes, threats of pandemics, droughts, and other natural events. In healthcare organizations, a crisis could involve reputational risk such as a high-profile lawsuit that impugns the integrity and character of a hospital, or a pandemic. In an academic setting, crises could include the death of a student, a shooting on campus, or a scandal involving a high-profile athletic department. Regardless of the crisis, the communications with the internal and external community are a critical responsibility of the leader.

TABLE 12.4. Example of a Communications Plan.

Topic	Objectives	Audience	Content	Method of Delivery	Timing	Person Responsible	Additional Costs
Ongoing information sharing strategic plan	Provide information about the status of the plan. To engage staff in implementation of strategic plan Recognize successes of strategic plan	All staff	Status of activities related to goals and progress metrics	Email Town hall meetings Video	Monthly	Dean, CNO with assistance from communications staff or administrative staff	None
Progress of the plan	Review the progress metrics of the plan Decide on adjustments to the plan	Leadership Team	Review specific metrics and discuss changes that may need to be made as well as changes in action plan	In-person or electronic meeting	Bi-weekly	Dean, CNO	None

Crisis communications are the strategies employed by the leader to prepare for an impending crisis, deal with the crisis during the event, and manage the post crisis period as the organization transitions to a new normal. The goals of crisis communication are many and include preparing the members of the organization for what is to come (and if the work of the organization will continue or be suspended), helping members address the issues that the crisis brings, protecting and preserving the economic and reputational resources of the organization (so that the organization will survive the crisis), and then preparing for back to normal operations once the crisis has subsided.

The communications landscape is complicated and will continue to get more complicated as technology evolves and the opportunity for misinformation and rumor grows. Today, everyone has a cell phone, the ability to take real time videos and photos, and share that with the world on social media outlets. The impact of social media can cause a firestorm that is not easily managed, so proactive approaches to a crisis are essential. The 24 hours news cycle adds to the ease of the transmission of negative information about an organization which could provide serious consequences that also need to be managed. Because the problem is complex, approaches to crisis communications are multifaceted and complex. There is probably no more important role for the leader than leading during a crisis.

Strategies for Managing Crises Communication

While it is unlikely there is a one size fits all type of crisis, there are several strategies that have been found to be effective in reducing the impact of the crisis on the members of the organization and the organization itself. Remember that, when a crisis occurs, every member of the organization feels the impact from the crisis and internalizes the impact of the crisis. For example, people might wonder if their job is secure or if the organization will continue to exist after the crisis is over. If there was an ethical lapse in an organization that spurred the crisis, employees might feel embarrassed by what has happened and feel that the external environment will see their whole organization, including them, as flawed. There may be conflict between members of the organization based on what each believes about who was "at fault" for initiating the crisis. In the case of a widespread infectious disease outbreak, hospital staff may worry about their own health, about infecting their families, and wonder when they will be able to return to a normal life. Whatever the crisis, people will view the magnitude, impact, and outcome through their own lens and will respond to it in a unique way. Leaders must be ready for and open to different perspectives, views, and reactions to any crisis.

Regardless of the type or scope of a crisis, members in the organization will look to the leader to be calm, poised, and project confidence, ready to make decisions to guide the organization forward. This does not mean that you can't be frightened about the crises and ask yourself if you are up to the task of leading others through a difficult, challenging, and usually emotionally laden event or set of events. However, nothing instills more fear in an organization than if the leader appears unprepared to lead, unorganized, and erratic. The calm, caring, empathic, and supportive demeanor of the leader will instill confidence in the members of the organization which will help to reduce the impact of the crisis. Even if the leader is unsure of the future, all communications should work to instill confidence in the staff and build trust in leadership.

One aspect of crisis management is for an organization to have a crisis management or emergency preparedness plan in place which establishes the potential response depending on the type of crisis. This becomes the starting point for invoking the response team, establishes an organizational framework depending on the type of crisis, and helps define the pre-crisis preparedness. Crisis communication activities can be organized in three categories: pre-crisis activities, crisis activities, and post-crisis activities as shown in Table 12.5.

Pre-crisis Strategies

Many organizations go through the motions of preparing for a significant crisis, thinking it will never happen and they will not have to launch the sequence of activities that have been developed as part of the risk management plan. But, these organizations thoughtfully and comprehensively develop continency plans. Preparing for a crisis and the communications that will necessarily flow from that difficult situation is critical to be able to quickly and effectively address the crises that is looming over the organization. Unless an organization develops contingency plans before the crisis occurs, they may be unable to effectively manage the crisis. Building an effective communication system that can be expanded in the face of a crisis will allow the organization to rapidly address the issues they will face as the crisis unfolds.

Consider the crisis associated with the pandemic of 2020. Without an effective communications structure in place, faculty, staff, and students in universities would not have been able to effectively exit the campus and reduce the spread of the virus in the university community. Hospitals would not have been able to communicate the processes and procedures for acquiring personal protective equipment or managing the staffing on the units. Communicating the change from in-person care to telehealth and how to manage that practice was essential to keeping health care available in the community. Letting all the healthcare workers know how to protect themselves, what special protocols to use, and how much they were appreciated was the result of having an effective communication strategy in place before the crisis occurred.

Before a crisis ever occurs, there are several strategies that an organization can do to get ready for such an event. Assessing where the organization's vul-

TABLE 12.5. Crisis Communication Actions.

Stage of Strategy Preparation	Strategies for Leaders
Pre-crisis Strategies	• Identify the organization's vulnerabilities/risks • Reduce risks as much as possible, communicate protocols, processes, and procedures • Create the structure for the communications team • Decide who will be the spokesperson • Establish notification and monitoring systems • Develop contingency plans for communication if everyone is separated • Build a social media presence to use during a crisis
Crisis Strategies	• Communicate, communicate, communicate • Make sure the communications are clear, consistent, and accurate • Create a staging plan for distribution of messages • Express empathy, sympathy, and support • Be authentic but express optimism • Be transparent about what you know and what you do not know • Deal with crisis but do not forget the daily operations of the organization • Gather information from as many voices as possible • Communicate both the what and the how of dealing with the crisis • Keep the web updated
Post-Crisis Strategies	• Assess the crisis situation. Complete an after-action review. Were you ready? What were the outcomes? Were the right people in place? • Continue communicating the important messages. • Let the community know what you have learned from this experience. What will you be taking into the future? What could have been done better? • Create a plan to assess and address the emotional impact of the crises.

nerabilities or risks lie helps the leader understand what protocols, processes, and procedures will need to be put in place to avoid or reduce the impact of the crisis. Communicating those protocols, policies, and procedures are essential so that everyone in the organization knows what to do when a risk arises. The process of developing a risk reduction plan might seem like time spent for work that will never be used but it is critical to have these plans in place when difficult times arise. The Jeanne Clery Disclosure of Campus Crime Statistics Act of 1990 (Jeanne Clery, 2018) was passed to improve campus safety for students and the entire community. It was named for a Lehigh University student who was murdered in her dorm room. Educational institutions are required by the Clery Act to have an emergency preparedness plan and make it available on their primary website.

Every organization should have a system that supports rapid notification of its members of essential information. In addition, the leader should be able to monitor how widely that information has been consumed. There are programs that provide data on how many of the messages sent have been open, for how long they were open, and if they were forwarded to others. These data provide essential information about the penetration of the messages being sent. The organization should also plan for alternate means of communication if the phone lines and cell phone towers are disabled. All of these approaches are organized in the risk management plan that is ready to be deployed in the face of a crisis. Implementing and periodic testing of an emergency notification system is another requirement of educational institutions defined in the Clery Act.

Today, most organizations have a social media presence which may be robust and informative, or merely a collection of out-of-date information. Building a social media presence that becomes a trusted and visible source of information before a crisis provides you with a platform where both the internal and external community will naturally go to receive information and updates about how the organization is managing a crisis. A strong social media presence will allow the organization to use social networking tools to communicate the same messages they are sending out via email or are posting on their website. This level of information distribution is essential, recognizing that today's consumers get information in many different ways. Building that robust information infrastructure before the crisis provides you with the avenues for communication when a crisis develops.

An important strategy is to assemble a communications team. This team should include the communications director, someone from the emergency response team, and the leader at a minimum. Often legal counsel will sit as a member of that team. Depending on the size of the organization, it is important to include someone from the organization whose advice is valued and trusted, or an informal leader who is looked up to by members of the organization. The key is to create a team of people who have exemplary communication skills, those who understand the nuances of the organization, and those who are team players.

It will be important for all leaders in the organization to speak with one voice. Deciding who will be the spokesperson for the organization is a critical first decision to be made by the crisis communication team if it was not made before the crisis occurred. Confusing messages from leaders, or the presence of multiple leaders saying different things, will only increase anxiety in the organization and result in people spending time trying to find out what is right and how they are being impacted. In a crisis, it is helpful for all communications to constituent groups within the organization to come through the CEO or chair of your communications team so that there are no differing messages from different leaders. This is not to say that one person should make all the decisions. Because a crisis often requires quick assessments and decisions, a leader should work with the leadership team to define roles and the decision-making responsibility for each member of the team. In a crisis, decision-making cannot wait for usual protocols and leadership team members need to understand their role in the crisis response plan. By having a point person supervise all significant communications to the community, discrepancies in policy and process can be identified before they are broadly distributed.

Crisis Strategies

One of the key principles in a crisis is that the organization should communicate-communicate-communicate. If an organization is not letting people know what the crisis is about, what they are expected to do and how the organization is responding, the members of the organization will create and perpetuate their own reality about the crisis. Again, the Clery Act requires educational institutions to communicate in a timely manner any events, internal and external, which may impact the safety of members of the educational community. Accreditation of hospitals, nursing homes and other agencies have standards requiring a crises management strategy that include having a communications plan.

Once the communications team is assembled, decide what the objectives for this team will be. At a minimum, this team should have the responsibility for creating the messages that will be sent out to the community, logging the information into a database so employees have easy access to the messages over time, and staging messages in a way that is most informative for the constituents. Receiving five messages in the span of an hour on one subject assures that none of them will get read. By staging them on separate times during the day or on separate days, if possible, chances increase that they will have an impact. Staging also means that the information from the parent organization may need to come out before the information from the unit of the hospital or school in a university. For example, the university president might send the deans an email describing the universities response to a crisis with directions to each dean to send a message to their constituency customizing the general direction to the unique aspects of the school. Staging will allow the president's message to go out first, followed by the dean's message.

A key to these communications is timing and transparency, letting people know what you know about the crisis and being honest when you do not know an answer. Certain communications need to be carefully timed based on the context of the crisis. The more one communicates, generally, the better. Transparency builds trust and trust builds confidence that their leader will lead them to a positive outcome. Members of an organization would rather hear their leader say they do not know than finding that what they were told was untrue. It is also important for a leader to help people understand that, at times, as a crisis is unfolding, what is true today might not be true in the future. For example, in the case of the COVID-19 pandemic of 2020, the processes and protocols for operation changed each day as we learned more and more about the infectious disease. Helping the members of the organization realize that you will be honest and transparent with them as information changes will help reduce their stress.

Knowing how frequently to communicate with the constituents is often a delicate balance. Too many messages distract people from focusing on their important work during this difficult time, too few messages and people feel isolated and they begin creating their own version of what is happening in the organization. In times of fear and uncertainty, people look to their leaders for guidance, reassurance, and meaning. They look for messages that are clear, concise, and accurate so there is no question about their role. The leader must be authentic in realistically recognizing the scope of the crisis, but optimistic to provide hope for the community that there are strategies that can be used to mitigate its effect. Being overly optimistic, dismissive, or too negative will cause fear and uncertainty in the community. A leader should err on the side of over-communicating rather than leaving the community with gaps in knowledge creating stress and fear for the future.

There are two kinds of messages that a leader can send to an organization in a crisis. The first kind of message is focused on guidance; facts and information that will help people do their job during a turbulent time. This might include changes in standard operating procedures, new rules and regulations, or new ways to conduct business. For example, in the pandemic of 2020, hospital leaders had to get information out to their employees about the epidemiology of the virus, the use of personal protective equipment, what to do if they had symptoms, and revised human resources policies and processes. In academia, faculty, staff, and students had to be informed of new approaches to delivering the educational material, the resources they had available to accomplish this goal, how clinical experiences were going to be addressed, and what the rules were for entering the campus. For example, one educational institution used the following Flow Chart in Figure 12.2 for faculty, staff, and students to let them know what to do when they were returning to campus. By providing specific and timely information, leaders help to allay the anxiety of their staff. Staff who know what they are expected to do and how to do it are better prepared to deal with a crisis. At the beginning of the crisis, these messages will come out daily, or more often if needed, and taper off as the crisis comes under control.

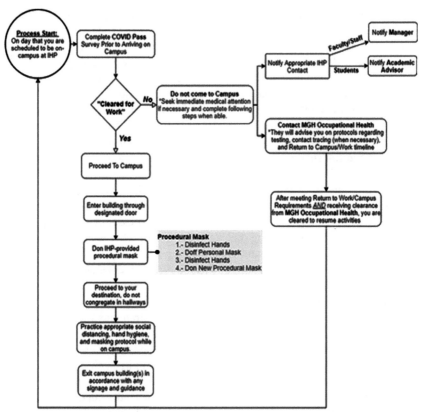

FIGURE 12.2 Flow Chart Example. (Used with Permission: Denis Stratford and Taylor Wallace; MGH Institute of Health Professions 2020).

The second type of message is one of inspiration, encouragement, and support for the work people are doing individually and collectively in turbulent times. This is more focused on the emotional intelligence of your community rather than protocols and policies. These messages should authentically relay the support and encouragement for the members of the organization. You might think that these messages are not as important as the ones that share information but for some of the staff, these messages are what keeps them engaged and moving forward in difficult times. For everyone, it humanizes the crisis and lets people know that they are not alone, and their feelings are shared by many. These messages tend to be more heartfelt, focused on the positive events that have happened in the organization, provide encouragement and thanks to the staff for their extraordinary work, and continue to stress that we are all in the situation together. These messages will come out less frequently than the informational messages but need to be included as an integral component of the communication plan. The objective of these messages is to allay as much anxiety as possible and recognize the difficult work that staff are doing.

In addition to the messages that you send to your organization, it is critical for the leader to keep stakeholders informed on a regular basis of how your organization is responding to the crisis. In academia that might be your external advisory board, dean's council, or philanthropy council. In the hospital setting, the external stakeholder might include donors, external advisory boards, or clinical partners. Messages to these groups are designed to keep friends of the organization informed about decisions made and potential challenges to be faced. By keeping the external stakeholders informed of how the crisis is being managed, the leader validates the importance of your most trusted colleagues and engages them in the future of the organization.

Depending on the nature of the crisis, the press might reach out about a difficult situation. In some organizations, there is an office for strategic communications that handles all these issues, and the leader should refer the situation to that office. In other organizations, the leader will be responsible for managing the crisis communication for the events that happen in their clinical department or school. For example, in academia, the press might be informed about a student who filed a Title IX complaint which addresses the protection of people from discrimination based on sex in educational programs or activities that receive federal financial assistance. The first thing a leader needs to do is to make sure their staff knows that the press is interested in talking about the situation, and they should not provide any information to the press. In addition, they should be informed that if they are contacted by the press, those requests should be referred to the department's communications director. In this case, Title IX is covered by the Family Education Rights and Privacy Act (FERPA) and faculty and staff are required to protect the student's privacy. In all cases, the leader will want to manage the message to the press in both content and timing. Speaking with one voice at this time is critical. The leader will engage the communications team to develop a plan for responding to the press that will include whether to respond at all and the content and timing of the message if a response is warranted.

If the decision is made to respond to the press, it is critical that the leader communicate with the key stakeholders first and then the media. Your internal community, board of trustees, or advisory groups should never read something in the newspaper before they have heard it from the leader. Once the internal stakeholders are notified, timeliness of communication with the media is essential. If the leader waits too long, the media may create their own version of the facts before the actual facts are revealed. The message to the press must be carefully crafted to provide facts without divulging any protected information. If mistakes were made, work with the legal counsel to determine how transparent you can be in admitting those mistakes in judgment or policy and communicating the steps the institution will take to address the problem so that it does not happen again. Once your message is crafted and approved by legal counsel, controlling the distribution to the media is critical to getting the message out and having it fade as quickly as possible. By sending out a press release to all media outlets at once, you can often reduce the number of days a story runs. By controlling both the message and the timing, the organization is able to reduce reputational impact and get back to normal operations as soon as possible.

The press is not the only source of external messaging leaders deal with today. Social media has transformed the way people get information because everyone has a cell phone to take photos and videos, and access to platforms that allows information to be shared broadly. In a crisis, administrative and organizational leadership will follow social media outlets but knowing which people within the organization have a large media impact can be helpful. These individuals can help identify the character of the information on the web as well as shape the message in a way that would be helpful to the organization. In the clinical setting, these individuals might be trusted nurses, aides, or clerical staff and in the academic setting it might be student government leaders or leaders of clubs on campus. These individuals need to be identified and prepared in advance of any crisis and helped to know the institutional messages that can and should be shared during the crisis phase. Using social media proactively is an effective tool in disseminating your story.

Throughout the crisis period, a leaders must be ready and open to listening to their constituencies. Members of your community who have complex life situations will respond differently to a crisis than perhaps the leader or the senior leadership team. For example, during the pandemic crisis, some nurses were afraid of bringing the coronavirus home to their children or elderly parents. Some staff, deemed essential workers, had preexisting conditions making them more vulnerable to the serious impact of the virus and feared being in the hospital. Still others were trying to manage childcare and work because schools were not in session. Just as with other areas of leadership, a leader should be making decisions about strategy based on data. By actively listening through focus groups, task forces, or surveys, the leader will have the data to create a plan to address the needs of the constituents. You might consider creating a "voice of the staff" or "voice of the faculty" task force that provides information to the senior administration about the issues faculty or staff are facing.

Once a plan to address those issues is created, communicating the message of support, understanding, and help can bring a community together during difficult times. By only listening to the senior administrative team, the leader gives the community the message they are not interested in the unique challenges that members of the community face.

While managing and communicating in a crisis can be consuming for a leader, it is critical to remember that the role of the leader is to lead all aspects of the organization, even in the face of a crisis. Diverting most or all attention to the crisis for a prolonged period of time will result in secondary crises being developed when the primary crisis begins to fade. Communicating to the community that there is work that is happening in the organization outside the specifics of the crisis can build confidence that a strong organization will exist when the crisis is over. Examples of business as usual in a crisis could be continuing with a building project, continuing with the promotion process for faculty or staff, or continuing with the hiring process for critical roles within the organization. Keeping the organization informed of the activities that cannot be done because of the crisis in addition to the ones going forward helps the organization stay focused on how it is achieving its mission.

Post Crisis Strategies

Communication with the community does not stop when the crisis is over. In fact, some of the most important communications will be when everyone feels like the acute crisis is over and the leadership must take the organization to a new normal. Often a crisis will allow a leader to make much needed changes in the organization that were resisted by members of the community before a crisis. For example, in a school of nursing, faculty might have been resistant to supporting clinical placements in telehealth or virtually. When the coronavirus became widespread, most in-person clinical placements were cancelled, and students were unable to progress in their academic programs. Faculty who engaged in telehealth practice found that students had a meaningful clinical education experience and learned a skill that will be critical to the future of healthcare delivery. These faculty will be the early adopters to transform the way we provide clinical education in health professions programs for the future.

Following a crisis, a leader will assess the crisis situation and the organization's response. What was the impact of the crisis on key elements of the organization such as reputation or finances? What was done well, and what could have been done better in responding to the crisis? What was needed for the organization to have a more responsive approach to the crisis? If there are changes in the financial health of the organization because of the crisis, the leaders should be ready to explain the impact of a budget deficit. Will there be layoffs or furloughs? What resources will be cut that affect the day-to-day work of the staff? Will benefits be affected? Will the impact be short term or long term?

The importance of honesty and transparency on these financial issues cannot be overstated. Reassuring the members of the community where possible and sharing uncertainties where they exist helps the members of the organization mitigate their anxieties about the future. For example, in response to the question about layoffs, a leader may say, "It is the organization's goal to not lay off anyone and we have no plans to lay off anyone at this time. If the financial health of the organization worsens, we will have to reexamine that strategy, but we are working hard to retain all of our employees." In this way, the leaders share their strong commitment to each member of the workforce but recognize that, if things change, the strategy might have to change. Communication to the community about the status of the organization, what was learned, and how the organization plans to use the lessons learned in the crisis to advance or even transform the organization is a critical element of creating an environment for healing.

Leadership in a crisis can be a determining factor in the success of a leader. How a leader communicates important messages of hope and resilience as well as operational changes will define how that leader is viewed by their organization. The three phases of crisis communication begin before a crisis is even known and continues through a period after the crisis is over. Communication at each step is critical to a successful outcome for the leader and the organization.

Consider: **How have you managed crisis communication or witnessed someone managing communications during a crisis? What worked and what did not work in the way you or the other person managed?**

COMMUNICATION AS A TOOL FOR ORGANIZATIONAL INTERVENTION

Although the examples of communication used throughout this chapter focus largely on the elements of communication among individuals and groups, it is critical to consider the impact the leader's communication has on the organization. You, as leader, convey an understanding of the organization's culture when you communicate, in written or verbal forms. Humility, respect, kindness, compassion, positivity, hope, and encouragement form the basis for informative, factual, data oriented and evidence-based messages. The late author Maya Angelou said, "People will forget what you said, people will forget what you did, but people will never forget the way you made them feel." That is another form of communication and the feelings you engender will spread quickly through an organization.

We have discussed many of the tools and methods that leaders need to do their work in organizations; however, how leaders communicate is both an art and a science. In organizational work, the leader has the responsibility to create a narrative about the meaning and purpose of the work of the organization especially in times of major organizational change, social unrest, economic strain and global health crises. Communication within an organization can help make sense of what's happening external to the organization and to also help shape people's understanding of why change is important internally.

Conveying how the efforts of employees are valued, or how the current conditions differ from past conditions will help set the context for change. It is through communication that the leader engages with others, creates urgency, shares a vision, establishes resiliency for challenging times, recognizes accomplishments, and celebrates success.

Communication skills are often honed over time and leaders understand that effective communication is essential for shaping the experiences of those they serve and those who they partner with to meet the organizational mission.

SUMMARY

Effective communication is foundational to being an effective leader. It is the means for building trust, conveying a vision and meeting the organizational mission. It is not an exaggeration to say that without well-honed and effective communication skills, there is no leadership. There are many elements of communication described in this chapter that a leader needs to consider. Effectively using the wide range of tools, methods and modes of communication, knowing your internal and external audiences, and communicating important messages more than once highlight just a few key points. Communications planning is essential to leading major organizational change and although effective communication is challenging, it is the bread and butter of leadership.

CRITICAL THINKING QUESTIONS

At the beginning of the chapter an academic and clinical vignette were presented. Please review the vignettes to address the following questions. The questions are specific to the vignettes.

Academic Vignette

1. What do you need to consider in developing your communication with different stakeholders of community leaders, faculty, and students? How will the content of the communication be different for each? What are the critical elements of your communication that need to be incorporated for each stakeholder?
2. How will you communicate the urgency of this effort through different communication modes, including person to person, individual emails, group emails, or group meetings?
3. What elements of communicating up, as well as difficult conversations, will be important in your communication with the dean and the VP?
4. You have noted that mounting the testing sites is urgent and that thinking about crisis communication planning will be useful. What is your plan?

Clinical Vignette

1. As chief nurse for the life care community organization, you know you have several constituencies to communicate with in responding to the threat of the hurricane. What are the critical communication considerations for each of the stakeholder groups?
2. How will you manage the conversation with the CEO to effectively communicate up, as well as use the elements of a difficult conversation?
3. What does your crisis management communication look like? How are you going to use the various modes of communication and what will the messages be? Which communications are the most critical?
4. Listening to others will be very important in managing this situation. When you have a sense of urgency, how will you manage to listen to others?

REFERENCES

Bernstein, J. (2016). The 10 steps of crisis communication. *Bernstein Crisis Management*.https://www.bernsteincrisismanagement.com/the-10-steps-of-crisis-communications/

Center for Creative Leadership. (2021). *What's your leadership brand?* Center for Creative Leadership. https://www.ccl.org/articles/leading-effectively-articles/whats-your-leadership-brand/

Cherry, K. (2019, September 28). *Understanding body language and facial expressions*. Verywellmind.https://www.verywellmind.com/understand-body-language-and-facial-expressions-4147228

Covey, S. (1989). *The 7 habits of highly effective leaders*. Franklin Covey Co.

Garland. P. (2019). *The Feedback Fallacy*. Harvard Business Review

Goleman, D. (1995). Emotional Intelligence: Why it Can Matter More than IQ. Bantam Books.

Jeanne Clery Disclosure of Campus Security Policy and Campus Crime Statistics Act of 1990, 20 U.S.C.1092(f) (2018).

Kahneman, D. (2011). *Thinking, fast and slow*. Farrar, Straus and Giroux.

Patterson, K., Grenny, J., McMillan, R., & Switzler, A. (2012). *Crucial conversations: Tools for talking when stakes are high*. McGraw-Hill.

Perlmutter, D. (2020). Admin 101: How good leaders say no. *Chronicle of Higher Education*.

Peters, T. (1997, August 31). *The brand called you*. Fast Company. https://www.fastcompany.com/28905/brand-called-you

Peterson, C., & Seligman, M. E. P. (2004). *Character strengths and virtues: A handbook and classification*. American Psychological Association; Oxford University Press.

Rath, T. (2007). *StrengthFinder 2.0*. Gallup Press.

Scott, S. (2004). *Fierce Conversation: Achieving success at work and in life one conversation at a time*. Viking.

Sorokowska, A., Sorokowski, P., Hilpert, P., Cantarero, K., Frackowiak, T., Ahmadi, K., Alghraibeh, A. M., Aryeetey, R., Bertoni, A., Bettache, K., Blumen, S., Blazejewska, M., Bortolini, T., Butovskaya, M., Nalon Castro, F., Cetinkaya, H., Cunha, D., David, D., David, O…. Pierce, J. D. (2017). Preferred interpersonal distances: A global comparison. *Journal of Cross-Cultural Psychology, 48*(4), 577–592. https://doi.org/10.1177/0022022117698039

Stone, D., Patton, B., & Heen, S. (1999). *Difficult conversations: how to discuss what matters most*. Viking.

Social Triggers. (2018, March 16). *How to use hand gestures in a powerful way when you communicate*. Social Triggers. https://socialtriggers.com/21-hand-gestures-for-powerful-communication/

Stratford, D., & Wallace, T. (2020). Concept Map Example. MGH Institute of Health Professions.

Uono, S. & Hietanen, J. K. (2015). Eye contact perception in the West and East: A cross-cultural study. *PLoS ONE, 10*(2), e0118094. https://doi.org/10.1371/journal.pone.0118094

Wikipedia. (2021). *Crisis*. Wikipedia. https://en.wikipedia.org/wiki/Crisis

CHAPTER 13

Creating High Performing Teams

ACADEMIC VIGNETTE

The college of nursing has been under scrutiny by the state board of nursing. The NCLEX pass rate plummeted from an average annual pass rate of 86% down to 75/76% in the past three quarters. The state board of nursing scheduled an on-site full survey that was to happen within 90 days. The dean convened the department leadership committee (DLC) which is made up of the department chairs and the administrative deans. This group of leaders meet bimonthly and they think of themselves as the dean's leadership team. Several of the committee members don't believe they communicate well with each other. There was a shared sentiment among some members that it was often hard to arrive at a decision. They frequently debated issues and couldn't reach a resolution. They have talked about the factors contributing to the decline in NCLEX scores but could not agree on an action plan because everyone saw the causes differently. They are all worried about the work that lay ahead and the short timeline, as well as the outcome of the visit. A possible outcome would be that the program be placed on probation. This would be very upsetting to everyone and would likely decrease interest in the program resulting in a decreased class size requiring budget cuts and loss of jobs. The ability to improve the NCLEX scores requires a high level of teamwork.

CLINICAL VIGNETTE

The nurse executive committee (NEC) of a large community hospital consisted of three associate chief nurses, two executive directors and the chief nursing officer. The committee members thought of themselves as a team that led nursing practice and patient care services operations. A sentinel event occurred a month ago that included a wrong sided chest tube placement in a patient being cared for in a medical unit. This error was reported to the Department of Public Health, the Board of Medicine, and The Joint Commission (TJC). NEC was one of several leadership groups across the organization that was preparing for the DPH site visit.

Generally, NEC members got along pretty well, and were able to come to decisions fairly rapidly. One major concern that many of the members had was that the follow through on decisions had fallen short. One member of the committee seemed to be favored by the CNO and this person often did not complete her work as planned. This created a great deal of frustration for the rest of the team members because her failure to complete the work reflected on the entire team.

INTRODUCTION

Teams are a way of life in healthcare. Teams are two or more people who work together toward a shared goal(s) and the accomplishment of the mission of the organization. A team can be a patient in the ICU with a nurse providing care. A team can be all of the nursing staff covering a specific unit, or people from different disciplines that provide care to a defined population. Having a team in which members have different skills, experiences, and knowledge provides a wider array of ideas that can be brought to bear on a decision.

There are many different types of teams that leaders either lead or are members of. Teams can be intra-professional or interprofessional. Intra-professionally there are nursing teams, physician teams, physical therapy teams, and so on. However, more attention has been given to the importance of interprofessional teams through efforts such as the National Center for Interprofessional Education and Practice, governmental agencies such as the Agency for Healthcare Research and Quality (AHRQ), the Institute for Healthcare Improvement (IHI), and many others that provide resources and opportunities to build effective teams. Such teams have often been referred to in the healthcare literature as interdisciplinary or multidisciplinary, but today, the widely accepted term for teams of providers and clinicians from a diverse set of professions is interprofessional (Freeth *et al.*, 2008).

Why Effective Teams Matter

Collaboration is a process and set of behaviors that team members use to assure shared decision-making. Assuring collaborative decision-making requires effective leadership that sets the stage for respect for each team member's role, knowledge, expertise, and skill. The team leader, in partnership with team members, develops a commitment to a well-defined goal. There is accumulating evidence in healthcare that teams are essential to providing high quality of care to individuals, families, communities, and populations of patients (Weiss and Tilan, 2014). The ability of the team to make good decisions effectively will have an impact on the quality of the product-educational programming or care delivery. We have a long history in the US healthcare system of highlighting the accomplishments of the individual contributor rather than the team contribution. This is not to say that individuals should not be accountable and recognized for their efforts and accomplishments; however, we have learned that creating a culture of safety is dependent upon effective teamwork.

Effective Teams

There are many models of team development and these can be introduced through team training programs. One that has been developed by the American Hospital Association, called "Video Triggered Teamwork Training," is a practical method of simulation-based training. Access to these team training modules can be found in the website www.aha.org/center/performance-improvement/team-training (AHA, 2021).

The aim of having high performing teams that make good decisions, manage conflict, and work well together is paramount in healthcare delivery today. Katzenbach and Smith (1993) in their classic and seminal book *The Wisdom of Teams* which remains highly relevant today, describe the team performance curve (TPC) representing the trajectory leading to a high performing team. The trajectory begins with a working group, characterized as a group of people coming together. The work of the group relies on the efforts of individuals independent of each other. This is followed by the pseudo team that is lower performing than the original group. This level of team performance is enmired in conflict that interferes with individual contributions of the group. Moving through this stage requires leaders to help the team focus on the goals, manage conflict, and begin to trust each other. The next phase is the potential team that is heading in the right direction but still needs clarity about the goals and how to work together. Katzenbach and Smith state that the, "steepest performance gain is between the potential team and the real team." When the real team stage is met, the team is committed to the goal, bring their complementary skills to reach that goal, and members hold themselves accountable for success, individually and collectovely. The real team can go even further to the "high performing" stage, in which team members are deeply committed to each other's development and the success of the team. Teams that are short lived or have high turnover will have great difficulty getting to the high performing stage.

Tuckman (1965), in another seminal contribution, is well known for his model of team development including the stages of forming, storming, norming, and performing. During the forming stage, team members are polite in

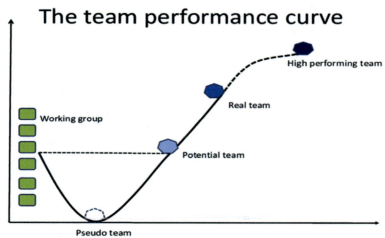

FIGURE 13.1 Stages of High Performing Teams. Katzenbach and Smith (1993).

getting to know other team members. At this stage teams often are not clear what the work of the team is, or what they are expected to contribute. The storming stage is when teams often flounder and fail. For instance, team members may question and disagree with the goals of the team. They may challenge the authority of the leaders and there may be conflict among team members. It takes an effective team leader to manage a team through this stage. During the norming stage, team members understand and work with the leader, resolve conflicts, and recognize the strengths that each team member brings to the team. During the performing stage, the team works collaboratively to accomplish their tasks to achieve the goals. Some teams are permanent structures within an organization, and others adjourn after completing their work. Adjourning may create a sense of loss for some team members, both in terms of the meaningfulness of the work and interactions with other team members. Helping team members anticipate the adjournment, as well as celebrating the accomplishments, are useful during this phase.

What Makes an Effective Team?

There are several models of effective teams. All are useful in thinking through what contributes to effective teams. We will discuss three models that we have found to be particularly useful.

Katzenbach and Smith Model

The first model is the Katzenbach and Smith model of team basics as noted above. In this model, the outputs are at the points of the triangle. (See Figure 13.2). The sides of the triangle are the major elements with the inner triangles being the behaviors necessary to achieve the elements. For instance, having problem solving ability along with technical and interpersonal capabilities are essential skills, and having those skills contributes to the collective work products and performance results.

Lencioni Model

To address elements necessary for effective teamwork, Lencioni (2002) identified five dysfunctions of a team that are presented in a pyramid, representing a flow of dysfunctions that lead to failure to achieve results. For team effectiveness, each dysfunction needs to become a team function. The dysfunctions include absence of trust (which is foundational to poor outcomes), fear of conflict, lack of commitment, avoidance of team accountability, and inattention to team results or objectives. See Figure 13.3.

Absence of Trust

The most important of the dysfunctions is at the base of Lencioni's triangle and is trust. In this model, trust is the critical element that is foundational to an effective team. Lack of trust will create fear of being vulnerable with oth-

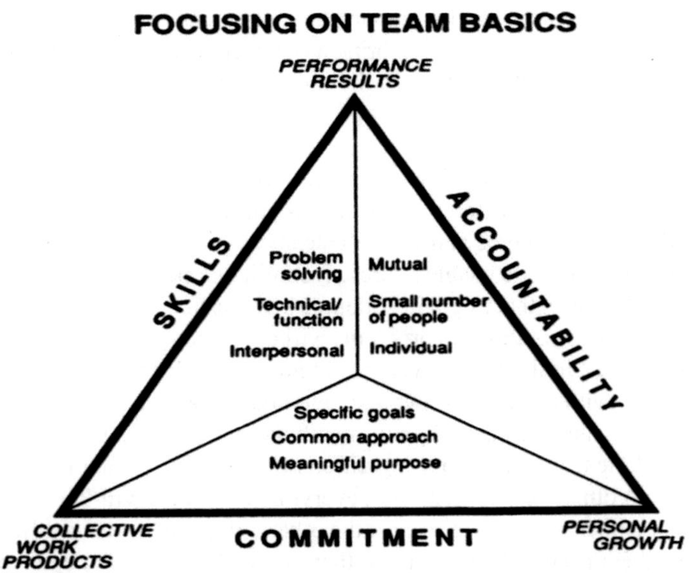

FIGURE 13.2 Model of Team Basics. Katzenbach and Smith (1993).

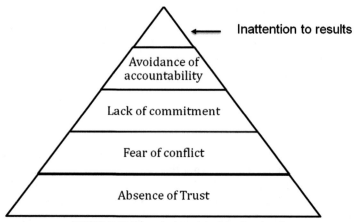

FIGURE 13.3 Lencioni Model of Dysfunctional.

ers, admitting mistakes, or asking for help. This creates an environment where small mistakes can lead to big problems, with people not being able to fully understand or execute what they are expected to do. The culture of a team that lacks trust is one that is judgmental, critical of each other, and competitive.

Fear of Conflict

Fear of conflict in the service of maintaining artificial harmony prevents open and critical conversations. We each bring a perspective to our work, whether in a clinical or academic setting, that is a lifetime of experiences that lead us each to contribute to identifying and solving a problem, establishing priorities, and creating processes that serve to better patient care and educational programs. Having honest and open discussions about important decisions is the way to get the best decisions. When team members feel safe to put their opinions forward to the team and examine the pros and cons, the team can make decisions and take effective action. If they are unable to present conflicting perspectives respectfully and accept decisions that might not support their particular positions, ideas can be stifled, creative solutions to problems will not be considered, and teams will be compromised in their effectiveness. Team members will create back channels and talk, with and about other team members, that impede open conversation with the team. Cliques of team members may form that will undermine the work of the team. We also bring different personalities that may come into conflict with others on the team. Not everyone on a team will like each other, but each member will need to respect the others. When personal conflict arises, team members need to feel confident that this will be managed equitably and respectfully by the members and the team leader.

Lack of Commitment, Accountability, and Results

When there is a lack of trust and avoidance of conflict, there will be a lack of commitment of team members to the team. The lack of commitment shows up in missed meetings, consistently coming to meetings late, and not completing work that was assigned or agreed upon to complete. Decision-making is compromised and there is ambiguity in the outcome of team meetings, especially who will do what and when. When there is a lack of commitment to the team, there will be a lack of accountability. Team members will be reluctant to call out other team members who may not be doing their fair share of work. If there is no accountability, why should I be accountable and have to pick up other people's work? The tip of the triangle captures the final outcome, which is inattention to results or the objectives of the team. This then may ripple through the entire team with even highly motivated individuals feeling that the team is ineffective and decide to participate in a limited way or not at all. The result is that the team does not meet the objectives, and patient care and student learning may be compromised. Table 13.1, includes actions team leaders might consider in avoiding or managing team dysfunctions. With each of the dysfunctions, leaders may need to work with individual team members outside of the group, and potentially remove them from the team if necessary.

Lombardo and Eichinger Model

Another model of team development was created by Lombardo and Eichinger (1995) and known as the T7 Model. This model is considered by many scholars to be the most comprehensive framework because it includes internal as well as external factors that contribute to team function (Korn Ferry Institute (2016). Each of the factors noted begin with T and therefore the name T7. The internal factors include:

- Internal Factors:
  —*Thrust*: the team has a common purpose team goal.
  —*Trust*: Team members can rely and have confidence each other including the leader.
  —*Talent*: The team members' collective skills can accomplish the goal.
  —*Teaming skills*: The team knows how to work together to solve problems, manage conflict, and move work forward.
  —*Task skills*: Team members can skillfully and successfully complete tasks.
- External Factors
  —*Team leader fit*: The extent that the leader can work effectively with the team to accomplish the goals.
  —*Team support from the organization*: Leadership of the organization

supports the work of the team with resources and decision-making authority.

While each team development model or framework provides a different constellation of factors important to team effectiveness, there are overlapping components and commonalities. These are trust, having clarity and commitment to goals, effective and efficient processes to do the work, accountability of individuals and the team, and having the right skills to get the work done. It may be useful to identify a model to move your team forward or to combine elements of different models. It is important and necessary work to develop trust and recognize that it takes time, thoughtfulness, and resources to build effective teams.

TABLE 13.1. Lencioni's Dysfunctions and Team Leader Actions
(Lencioni, 2002).

Lencioni's Dysfunctions	Leader Actions
Lack of Trust	• Role model asking for help • Admit mistakes • Support team members to admit mistakes and ask for help • Do team building exercises requiring trust • Share stories of team trust and distrust
Fear of conflict	• Help team members know what healthy conflict looks like • Share stories of conflict management • Create a situation that should generate conflict and then debrief • Acknowledge when teams manage conflict well
Lack of commitment	• Set clear expectations for actions needed by each team member; who, what, when, and where • ·Ensure each team is heard • Ensure decisions are transparent
Avoidance of accountability	• Provide feedback on work accomplished and goals met • Have consistent progress reviews • Keep team members to agreed-upon deadlines • Support team members providing feedback about a team member not being accountable; focus on the task not the person
Inattention to results/objectives	• Begin with building trust

CRITICAL SKILLS OF A TEAM LEADER

Build Trust

Building trust is critical as noted in each of the models above. A climate of openness, trust, and forthright communication is the basis of highly effective and collaborative teams. Teams that are composed of leaders and followers who see themselves as interdependent are teams that innovate, continuously learn, and try new things together because they are curious and willing to work together to solve problems.

Trust is earned. Many leaders believe that people should trust them because they are in a leadership position. Unfortunately, there are also leaders who believe that creating a competitive environment to keep people off balance will create innovation. Most people are willing to give leaders an opportunity to prove themselves. In order to earn trust, there are several critical actions that leaders need to take. Leaders will earn trust through creating a safe team environment, knowing each of the team members, being honest, being consistent, keeping their word, acknowledging mistakes, facilitating constructive team dynamics, and not playing control games.

Create Psychological Safety

Leaders should routinely frame the work of the team in a way that explicitly acknowledges that team members are interdependent and that they need each other to perform well. Helen Keller noted the importance of working together in her quote, "alone we can do so little; together we can do so much." A major component of team effectiveness is that the diversity of team members is embraced and enabled to share a wide array of ideas that drive teamwork. To do that, psychological safety must be attended to by team leaders so that it is the norm for team members to be themselves, ask questions, express concerns, and even make mistakes. Psychological safety establishes a shared belief among team members that interpersonal risk taking is encouraged. This is role-modeled by the team leader in their expression of fallibility. It can be defined as, "being able to show and employ one's self without fear of negative consequences of self-image, status or career" (Khan, 1990, p. 708).

Amy Edmondson (2012) describes leadership actions that promote effective teaming and include: framing the work for continuous learning; making it psychologically safe to ask questions and pose alternatives; and conveying that mistakes happen and when they do, the team will learn from them. Leaders communicate and hold up the purpose of the team, the "why we are here, what is the work, and why it is important." Leaders model their own fallibility and routinely relate that they cannot be effective without the team as a whole.

Leaders encourage boundary-spanning beyond traditional silos through inter-disciplinary collaboration.

This mindset sets the stage for teams realizing that taking risks is expected and encouraged. Risk taking in organizations is based on the trial of ideas. Nothing is improved without change, and change always carries some degree of risk, especially the risk of failure. Failure is important. The possibility of failure increases with the degree of risk, but a safe environment supports risk taking. We learn from failures more than we learn from successes because it causes a deeper emotional response, triggering reflection and analysis. We are beginning to recognize the importance of failure and learning from the failures. The CEO of Fahrenheit 212 (consulting company to the Fortune 500) Mark Payne has suggested that 90% of ideas fail (Fisher, 2014). That number is likely high, others have estimated the failure rate of change to be 50–70%. Whatever the actual rate is, a lot of ideas fail, but they can inform future change.

While the notion of psychological safety seems common sense, there is a range of work environments with many organizations having a culture of quality, safety, innovation, and support for workers, while others have a sick work environment that is toxic and negatively impacts the viability of an organization (Harder Wagner & Rash, 2014). Some work environments are hostile when a person in power, even if informally conferred power, creates an environment that is difficult or uncomfortable for another person to work due to discrimination. A RAND report found that 20% of workers report recent abuse or harassment at work (Maestas *et al.*, 2017). There is no place in the work environment for a leader to tolerate a toxic employee, a bully, someone who harasses others, or someone who discriminates against others. Northouse (2021), in his 4th edition of his highly acclaimed *Introduction to Leadership* book, added a chapter for the first time on destructive leadership. He provides readers with not only the damaging traits and behaviors of such leaders, but also provides a leadership instrument at the end of the chapter for readers to take when they are either a potentially destructive leader themselves, or they work in a team or organization under the direction of one.

Consider: **When have you felt psychologically unsafe in a team meeting? What could you do about it now that you are aware of the steps team leaders need to take to assure psychological safety?**

Today, team leaders have become more aware of the need to continually assess team dynamics as it relates to team members potentially marginalizing other team members. In healthcare and academic organizations, hierarchies are present and role groups may not experience equity and equality. This often plays out by one member of the team who has a higher rank minimizing the contributions of others in lower role ranks. This is often experienced by some team members as microaggressions which are commonplace, brief behavioral indignities that may be unnoticed by many but are experienced as hostile and derogatory. Abram X. Kendi (2019) has reframed this term in the context of racism as racial abuse. It is the accountability of the team leader and team members to assure that these behaviors are addressed and eliminated.

Know the Team

Trust within a team is built on each team member knowing the other and members knowing the leader. Even if people have worked together, they may not know that person. We all make assumptions about others, seeing others through our own lens. Getting to know other team members cuts through the assumptions to a more accurate understanding of a person. A leader needs to know each team member and their strengths and weaknesses. Observing interactions of team members will yield much information about the trust level in a team. Do team members make eye contact? Is there silence when asking for feedback? Do team members roll their eyes when ideas are presented? Do you sense that there is a trust problem? There are numerous team assessments that can be used to provide information about the level of trust. Exercises to enhance trust include having each person share with the group a personal dream or goal. Having social events with the specific purpose of team members getting to know each other outside of work can be very useful. In addition, using personality type assessments such as The Myers Briggs Inventory (Briggs, 1987), The DiSC Classic 2.0 (2003), and The Gallop Strength finders (Rath, 2007) and emotional intelligence assessments (of which there are many), are useful to provide professional development, reflection opportunities and insights into how team members can work more effectively together.

Be Honest

"Lying is incredibly common in everyday life and rampant among leaders of all sorts of organizations, including some of the most venerated leaders and companies" (Pfeffer, 2015). Honesty is a critical component in building trust. There are models that help leaders consider their intentions and other components of credibility, which Covey calls the four cores of credibility (Covey, 2006). He describes how trust is built and maintained between individuals and in groups. Four cores of credibility are at play in developing and maintaining and/or recovering trust. The first core of credibility is integrity, which is defined as acting in accordance with your values and beliefs. The second core is intent, which has to do with one's motives, agendas, and resulting behavior. Trust grows when motives are straightforward and based on mutual benefit.

These two cores comprise one's character. The third core is capabilities, which are the abilities one has that inspires confidence (e.g., talents, attitudes, skills, knowledge, and style). The fourth is results, which refers to one's track record and performance in getting things done. These two cores comprise one's competence.

It is important to understand the relationship among the components of credibility that are foundational to a leader's behaviors. We see evidence of this in politics, the media, and in organizations. For instance, we hear about fake news on a daily basis. We know that some leaders in all sectors lie. Even though there are now fact checkers to provide input on the validity of statements in the media, only 29% of those surveyed believe the fact checkers (Rasmussen Report, 2016). More people are getting their news and information from social media sites that at times have little interest in monitoring posts for truth. They promulgate conspiracy theories and lies. A recent study by faculty at Stanford found that college students had little skill in differentiating truth from lies on social media sites. Lying is so prevalent that there has emerged a Pro-Truth Pledge and commitment to a set of truth-oriented guidelines (Tsipurksy, Votta, and Rooswe, 2018).

Leaders of all types lie to create a perception of success, to look better than they are, and cover up problems. Philip Morris USA Inc, for years, lied to the public and government agencies about the effect of smoking on health (Gratale *et al.,* 2019). It took decades of work to change the public beliefs about smoking.

For a leader to move a plan forward, honesty is essential to creating trust needed for setting goals and creating a plan for the organization. Honesty needs to be coupled with transparency. Keeping people accurately informed to the best of a leader's knowledge is critical. The more transparent and truthful a leader is, the more trust is built. An area that tends to create angst and rumor is the state of finances of an organization. Although some leaders in the past have held financial information close to the vest, today, best practices, partly driven by regulators and the law, is to publicly report financial information to both internal and external organizational stakeholders. If an organization publicly reports financial information, the information should be organized and shared with employees before it becomes public. Financial transparency and honesty are an ethical responsibility. Without honesty, the way forward may be built on sand and trust will be greatly compromised.

Be Consistent in Your Visions and Goals

In building trust, consistency of vision and goals helps your team know the direction of the organization. Some leaders are known to have a vision of the day or be indecisive about a vision and goals, leaving team members struggling to figure out what direction the organization is heading. It is as if a new vision and/or goals are discussed at every meeting based on who the leader talked to most recently or what article he/she read. A consistent vision and goals are critical to creating a sense of stability in order for people to trust that the leader knows where to take the organization in order to be successful. Having a consistent vision does not mean that strategies or tactics are not open for change, it means that there is at least a direction that everyone can count on to work towards.

Keep Your Word

Leaders gain trust when they do what they say they are going to do. However, demands on leaders can be non-stop and promises can fall to the bottom of the to do list, particularly if they do not fall into the critical category of work. There are many things that need to be tended to by leaders that are priorities, and in order to keep their word, they should delegate the work if possible so that it gets done. Also, be realistic about your daily calendar. Build in time for email responses, lunch, or performance review follow-up. You are the only one who can manage your time realistically and effectively.

There are key elements in keeping a promise or keeping your word. Define the promise, let people know when to expect the promise to be kept, and when it has been kept. If a leader cannot keep his or her word, then followers need to understand why not. Any deviation from keeping your word can result in a loss of trust. Trust is easily lost and difficult to rebuild. Surprisingly, leaders often feel that they do not need to explain a failure to keep a promise or feel embarrassed that they did not follow through. This may be couched in the thinking that they do not owe their followers an explanation because the issue is not really important, or simply because they are the leader. One of the most common breaches of trust includes sharing information that had been promised to be confidential. Once a leader has breached the confidence of one person, it will become general knowledge and trust will be compromised. Others will be careful in what they say, and a leader may not get honest information.

Promises need to be based in reality in order to be kept. It may be that you communicate to a team member that, ". . . at this time, this is what I plan to do… and I will let you know if I need to change this plan." An example of the consequences not being realistic is telling an employee that because they have done an outstanding job, you are going to advocate for a significant salary increase or promotion. This may take the shape by the employee being scored as excellent in all categories of annual evaluation. You put forward the request, and the HR department lets you know that the salary increase requested is excessive and will not be approved. The employee is on the low side of the pay scale, and you believe that the request is reasonable, but you are distracted by other events that are high priority and you do not get back to HR with further documentation for the raise. The time frame for the raise is closing and you do not have time to work with HR for the higher raise, so you give the employee the average pay raise but do not inform the employee of this because vacation schedules and meetings away from the office limit the time to meet. The employee feels that you have been dishonest and begins looking for a new job. In keeping your word, at the very least the employee should have been informed of the response from HR and what the plan is to move the request forward to have a different strategy to increase the salary.

Acknowledge Your Mistakes

No one is perfect; humans are fallible. It is very heartening to team members for leaders to acknowledge a mistake, be transparent about it, and apologize. When team members see a leader share a mistake, it makes it more likely that they will share mistakes and problems leading to a stronger organization. By acknowledging mistakes, team members will feel more comfortable to speak up to identify an issue, raise a concern, and solve a problem together. Leaders are closely scrutinized and talked about by nearly everyone in an organization. So, owning up to mistakes helps build trust, provides a role model for the team, and shows integrity. Leaders often think that they have to be right all of the time because they are the leader, and that people depend on them to have the answers. They may also feel that if they admit they are fallible or appear vulnerable, that they will be perceived as a weak leader. While there are many contextual issues involved in making a mistake, admitting it and apologizing is the best road to take. Apologies go a long way to having people perceive a leader more positively.

Consider: **Can you think of a situation in which you would now apply this new information?**

Avoid Playing Games

Most of us do not start out thinking that we can engage in game playing to accomplish our goals. In designing a way forward, the full team needs to be engaged in decision-making that leads to the team goals. This cannot happen if the leader engages in game playing. Two common examples of game playing include "King of the Mountain" and "Simon Says." King of the mountain is when the leader has to be the top person and makes it known that his/her opinion and decision-making is the rule by which everyone will play. The king will push members of the team down the mountain in order to have control of the mountain. A leader who needs to be king of the mountain does not develop individuals on the team and ensures that they have limited opportunity and always know who the king is. However, people will spend time and energy in finding ways to dethrone the king.

Another game that leaders play is Simon says. In this, as in the childhood game, members of the team are expected to do exactly as the leader says, if the leader says be quiet, the follower needs to be quiet. If the leader says admit fifty students even if there are only faculty and staff to support 30, it must be done, or the person is eliminated from the team. While king of the mountain and Simon says have similarities, they are both destructive forms of leading teams and undermines trust. Leaders who employ these behaviors are conveying that not only are ideas of others not valuable but the people themselves are not valued. Leaders that play these games will have discouraged and unengaged people as part of their team.

Inspire

Inspiring a team is to reach team members at an emotional level. Inspiration links the work of the team to the values of the team member and to what they define as meaningful work. Part of the leader's responsibility is to frame and to consistently reinforce that the work is important and meaningful. In addition, teams are inspired when they are recognized for the important work they have accomplished. As the team is moving forward toward a goal, inspiration takes form in communicating positive feedback to the team. Team members are inspired when a lot is expected of them, the team leader is elbow-to-elbow alongside their team members, and the team leader incorporates suggestions and innovations by team members.

Communicate

Given that one of the elements of an effective team is communication, the ability to effectively communicate is an essential skill of a team leader. See Chapter 12 for a more extensive discussion of communication. The leader needs to know what to communicate, when to communicate, and the purpose of the communication. One of the most essential skills in communication for leaders is listening. Leaders need to listen to the team members. Listening is one of the skills we know is essential but can be challenging. Part of the challenge is that leaders tend to think they need to have the answers and should communicate this, while often the answers lie with listening to others. In addition, getting buy-in to the work of a team is built on team members feeling valued, and feeling valued is related to being heard. Being attentive to the words, body language, and facial expressions of team members provides important information about the dynamics of the team. To listen, leaders need to pay attention and be present. This takes work, practice, and is a key skill in creating an effective team. Modeling for others that not knowing is acceptable, leaders will often say, "I don't know the answer to that question, but I will find out and get back to you."

Demonstrate Confidence

Leaders need to know what they are doing and be seen as confident in their ability to lead. Team members will know immediately if the team leader is confident or not. It is a rare situation in which the team leader is the most knowledgeable person about all aspects of work to be done. Being confident is not about being the subject matter expert, it is about being confident and competent in leading. Covey (2006) described credibility as one of the key competence capabilities in addition to intent, integrity, and results.

Leaders know the strengths, talents, challenges, and weaknesses of each team member. It is being confident in your ability to coordinate, facilitate, hold members accountable, and move the work forward. Being confident means recognizing which team members have the skills and abilities needed to get the work done and those who need further development. Leaders effectively orchestrate the work.

Delegate

A leader does not do all the work. A leader knows how and to whom to delegate. The first principle of delegation is to choose the right person to whom to delegate. The person should have the competencies (knowledge, skills, and attitudes) to accomplish the delegated work. If the person does not have the skill set needed, the team leader will develop a professional development plan for those individuals. There are times that you will need to support and teach the person in order to be successful by identifying resources that will be useful for the person to learn about. In addition, it is important that the person is interested in and hopefully even passionate about the delegated work. If you assign someone a task and they are resistant to doing it, the work will be compromised. The person will need to know the reason for the delegated activity. Reasons may include needing to offload work that is more aligned with the designee, or it may be part of a professional development plan for the person to develop new competencies. In delegating, the task needs to be clearly described with specific expectations defined. If you want the work to be done in a specific way, that needs to be very clearly explained. If resources or access to specific information are needed to be successful, make sure they are available. Delegation also requires the leader to give the authority for completing the task. Delegation often fails because people have the responsibility for accomplishing a task, but not the decision-making authority to hold others accountable. Giving authority may feel like sharing or completely relinquishing control. However, leaders remain ultimately accountable for the work delegated, and should be kept informed of progress to ensure accountability. It is always important to recognize the work done through delegation and to say thank you to the person-both publicly and privately.

Negotiate

Effective leaders find themselves in situations in which negotiation is required, both in formal and informal ways. Negotiation is defined by Ury (1981) in his landmark book, *Getting to Yes*, negotiation as reaching wise and fair agreements efficiently and civilly. Negotiation is a process between two or more people. The aim of negotiations include compromise to meet a mutually acceptable outcome.

Labor contract negotiations are a common formal process that nurse leaders in unionized organizations, both academic and service, participate in and/or lead. These negotiations can be contentious or not depending on the timing, context, and leadership.

A leader who is unable to identify points of conflict and be able to work through those conflicts with members of the organization will not be effective in their role. Consider how ineffective a leader would be who is unable to negotiate with team members or their own supervisor. Developing and honing negotiation skills are important to developing and sustaining productive teams. One of the key principles in any negotiation is that both parties leave the negotiation feeling they received a reasonable deal. The best negotiations are the ones in which there is mutual benefit. There are several approaches and strategies that are useful in the negotiation process.

- *Know what you want in the negotiation.* This is the most fundamental rule of negotiating. A leader needs to be clear on the most important gains, whether they are negotiating for more resources, personnel, or decision-making participation. In each instance, going into the negotiation knowing what the best outcome is, as well as what an acceptable outcome of the negotiation could be, is critical to be able to frame your request. If additional resources for a more effective clinical service or educational program is the critical issue, know the amount needed and have a compelling rationale.
- *Know as much as you can about the party with whom you are negotiating.* Going into the negotiation process with a complete picture of the situation you are negotiating, from the perspective of the opposing side, will put you in a much stronger position. Knowing the priorities of the person or groups you are negotiating with as well as the constraints they face will give you critical information in approaching the negotiation.
- *Harness the power of silence.* It is human nature for some people to get into uncomfortable situations and feel they need to fill up every moment of si-

lence. Expert negotiators know that silence can be their ally by encouraging the opposing negotiator to begin talking, and perhaps make concessions that they would not otherwise make. Dr. Ed Brodow (2021) suggests that a good negotiator follows the 70/30 rule; listen carefully 70% of the time and speak 30% of the time. By asking a lot of open-ended questions and listening carefully to the response, the opposing negotiator will reveal information that will be helpful in the negotiation.

- *Show how making this deal will improve the opposition's position.* Having the opposing side's view, negotiators are able to frame their arguments in a way that makes the proposal too good to pass up. Understanding the pressures the opposing side is under helps to show how your proposal minimizes or reduces those pressures. There will be times when you have to give a little if the opposing negotiator has also given a little. By showing your willingness to be flexible, when the opposing side has demonstrated their willingness to be accommodating, the outcome will likely be more satisfying to both parties. As previously stated, the best negotiations are when both parties believe they have received a good deal.

- *Do not paint yourself into a corner.* There are two important elements related to this strategy. First, a good negotiator will never wield threats that they know they will not be able to implement. For example, if you say that you will be unable to stay at the organization if your demands for additional resources are not met and your opposing negotiator says they are unable to meet them, you are left with two very challenging alternatives. You may choose to leave the organization even though you might not have a better offer, or if you stay, you will have to overcome the credibility issue of making an idle threat. If an increase in resources is critical for remaining at the organization, have a good alternative option if you cannot come to an agreement. Knowing that you have explored other positions and there are exciting options available will give you the inner strength to negotiate from a position of strength.

The second aspect of this strategy is to remember that negotiations take time, and a good negotiator will have patience with the process. If you go into the process with a short timeline, the opposing negotiator will sense your time pressure and be less likely to offer what is being requested. If you are flexible about time, others might feel like they have to make concessions in order to close the negotiation. The ability to be patient can often make the difference between a successful and failed negotiation.

Manage Conflict

Conflict is inevitable in teamwork. It is always useful to prevent conflict (not at the expense of a high performing team) rather than having to address it.

Anticipating situations in which a particular decision will be viewed very differently by individuals or groups is critical. Anticipating conflict will provide the opportunity to lay the groundwork to prevent conflict and, to the extent possible, include all groups in a decision that may end up contentious. There is no way to prevent all conflict in the workplace and the effectiveness of the team depends on how conflict is managed by the leader. Disagreement about ideas that is done respectfully is not conflict. Conflict carries a highly charged emotional response to another person or situation. Common sources of conflict include (Elorus, 2018):

Leadership Style

This source of conflict is common when leadership changes and the style change can be confusing to team members. One leader may have trusted the team members to do what they needed to do, and the new leader may be a hands-on leader that is interpreted as not trusting the team members. There may also be strong feelings related to the previous leader leaving. Leaders need to explain their style to the team, as well as build trust and be willing to make changes in their leadership style.

Personality Differences

There are no two people who think exactly alike or work in the same way. We interpret people's behavior and communication through our own lens and may assign intentions to another person that are completely off base. Providing the opportunity for team members to get to know each other as people and not just workers is usually helpful to manage conflict related to personality.

Accountability

We all tend to look outside of ourselves when something goes wrong, such as, "It is the other team members that did not get their work done in time." The blame game needs to be managed by understanding the barriers to getting work done and helping people manage their responsibilities. Team members need to be accountable.

Cultural Conflicts

Conflicts related to values and beliefs lead to misunderstandings and the lack of appreciation of how culture has influenced work style. The leader needs to help members focus on what is shared rather than what is different, while helping all members to understand that everyone is different.

Working Style

Some people immediately begin to tackle their team responsibilities and others may tend to think through the details of what they need to do and take longer to complete work. In other words, people may have different rhythms of work in terms of speed and intensity. Leaders will need to help the group focus on the work accomplished when it is due, rather than how a particular team member got there. It may be important for there to be at least compatible work styles among team members.

The Thomas-Kilmann Conflict Model and Instrument

The Thomas-Kilmann Conflict Model (Kilmann, 2011) provides a useful way of understanding conflict management styles. See Figure 13.4. This model is based on the continuums of assertiveness and cooperativeness identifying five styles of managing conflict. The competing style, having high assertiveness and low cooperation, could be reflected when someone feels strongly about a principle, value, or idea, or when they just want to have their way. The accommodating style is high cooperation and low assertiveness. There may be important reasons to strongly cooperate, such as times of major challenges. However, people may cooperate but feel angry or uncomfortable doing this, or not feel empowered to assert their position on an issue. Avoiding style may be useful when emotions are high, and taking a step back and coming back to an issue at a later time will give everyone a chance to lower the emotional level. However, this style could also present itself as being ineffective, being fearful

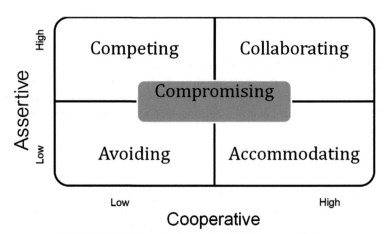

FIGURE 13.4 Thomas-Kilmann Conflict Management Styles.

to state a position, or not caring about an issue. Compromising is at the center midway of assertiveness and cooperativeness. It is when both parties are willing to give something up to gain something. It is splitting the difference and often useful for a quick fix to a conflict. Collaboration is when both parties expect that they can work out a way for each to get what they want. It takes significant conflict negotiation skill and creativity to think differently about the possible outcomes. It is critical for the team leader to know their predominant style as well as each team member's predominant style. An effective leader can move between styles depending on the situation and desired outcome.

Conflict is going to occur among team members and between team members and the leader. When conflict is between a leader and team member it may be useful to recognize it within the team but meet with the individual's outside of the team meeting. There are many resources that may be useful. We have found that having all team members read Patterson's (2012) *Crucial Conversations* and Scott's (2002) *Fierce Conversations* is very useful in helping the team understand and manage conflict.

Be Accessible and Available

Accessibility and availability to team members are important behaviors. We learned that having some boundaries about this is crucial. Accessibility is based on open and honest conversations, mutual feedback, and non-hierarchical relationships that contribute to trust, improve communications, and create greater team effectiveness. Accessibility requires availability. Availability is setting aside time and method for communication. It requires letting people know what tools you find useful for communication—in person, email, text, phone, or/and internal communication system. It also requires letting people know specific times you will plan on being available. Specifying your availability will help to manage the drop-in interruptions that can derail your work that needs to get done. Often just knowing the leader's willingness to be available and accessible reassures team members that you are engaged and feel the work of the team is important. This mindset is at the foundation of what some leaders ascribe to, the idea of leaders serving followers or servant leadership. Servant leadership emphasizes that leaders be attentive to the concerns of their followers, empathize with them and nurture them. (Northouse, 2019).

Be Accountable

As a leader, you hold members of your team accountable, but less frequent is the leader accountable to the team. In most organizations, a leader is accountable to a higher-level leader or a board, but not to the team. Accountability should include being accountable for the work getting done as well as your leadership of the team. Creating metrics that are shared with the team, or better yet, co-created with the team is important to developing and continuing trust. The process of being accountable to your team will give everyone a sense of your commitment and transparency in terms of your contribution to the effort. Accountability includes elements such as: vision is clearly communicated; opinions are solicited; team members feel safe to speak up, be themselves, and disagree; and team members feel they share in the decision-making.

Build Your Team

The nature of teams, whether in the service setting or in the academic setting, is that they are dynamic. Team members come and go and team objectives and priorities change based on the needs of the organization and its customers. While leaders often head teams that are already formed, leaders can reform the team with some members staying and others leaving or disbanding a team and starting over. Having the right people on your team is critical. As referenced earlier, Jim Collins (2001), in his now classic book *Good to Great*, recognized that organizations that went from good to great got the right people in the right seats on the bus.

It is essential to identify the knowledge and skills needed for your team to be successful. It is also essential to have people who know how to work with others. While every team needs to be intentionally developed, this process can be greatly helped if the individuals are committed and able to work effectively in teams.

Match Strengths to Responsibilities

The team members who will be leading the path forward will need to have their responsibilities match their talents and strengths. The major premise of Buckingham & Clifton's best-selling book (2001) *Now, Discover Your Strengths*, is that if leaders and team members start with knowing the strengths of individuals and build teams with that in mind, the rest will fall into place, including matching clearly defined scope of responsibilities for team members. When there are no clearly defined role responsibilities, confusion occurs, creating inefficiencies in the organization and frustration among team members. Team members often feel that they do not know who is supposed to be doing what. It is very useful to include the team members in defining roles and expectations. This can be done through team meetings with a specific focus on defining who is going to do what and when. A leader should weigh in on the role definitions based on their knowledge of the team members' skills and interests.

A challenge within any team is matching the team members' interests to the needs of getting the work of the team done in service to the organization. Some team members may be very good at certain activities but may feel bored with continuing to do the same old thing. Each team member's preferences and interest in professional growth need to be taken into consideration. When possible, an agreement should be made that if the team member will take on the responsibility that they are good at but reluctant to do, they will be given a responsibility that is consistent with their area of interest at a later date. Matching the team member's interest to their scope of responsibility is critical in keeping talent in the organization, as well as expanding the talent and skills of each employee. If the interests of a team member are not consistent with the needs of the organization, there should be a plan to help that person move, to another department in the organization or to a different organization altogether, in order to continue developing. It is far better for an organization to keep talented people in the organization even if moving that person to a different unit is a loss for that unit

Develop the Team Through Learning

An approach to increasing effectiveness within teams that has a history in healthcare and other high-risk industries, like the airline and nuclear industries, related to creating a highly reliable organization imbued with a culture of safety, is called "team training."

Teams develop normative behaviors over time and roles of team members evolve, but not necessarily always in a positive and effective way. For this reason and more, team training has become the norm in healthcare settings today, less so in the academic and business setting, but the principles would be as useful there as well. Team training is a set of approaches and methods for assuring and optimizing effective communication, coordination, and collaboration. Team training provides a structure for developing behavioral expectations, practicing them, and evaluating them over time as the agreements among team members are integrated into the everyday practice setting (Weaver, Dy, and Rosen, 2014). Team members exchange information, behavioral modeling, and simulation in a synchronous classroom or virtual setting using KSAs (knowledge, skills, and attitudes) as a competency framework, and then transfer this into highly effective team performance.

But, before the onset of team training in healthcare delivery, team building was the norm. The major premise driving team training programs is that teams have purpose, and in order for teams to function effectively, team members need to be in alignment with the organization's definition of the purpose of any given team. Team members need to be both organizationally minded and team oriented in this framework.

Thiel *et al.* (2019) propose five team building essentials:

1. *Clarity*: Team members know and appreciate the purpose of the team's role in the organization.

2. *Relevance*: The goals and purpose of the team are shared by the individual team members.

3. *Significance*: What the team members do each day, their objectives make sense and sufficiently guide their attitudes, commitment, and daily work.

4. *Achievability*: What is expected of team members is believed to be realistic and achievable.

5. *Urgency*: There is a shared commitment by team members to work efficiently together to meet the team's purpose and objectives.

The Princeton Management Consulting Group offers a free Blind Spot Survey tool to help leaders understand blind spots about yourself, your team, your organization and your market. It is self-scored and can be accessed at; *http://princetonmc.com/wp-content/uploads/leadership_blindspots_survey.pdf.*

Change the Composition of the Team When Necessary

While you may have had the right people in the right positions at the beginning of the process to define the vision and goals, with time, there may be a need to refine the team. However, in Jim Collin's (2001) example of the bus, once the bus is moving forward it may become apparent that some people on the bus may need to get off the bus and others added. Removing people who have been part of the visioning and planning is difficult. In some cases, people may have the insight that they are not the right people to carry the vision forward, but the reality is the leader may need to make the change. There are many situations where a team member wants to be off a particular team, and that will be an easier change for a leader to make.

Making personnel changes is a challenge that leaders may not look forward to doing. Many times, there is a positive history of working together, and there may be a friendship. Ensuring you have the right people in place is the only way that a leader will get the organization to achieve the vision. There are several reasons to remove people from a team. These include the team member not being on board with the vision and priorities and creating barriers to moving forward. The member may not follow through on the work responsibilities or may create difficult team dynamics limiting the ability of the team to problem solve effectively.

Removing people from a team must be done respectfully and as compassionately as possible. There are many considerations, including whether to keep the person within the unit in a different position, move the person to a different unit within the larger organization, or terminate. In addition, there are rules about relieving people of the job they were hired to do. If the organization is unionized, there are also rules about how someone is either fired or moved to a different position. Working with the HR department will keep informed of the legal and regulatory issues associated with this transition, as well as give you advice about strategies you can use to make the change. Whatever the challenge, if there is even one person who is not the right person, that person can have a profound effect on limiting the group's movement forward.

In moving a member off the team, the leader needs to consider several questions. First, what has been the history and service to the organization to date? Elements that go into considering the history include:

- How long has this person been with the organization?
- How near are they to retirement or other personal major life events that may impact their perspectives about a major transition?
- Is there a skills gap that could be addressed?
- Is there a fundamental disagreement about the direction of the organization?
- Is the person committed to the well-being of the organization?

Based on the responses to these questions, a decision can be made about how to proceed. There may be concerns by the team member that include salary change, status within the organization, and concerns about future employment. The most challenging to manage is the emotional response, including anger and embarrassment about being perceived as not good enough. While the team member is responsible for their own emotional response, the leader needs to be prepared for the emotions, keeping in mind that every team member change carries an emotional response. The leader can offer the team member coaching or counseling if available within the organization. If the leader is unprepared for this, or uncomfortable dealing with a range of emotions, it is wise to seek advice from a coach, colleague, or other professional.

Evaluate Team Effectiveness

Team training scholars (Agrawal, 2014; Katzenbach and Smith, 1993) propose the Five Cs of Effective Teamwork model for evaluating a team's effectiveness. Do team members believe they have the following?

- Common goals,
- Commitment to other members of the team and to the work of the team,
- Competence in their function and roles,
- Communication that is timely and respectful, and
- Coordination that includes the necessary resources, technology, and people to do the work?

Many healthcare organizations are led by an interdisciplinary dyad or triad such as a physician and nurse, a nurse and administrator, or all three. When this is the case, work by leaders is required ahead of the work by teams in evaluating team effectiveness. Effective team leaders guide their teams by using principles of psychological safety (Edmundson, 2012): being sensitive to the interests, needs, and motivations of team members. They address conflict head on in a serene but assertive manner and model a shared purpose and interest in resolving conflict using the shared team wisdom. Applying these principles assures that when conflict arises, team members can creatively and consistently drive toward resolution with the facilitation and guidance of team leaders. This work takes time and cannot be accomplished while performing the routine functions of the team. Therefore, routinely meeting off-line or at special planned meetings are essential to accomplish this important work.

Capitalizing on relationships among team members to advance high performance teamwork is the aim of "relational coordination" a term coined by organizational scholar Jody Hoffer Gittell (2009). To foster high performance teamwork, organizations and leaders create structures and processes that drive effective and positive relationships among team members in a systematic way. Her contention is that through relational coordination work practices (Gittell, 2009) extraordinary results can be achieved. These work practices and related processes are illustrated in Figure 13.5.

Given the dynamic nature of teams, it is essential that organizations develop strategies to ensure that team norms, expectations, and standards are continuously monitored, upheld, and improved. Some organizations develop their own homegrown approaches based on best practices to develop protocols and agreements to address team members' roles, responsibilities, and behaviors,

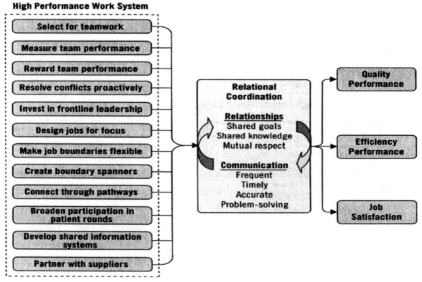

FIGURE 13.5 How High-Performance Healthcare Works (Gittell 2009, pg. 53).

and then develop a program to disseminate and implement these team member expectations across the organization, practice by practice (Weaver, Dy, and Rosen, 2014).

Periodically assessing how team members perceive the effectiveness of their teamwork is one way of checking in on the health of a team. One group within the National Health System in Great Britain developed and made public a tool that examines the perception of team members of the effectiveness of the team and includes the scoring rubric for the areas of: purpose and goals, roles, team process, team relationships, intergroup relations, problem solving, passion and commitment, skills and learning as well as a total score (London Leadership Academy, 2020).

SUMMARY

Essential work in organizations occurs not through individuals working alone to carry out essential functions or solve important problems, but rather through people working and learning collaboratively in teams. We often mistake groups of people as teams. However, there is a process of team development that has been described that moves groups to high performing teams. There are numerous models of team effectiveness, and we presented three common models. These models have common themes that include trust, communication, respect, necessary skills, and accountability. There are important skills that team leaders need to bring to create and lead effective teams. Leaders need to build trust, communicate, inspire, delegate, manage conflict, be accessible and available, and be accountable. They also need to know how to build an effective team, as well as change the composition of the team as the work and skills needed may change. Leading a team takes work and thought to move a group of people to a high performing team.

CRITICAL THINKING QUESTIONS

At the beginning of the chapter an academic and clinical vignette were presented. Please review the vignettes to address the following questions. The questions are specific to the vignettes.

Academic Vignette

1. Select a model of team effectiveness (i.e., Katzenbach and Lencioni, T7) and analyze the inability of the academic team to make decisions. Describe how the challenges in the scenario fit with the elements of the model.

2. Describe how the academic leadership team can begin to build open communication and trust with one another. What actions can the leaders take to facilitate improving communication?

3. With the information provided to you, what would you assess as the level of trust present in the academic team? If limited, how might the leader build trust? What are the constraints on building trust?

4. You decide that some members of your academic leadership team are not performing in a way that you need them to perform. They obstruct movement in decision-making and you need to replace them. You have had a conversation with each of them about their tendency to derail decisions that are important. What steps will you take to make the necessary change?

5. How do the five Cs of effective teams apply to the academic leadership team? What is the most important C for the dean to focus on? What actions would you take to improve the effectiveness of the team?

Clinical Vignette

1. What stage of team formation do you believe that the clinical team represents? How can you move the team to be a high performing team?

2. Based on the Lencioni or the T7 model of team effectiveness, what dysfunctions need to be addressed in the clinical team?

3. What learning experiences do you think team members would benefit from to become a high performing clinical team?

4. What leadership characteristics might the chief nurse need to work on to be more effective with her team?

5. How might the level of trust be compromised in the clinical team? How can trust be built within the team?

6. What conflict management approach does the CEO seem to have? How might this shift?

REFERENCES

Agency for Healthcare Research and Quality (AHRQ). (2021). *Pocket guide: Team STEPPS*. Agency for Healthcare Research and Quality (AHRQ). https://www.ahrq.gov/teamstepps/instructor/essentials/pocketguide.html

Agrawal, A (2014). *Patient Safety A Case Based Comprehensive Guide*. Springer Publishing

American Hospital Association. (2021). *AHA team training*. American Hospital Association. https://www.aha.org/center/performance-improvement/team-training

Brodow, E. (2020, December 9). *Ten tips for negotiating in 2021*. Ed Brodow. https://www.brodow.com/Ten-Tips-For-Negotiating by John Wiley and Sons

Clifton D. & M. Buckingham, M. (2001). *Now Discover Your Strengths*. Gallop Press

Collins, J. (2001). Good to Great. *Why some companies make the leap and others don't*. Harper Business

Covey, S.R. (2006). *Speed of Trust, the One Thing That Changes Everything*. Free Press

Edmundson, A. C. (2012). *Teaming: How Organizations learn, innovate and compete in the knowledge economy*. Harvard Business School.

Elorus Team in Workplace. (2018, May 11). *Causes of workplace conflicts explained: Reasons, types and signs*. Elorus. https://www.elorus.com/blog/causes-of-common-workplace-conflicts-explained/

Fisher, A. (2014, October 7). Why most innovations are great big failures. *Fortune*. https://fortune.com/2014/10/07/innovation-failure/

Freeth, D., Hammock, M., Reeves, S., Koppell, I., & Barr, H. (2005). *Effective interprofessional education: Development, delivery and evaluation*. Blackwell Publishing.

Gallup. (1999). *Clifton Strengths Assessment*. Omaha, NE: Gallup.

Gittell, J. (2009). *High performance healthcare*. McGraw Hill.

Gratale, S., Sangalang, A., Maloney, E., & Capella, J. (2019). Attitudinal Spillover from Misleading Natural Cigarette Marketing: An Experiment Examining Current and Former Smokers' Support for Tobacco Industry Regulation. *International Journal of Environmental Research and Public Health, 16*(19), 3554; https://doi.org/10.3390/ijerph16193554

Harder, H., Wagner, S., & Rash, J. (2014). *Mental illness in the workplace: Psychological disability management*. Ashgate Publishing Ltd.

Kahn, W. A. (1990). Psychological conditions of personal engagement and disengagement at work. *The Academy of Management Journal, 33*(4), 692-724. https://doi.org/10.5465/256287

Katzenbach, J. R., & Smith, D. K. (1993). *The wisdom of teams: Creating the high-performance organization*. Harvard Business School Press.

Kendi, I. (2019). *How to be an antiracist*. Bodley Head.

Kilmann, T. (2011). *Celebrating 40 Years with the TKI Assessment A summary of my favorite insight*. https://kilmanndiagnostics.com/wp-content/uploads/2018/

Korn Ferry Institute. (2016). *Driving team effectiveness: A comparative analysis of the Korn Ferry T7 Model with Other Popular Models*. https://www.kornferry.com/content/dam/kornferry/docs/pdfs/driving-team-effectiveness.pdf

Lencioni, P. (2002). *The five dysfunctions of a team: A leadership fable*. Jossey-Bass.

Lombardo, M. M., & Eichinger, R. W. (1995). *The Team Architect® user's manual*. Lominger Limited.

London Leadership Academy. (2020). *Team effectiveness questionnaire*. London Leadership Academy. https://www.londonleadershipacademy.nhs.uk/sites/default/files/Team_effectiveness_diagnostic-LAL1.pdf

Maestas, N., Mullen, K. J., Powell, D., von Wachter, T., & Wenger, J. B. (2017). *How*

Americans perceive the workplace: Results from the American working conditions survey. RAND Corporation. https://doi.org/10.7249/RB9972

Northouse, P. (2019). *Leadership Theory and Practice.* Sage Publishing

Patterson, K. (2012). *Crucial conversations: Tools for talking when stakes are high.* McGraw-Hill.

Pfeffer, J. (2015). *Leadership BS: Fixing workplaces and careers one truth at a time.* Harper Business.

Rasmussen Report. (2016, September 30). *Voters don't trust media fact-checking.* Rasmussen Report. https://www.rasmussenreports.com/public_content/politics/general_politics/september_2016/voters_don_t_trust_media_fact_checking

Rath, T. (2007). *StrengthsFinder 2.0.* Gallup Press

Scott, S. (2002). *Fierce conversations: Achieving success at work & in life, one conversation at a time.* Viking.

Thiel, C. E., Harvey, J., Courtright, S., & Bradley, B. (2019). What doesn't kill you makes you stronger: How teams rebound from early-stage relationship conflict. *Journal of Management, 45*(4). https://doi.org/10.1177/0149206317729026

Tsipursky, G., Votta, F., & Rooswe, K. (2018). Fighting fake news and post-truth politics with behavioral science: The pro-truth pledge. *Behavior and Social Issues,* 27, 47-70. https://doi.org/10.5210/bsi.v.27i0.9127

Tuckman, B. W. (1965). Development sequence in small groups. *Psychological Bulletin, 63*(6), 384-399. https://doi.org/10.1037/h0022100

Ury, W. (1981). *Getting to yes.* Harvard Business School.

Weaver, S. J., Dy, S. M., & Rosen, M. A. (2014). Team-training in healthcare: A narrative synthesis of the literature. *BMJ Quality & Safety, 23*, 359-372. https://doi.org/10.1136/bmjqs-2013-001848

Weiss, D., & Tilan, F. (2014). *The interprofessional healthcare team: Leadership and development.* Jones and Bartlett

CHAPTER 14

Change and Innovation

ACADEMIC VIGNETTE

Financial woes plagued the school of nursing at Fairport University. For five successive years, the school drew on its reserves to close with a balanced budget at the end of the fiscal year. The reserves will not cover two more years of loss. As the leader, you enlist the help of the school's financial team to understand what is at the root of the financial losses. The team noted that the various units in the school used different record keeping practices, with some noncompliant with the university policies. The practices were too varied to impose a simple solution. At the annual retreat of the leadership team, the urgency of the problem was presented, and a plan was developed in which the units would participate in a group level data review. The review process would also include education about required university fiscal policies and include the unit leader as well as the financial leader in each unit. The agreement was uniform and enthusiastic. The lead financial officer was put in charge of convening the group and leading the project. Over a series of meetings, the lead financial officer explained the need to adjust the operational plan based on perceived differences among the units. At the end of the next fiscal year, the financial officer reported that the groups were unwilling to cooperate, and the deficit funding continued.

CLINICAL VIGNETTE

In cooperation with the dean of the school of nursing, the chief nursing officer (CNO) agreed to establish a unit supporting the translation of evidence into practice. Office space was located, and staff were hired to support collaborations between faculty members and practicing staff nurses. Staff members included statisticians, editors, and experts who could advise on study designs. A librarian was hired to assist with locating evidence. The dean, recognizing gaps in the expertise of the faculty, hired several nurse consultants to address topical areas of clinical interest to the practicing nurses. Monthly meetings were scheduled for the oversight team, including key staff members, the dean, and the CNO. By the fourth month, the CNO began missing the meetings. Initially, everyone understood that there are emergencies that are unanticipated, and the dean made sure that the CNO was updated on the business of the meeting. A pattern developed wherein the CNO would miss a meeting, then attend the next meeting and ask that all decisions made in her absence be reviewed and reconsidered with her input. At first, the group was patient with these requests, but over time frustrations grew. The development of a clear set of priorities that could improve care outcomes and value languished. The attendance of other team members fell off, and the work of the unit was carried on by a small group of staff who faithfully reached out to the nurses they knew. The original promise of the initiative seemed unattainable.

INTRODUCTION

"If you want to truly understand something, try to change it."— Kurt Levin.

The preceding chapters have addressed the elements and features of the organization, as well as some of the essential actions required to lead an organization. Each of these is important to understand the organization, assess the organization, and evaluate its response to external events and leadership interventions. Recall that the work of leadership, as we have defined the term, involves engaging the component parts of an organization toward productivity, innovation, and decision-making that creates an impact that is greater than the component parts. In order to accomplish this, the primary objective of leading is to manage change. For this reason, the information in this chapter is critical to understanding how to lead. The organizational dimensions previously described guide the leader's understanding of the organization; however, these understandings are in the service of the leader's ability to effect change. Organizations that fail to change, and that do not renew themselves, are destined to fail (a key principle of systems theory), and a major tenet of the humanist author John Gardner (1995). Collins (2009) describes the hubris born of success as the beginning step toward organizational failure.

Driving Change in Organizational Culture

Culture and change are closely related. Successful change must be culture-sensitive and changing culture is among the most difficult of changes to accomplish. Malcolm Baldridge is famous for saying that, within organizations, "culture eats strategy for breakfast." He rightfully points out that a leader can have the best strategies for implementing a change, but unless the organizational culture is fully understood, the strategy is at high risk of being ineffective.

Some cultures prioritize stability, while others emphasize flexibility and an openness to change (Groysberg *et al.*, 2018). The former relies on rules, standardization, hierarchies, and predictability, while the latter values autonomy, competition, and the integration of individual action. Although we have argued that nurses in academic and clinical organizations can benefit from use of the same principles in leading their respective organizations, the qualities of the academic and clinical organizations display cultural differences. The tendency for academic organizations to devalue hierarchy and encourage individual creativity and autonomy often contrasts with the clinical setting, in which consistent practice and reliable results are a requirement. These differences are important to recognize. Each type of organization requires high quality outcomes but the balance between independence and conformity vary.

Increasingly, attention has been focused on building an *adaptive culture*. Heifetz, Grashow and Linsky (2009) described five characteristics of the adaptive organization: (1) naming the elephants in the room; (2) conveying that the responsibility for the organization's future is shared; (3) expecting independent judgment; (4) developing leadership capacity; and (5) institutionalizing reflection and continuous learning. The adaptive culture can embrace changes that are needed to thrive in the ever-changing world. While many descriptions of cultures are general enough to encompass several major ideas, high performing cultures usually embrace being a learning organization, creating a positive work environment, enhancing quality and safety, and being innovative as demonstrated in Figure 14.1.

Being patient with the change process, or at least attuned to the organization's appetite for change, is a critical element of success. Although cultural changes often proceed slowly, some occasions call for rapid change, which can be met with resistance unless the need for the change is urgent and clearly and convincingly communicated to all staff. Urgency will be described in more detail as a condition that helps to drive change.

A significant change in an organization's structure, leadership, or membership can influence organizational culture. For example, if a large academic health center were to create an extended affiliation with a series of community hospitals, the nurse and physician providers in each entity could experience disruptions caused by differences in culture and expectations. Nurses in the community hospital accustomed to practicing to the full scope of their legal authority might find the academic health center physicians expecting a greater level of consultation and deference from nurses. In an academic setting, if a new dean with significant experience leading a nimble and well-resourced

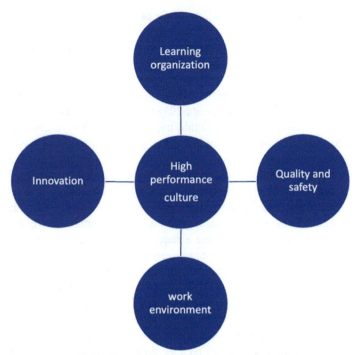

FIGURE 14.1 Elements of a High Performing Culture.

organization joins a large, public school with many layers of approval and policies, expectations about response time and the pace of change could be challenging. Structural and leadership changes present the opportunity to change
culture.

Changing the Culture

Organizations operate within an ever-changing environmental context.
Change is a process, not an event. We experience change in all aspects of our
lives, personally and professionally. The changes that have occurred across
your lifetime have been significant, but the changes across the last several years
have been breathtaking. For instance, in the post pandemic world, we are likely
to rely more on online technologies for shopping, working, and communicating
with our friends and families. In healthcare, these changes were implemented
rapidly (e.g., telehealth) and are likely to continue well beyond the pandemic.
But the ways in which such changes rolled out were heavily influenced by the
organizational cultures in which the changes were implemented. For instance,
a healthcare setting where clinical researchers were accustomed to solving

problems through innovative thinking, research laboratories used their own resources to develop testing kits for COVID-19 that were otherwise unavailable. In academic settings where the innovative cultures had established high quality online educational delivery approaches, the transition to remote education was far easier than in schools where traditional in-classroom methods were believed to represent the hallmark of high-quality education. Procedures, technology, work processes, and policies that govern clinical care are changing at an ever-increasing pace. The same is true for nursing education, where the use of technology, notably high-fidelity simulation, has replaced the old nursing arts laboratory and approaches to complex problem solving in teams has replaced the individualized skill of rote memorization.

Consider: **How would you describe the culture of the organization you currently work in? Have you ever been involved in changing an organizational culture?**

Organizations that are not adapting to the ever-changing environment often have a culture that supports the status quo and are at high risk to fail in the complex and quickly changing world in which we now live. Conditions supporting stagnation include: (1) the failure to perceive external changes; (2) the failure to examine internal beliefs; and (3) the failure to collect and review data about performance. Insularity and self-satisfaction put organizations at high risk for stagnation. For instance, hospitals that prepare the future workforce without consideration of new models of care or changing patient demands will find themselves out of step with the future. Schools of nursing might hold onto course content without substantially revising the curriculum to match current practices in the healthcare system. Organizations need to be responsive to the ever changing world and the faculty members of those organizations also require exposure to new ideas and opportunities to develop new skills.

Another contributor to insularity is past experience, and notably difficult or threatening experiences. For instance, when financial hardships affect organizations and result in cutting budgets and reducing personnel, these difficulties stay in the institutional memory of the organization. Then, when faced with similar circumstances, the past experiences and related outcomes reawaken old anxieties and the previous way of addressing the problem can emerge as the only way. After having cut positions and budgets, it may be difficult to convince people to try a new strategy to address the budget shortfall, such as bringing in new revenues and growing out of the deficit, rather than cutting back. The objective of leading is to move the organization forward toward its future and toward greater efficiency, effectiveness, and quality of work. Therefore, organizational leaders must be attuned to culture when considering the management of change. In healthcare and in higher education, a culture that values challenges, risk-taking, innovation and an engaged workforce will win out.

Resistance to change as noted in the example above is often due to fear: fear of job loss, fear of the unknown, fear of many different things. Often people do not recognize their fear when they resist change. Everyone creates stories about why the change cannot work or why leaders cannot be trusted, without recognizing that the genesis of these stories is their own fear. Leaders need to anticipate people's fear when engaging in culture change. Changing a culture requires numerous different interventions that take place over time. This gives leaders the opportunity to address people's fear. The context of the changing culture can either generate fear or alleviate it. If a leader approaches culture change from a negative perspective, such as basing the change on employees not being productive and needing to increase productivity or decrease budget as in the above example, the response will be fear leading to distrust and resistance. If the change is put into the context of creating better systems through greater support and resources for employees, the response will likely be much more positive.

Culture of Innovation

Some organizations are known for their innovation. The Ekvall model provides context for the interaction of creativity and innovation (Ekvall 1996). Creativity in this model recognizes the individual and team creativity comprising task motivation, expertise, and creativity skills. This feeds innovation within the work environment and recognizes the importance of resources,

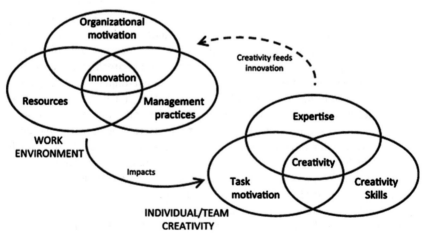

FIGURE 14.2 Ekval Model of Innovative Culture.

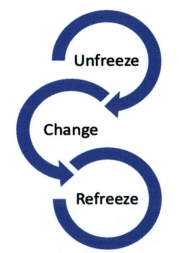

FIGURE 14.3 Lewin's Theory of Change.

management practices, and organizational motivation to support innovation. See Figure 14.2. While there are several models depicting elements important to innovative cultures, we have chosen this one because of the clarity of interaction at the individual and team level with the work environment.

Theories of Change

Theories of organizational change provide a structure for understanding the factors influencing change as well as the strategies used to promote organizational change. The most notable theory of organizational change in the social and behavioral sciences is Lewin's Theory of Change. According to Lewin (1947), change can be thought of as having three phases: unfreezing, changing, and refreezing. See Figure 14.3.

In other words, patterns must be stopped and new ways of organizing or being are discussed and adopted. Once implemented, the new ways of behaving need to be reinforced to sustain the change. Importantly, in order to guide change, the leader needs to understand what driving and restraining forces are influencing change. Those underlying forces need to be identified and moderated to ensure that the driving forces overcome the restraining forces. For example, an academic organization proposes to implement a new doctoral degree program and close a program that offers a master's degree. Although the match to the mission, vision and values statements is strong, the faculty members oppose this change. A significant underlying barrier is the fact that many of the faculty do not hold doctoral degrees and their continued employment could be at risk. In order to advance the agenda, the leadership team must find ways to improve access to the doctoral degree for employees who want to remain at the school. For others, articulating a set of roles and responsibilities that will not require the doctoral degree may be enough to assure their commitment to the change in program offerings.

A second theory of change that offers a more granular view of the process of change was proposed by Kotter (1996). Kotter's Eight Stage Process of Creating Major Change Model shown in Figure 14.4 recognizes the ubiquitous nature of organizational change and has identified eight steps that guide the leader toward successfully implementing change to a point of institutionalization.

Creating a sense of urgency for change is a foundational step in the change process with the work of coalition building and creating and communicating a vision following soon afterward. Kotter has emphasized the importance of the sequence to success in change management. Engaging the community, creating a vision or story about the change, and communicating are essential to successful change. Listening to employees' concerns and addressing them in a non-threatening and constructive way will help them see the opportunities created with this change. Kotter suggests that ideally, at least 75% of the organization should be favorable toward the change before moving on to the next steps (Kotter 1996). Creating 75% worth of support can take time.

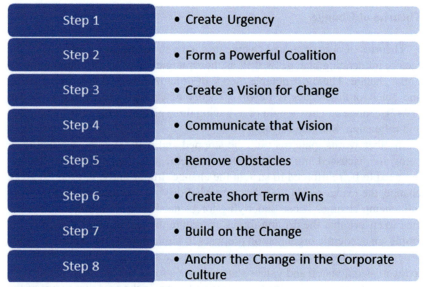

FIGURE 14.4 Kotter Eight Stage Process of Creating Major Change Model (Kotter [1996]. Leading Change. Boston: Harvard Business School Press, page 21).

Kotter suggests building a powerful coalition as the second step of the change process. The coalition includes employees with influence in the organization. This influence may not always be reflected in a formal title but will be individuals in the organization that others look to for wisdom, insights, and constructive thinking. By creating this coalition, the change may be discussed in both formal and informal settings, allowing for momentum to build.

Steps 3 and 4 relate to creating and communicating the vision. This is where the role of the leader is critical as both a visionary and a communicator. It is imperative that the leader has a clear vision of what the change is and why it is necessary. Linking the vision to the values of the organization and its mission will demonstrate its relevance in the organization. Being able to clearly articulate the importance of the vision as an integral part of the operations of the organization is critical. Employees will look to the leader to be consistent in their message and honestly and transparently discuss issues raised. A leader who does not consistently demonstrate commitment to the change will not be successful in its implementation.

Step 5 of the model involves empowering others to act, for instance, by removing obstacles or publicly encouraging the risk-taking that will support the change. One of the most important tools for a leader in an organization when executing a change is to identify and remove the obstacles that are preventing success. While members of the organization want to implement a change, they might face challenges that they do not know how to solve or lack the connections or organizational power to address. The leader's help in these situations will significantly affect how the change will progress. Step 6 involves recognizing and celebrating the progress seen in meeting short term goals. Celebrating these achievements lends visibility to the successes and builds momentum. Demonstrating success, even small successes, can help to win over those who remain skeptical about the benefits of the change.

Step 7 involves consolidating the change and producing more change by adjusting prevailing policies and adding more like-minded individuals to the change team. If the leader fails to continue to steward the change, members may easily fall back into the old ways of doing business. The final step, Step 8, involves anchoring the change in the organizational culture. The work of this stage involves connecting the new behaviors or structure to the new successes or productivities.

DIFFUSION OF INNOVATION

Roger's Model of Innovation Diffusion

As Kotter's theory of change proposes a process to ensure organizational change, Roger's (2003) theory proposes the process of diffusion of innova-

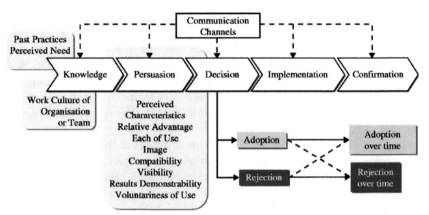

FIGURE 14.5 Stages of Rogers's Diffusion of Innovation Model. Source: Rogers (2003).

tion. His book *Diffusion of Innovation* explains how new ideas and technology spread through an organization. We know that all changes are not accepted, nor do all changes roll out at the same rate. Rogers's theory offers an explanation of the factors for consideration. Adoption of change is a process that begins with the awareness that the innovations exist (*see* Figure 14.5). This stage, known as knowledge/awareness, sets up the possibility of change but lacks the depth of understanding what would drive the change. Persuasion follows with those who favor the change, do the work of informing and persuading others. The next stage involves actually making a decision, which is done by an individual or a group. Movement at this stage is influenced by the balance of the personal characteristics of adopters (early or late) and the degree of change required of affected individuals. Once a decision is made to adopt, the implementation stage follows. During implementation, participants try out aspects of the change and evaluate its utility. Proposals for further adaptation may emerge. Confirmation/continuation completes the process with the individual, group, or organization accepting and agreeing to continue the change. The rate of change is influenced by opinion leaders, as well as the price of conforming or non-conforming to the proposal for change. While adoption is the term generally used to describe an individual's change, diffusion refers to the group's response to implementing the change.

Consider: **Think about a time when you were enthusiastically engaged in a plan for change and realized that you seemed more enthusiastic than others. How did this make you feel? What did you do when you felt that way?**

A number of factors have been shown to influence the rate of diffusion. Organizations that are smaller in size, less centralized, less complex, highly interconnected, and with resources that are not already committed have an easier time integrating innovations. The adoption of an innovation is largely dependent on how the innovation is aligned with the organization's core values and culture.

Champions are needed to increase the potential for success of the diffusion of innovation within an organization. As with any organizational change, having individuals who hold some organizational stature and are willing to keep the idea energized will increase the likelihood that a change will be successful. For example, these may be individuals who can influence others to think favorably about a change, or they might be people with formal authority who have the opportunity to provide formal rewards for people who adopt an innovation. Greenlaugh *et al.* (2004) built on Rogers' and others work in diffusion theory and developed a model for diffusion in service organizations which includes nine components: (1) innovation characteristics; (2) adoption by individuals, (3) assimilation by the system (system planning and decision-making); (4) diffusion and dissemination (use of opinion leaders, champions and type of program); (5) system antecedents for innovation (structure and culture); (6) system readiness for innovation including tension, fit, support, advocacy, and time resources; (7) outer context: interorganizational networks and collaborations; (8) implementation and routinization (leadership and management); and the (9) linkage of components of the model (White, Dudley-Brown and Terhaar, 2020 pg.40).

As with the Diffusion of Innovation model which notes that champions can accelerate the spread of change, Greenhalph *et al.* (2004) systematic review of diffusion of innovations in health services organizations model identifies a broad range of contextual considerations. These include antecedents to the innovation, qualities of the innovation, communication regarding the innovation, the readiness of the system for the innovation, and the process of implementation (Greenhalph *et al.*, 2004, p. 595). This systematic review provides a high level of specific, research-based direction for understanding innovations in the health sector.

MORE ON INNOVATION

Since the introduction of the notion of disruptive innovation by Clay Christensen and colleagues (1995), leaders have been more attuned to the ways in which innovations can result in complete overhauls of the standard ways of operating. A disruptive innovation can be described as the introduction of a new technology or practice so radically different that it results in significantly different changes. For instance, at its introduction, online education threatened to disrupt the usual face-to-face approach to higher education. Once nurse practitioners and other advanced practice providers were widely accepted, some believed that their introduction would radically change the ways in which care would be delivered. Christensen and colleagues (2000) proposed an approach to organizing healthcare delivery that would have rationalized the delivery system into centers or focus factories, where specialized activities would take place. Surgery or diagnosis might occur there, and treatment plans could be administered elsewhere, with reliability and higher value. A major difference between innovation and change is the degree of creativity and difference seen in innovation, and the certainty of the consequences of innovation. Change that displays high levels of creativity, including disruption to the status quo, constitutes innovation.

A deep understanding of innovation is often attributed to the work of Tom Kelley (2001) and the IDEO group, in their description of design thinking. Kelley and colleagues propose that the design process begins with an empathetic eye, that is, developing an understanding of a problem from the perspective of the other. A series of steps follow, including brainstorming on possible solutions, prototyping solutions, and revising in a rapid cycle. The design thinking process has been applied to a broad set of activities, including the redesign of physical space, development of gadgets, and helping people think about their careers. Although trendy in Silicon Valley and taught in higher education classrooms, nurses will recognize the similarity of the design thinking approach to a process common in the clinical care delivery setting: the Plan, Do, Check, Act cycle. Originally proposed by the industrial engineer, Walter Shewhart, as the Cycle for Continuous Learning and Improvement, and later popularized by Deming as the PDSA cycle (Deming, 2000), this approach is used for rapid cycle response to implementing and evaluating change.

Consider: **Have you ever been involved in a project that introduced an innovation and never really got off the ground? How would you think about your experience in light of the Diffusion of Innovation theory?**

Weberg (2017) has discussed the leadership of innovation. He acknowledges that hierarchy may be needed to provide structure within organizations, but that innovation lives on the edge of chaos. Innovation cannot occur in overly structured environments, nor can it thrive in overly chaotic ones. The importance of culture emerges again. Teams that are successful in innovation are teams that challenge the status quo, embrace the ideas of individual members, and work around outdated structures to develop innovations. Good ideas can come from anyone on the team. Leadership is not responsible for developing all the innovations but supports the process of innovation through conflict management and relationship development.

CLOSING THOUGHTS ON CHANGE AND CULTURE

Changing a culture is like changing the course of a large ship. The action does not happen quickly and must be carefully planned. The work may involve a needed alignment with the MVV of the organization. Publicly recognizing and honoring the positive performances of the faculty or staff and the constructive elements of a culture can drive change. Engagement of the members of the community and the key opinion leaders is essential.

Katzenbach, Steffen & Kronley (2012) told the story of John Rowe's arrival as Aetna's CEO in the early 2000s. Aetna was losing customers, the stock price was falling, work was siloed, and workers were discouraged about their futures and that of the company. Rather than telling everyone what needed to change, Rowe engaged the organization in a process of problem solving and strengthening the organization. Five principles of culture change emerged from this work:

1. Match strategy and culture: In every culture there are elements that work. Trying to impose cultural change without connection to current culture will result in failure. For instance, if there is a strong sense of customer service, build on that rather than trying to instill a cultural value of increasing income. The increased income will likely follow better customer service.

2. Focus on a few critical shifts in behavior: Coming into an organization and thinking that you will blow up the organization and turn it around is very unlikely to be a successful strategy. Identifying behavioral strengths of an organization, such as high commitment to engaging in quality improvement activities, can be the basis for creating additional behavioral changes. Building on the quality improvement commitment could then extend to identifying ways of translating that into creating patient centered care or student-centered learning. Being able to build on strengths that already exist will make culture change much more likely.

3. Honor the strengths of the existing culture: People in an organization usually have a level of allegiance to the organization, even if it is a dysfunctional one. Being critical of past leaders or current ways of doing things will create an immediate resistance to any proposed change. Honoring what has been accomplished and organizations strengths reinforces staff feeling recognized and valued.

4. Integrate formal and informal interventions: Formal interventions can include changes in policies/procedures, changes in structure of the organi-

zation, changes to incentive systems, and others. Formal interventions are not enough to be successful and need to be coupled with informal interventions such as setting up small group lunches to talk about how things were going in different parts of the business, doing walk arounds, engaging all levels of staff to talk about their understanding of the mission, and values of the organizations. The informal interventions reinforce the formal interventions and give staff the opportunity for input and to feel valued.

5. Measure and monitor cultural evolution: Consistent monitoring of the culture provides an early detection warning system of impending problems within the organization, as well as serving as benchmarks of progress for culture change.

SUMMARY

Effective leaders understand the prevailing culture as prerequisite to undertaking change. Culture, as the sum of beliefs, values and conventions that guide behavior can be changed. The purpose of culture change is to improve the effectiveness and efficiency of organizational structures, processes, and outcomes and to create a more engaged workforce within a respectful and inclusive work environment. Cultures contribute to the subjective experience of the workforce and the ability of organizations to achieve results. Envisioning, implementing, and managing a shared vision for an improved culture is a major responsibility of the leader. The culture-sensitive leader will also understand that managing or guiding change is a process that includes a set of stages and intentional leadership actions. The distinction between change and innovation relates to the degree of creativity contributing to the proposed revisions and the certainty of the outcomes. True innovation requires the support of specific leadership actions, including conflict management and relationship building.

CRITICAL THINKING QUESTIONS

At the beginning of the chapter academic and clinical vignettes were presented. Please review the vignettes to address the following questions. The questions are specific to the vignettes.

Academic Vignette Questions

1. How did the prevailing culture of Fairport University contribute to the outcomes in this vignette? Can you hypothesize about the culture of this organization?

2. In the context of managing change, how did the dean's actions contribute to the failure of this project to move forward?

3. How might you have led the change in financial accountability to produce the desired outcome?

Clinical Vignette Questions

1. What observations can you make about the prevailing culture? How did the introduction of new providers change the culture of the team?

2. What signs suggested that the team collaborations were at risk? When did these appear?

3. What change management activities might have been employed to strengthen the academic-practice collaboration? When would you have tried to intervene and how?

4. Given the state of the collaboration and the significance of the proposed work, what leadership efforts would you bring to the collaboration now?

REFERENCES

Batras, D., Duff, C., & Smith, H. B. (2014). Organizational change theory: Implications for health promotion practice. *Health Promotion International, 31*(1), 231-241. https://doi.org/10.1093/heapro/dau098

Christensen, C., & Bower, J. (1995). Disruptive Technologies Catching the Wave. *Harvard Business Review, 73*(1), 43-53.

Christensen, C. M., Bohmer, R. M. J., & Kenagy, J. (2000). Will disruptive innovations cure health care? *Harvard Business Review, 78*(5), 102-112, 199.

Collins, J. (2009). How the mighty fall. HarperCollins Publishers Inc.

Cooke, R. A., & Szumal, J. L. (2000). *Handbook of organizational culture and climate.* Sage Publications.

Deming, W. (2000). *The new economics: For industry, government, education.* (2nd Ed). MIT Press.

Ekvall, G. (1996). Organizational climate for creativity and innovation, *European Journal of Work and Organizational Psychology, 5*:1, 105–123, DOI: 10.1080/13594329608414845

Gardner, J. (1995). *Self-renewal: The individual and the innovative society.* WW Norton & Co.

Greenhalph, T., Robert, G., MacFarlane, F., Bate, P., & Kyriakidou, O. (2004). Diffusion of innovations in service organizations: Systematic review and recommendations. *Milbank Quarterly, 82*(4), 581–629. https://doi.org/10.1111/j.0887-378X.2004.00325.x

Groysberg, B., Lee, J., Proce, J., & Cheng, Y. (2018). The leader's guide to corporate culture: How to manage eight critical elements in organizational life. *Harvard Business Review, 96*(1), 44–52.

Heifetz, R., Grashow, A., & Linsky, M. (2009). *The practice of adaptive leadership*. Cambridge Leadership Associates.

Katzenbach, J. R., Steffen, I., & Kronley, C. (2012). Cultural change that sticks. *Harvard Business Review, 90*(7-8), 110–117, 162.

Kelley, T. (2001). *The art of innovation: Lessons in creativity from IDEO, America's leading design firm*. Random House.

Kotter, J. P. (1996). *Leading change*. Harvard University Press.

Lewin, K. (1947). Group decision and social change. In Newcomb, T. M., Hartley, E. L. (Eds.), Readings in social psychology (pp. 330–344). New York, NY: Henry Holt.

Mind Tools. (n.d.). *Lewin's change management model* [LAA1]: *Understanding the three stages of change*. Mind Tools. https://www.mindtools.com/pages/article/newPPM_94.htm

Rogers, E. (2003). *Diffusion of innovation*. Free Press.

Weberg, D. (2017). Innovation in action: Innovation, culture and leadership synthesis. *Nurse Leader, 15*(4), 241.

White, K., Dudley-Brown, S., & Tehar, M. (2020). *Translation of evidence into nursing and healthcare* (3rd Ed). Springer Publishing.

The Leader

CHAPTER 15

The Leadership Checkup

ACADEMIC VIGNETTE

Dr. Emma Blair's transition from the role of Chief Nursing Officer within a large medical center to the role of Dean of the School of Nursing at Covington University was causing her some anxiety. She had been at the medical center for many years and was now faced with an unfamiliar environment. The change in roles was something she had wanted for some time; but now that she was in the new role she was concerned that she may be lacking some critical skills. She outlined a course of action that would engage the faculty and staff in a series of brainstorming sessions to develop priorities for the school and explore plans for assuring leadership could bring excellence to the school. She felt confident in her ability to create and manage systems; she now needed to put that skill to work within her new environment and harness the knowledge of the faculty and staff to build a cohesive group with opportunities for strengthening the school. Her leadership talent was excellent, she just needed a checkup on how to manage in a new environment.

CLINICAL VIGNETTE

During the long days, weeks and years of COVID-19, the burden on management and staff at Bayview Community Hospital was severe. Nearly every unit along with the emergency room were trying to cope with 60% staffing to care for very sick patients. Individuals who had scheduled procedures requiring a hospital visit were postponed. Morale was low and burnout was high. The leadership teams for medicine and nursing were at their wits end. How would they continue to manage the hospital and provide critical patient care if they couldn't secure additional staff. Leadership called together all of the senior staff and asked them to assist in developing a plan of action. Although no one really had time to spend on planning; all of the senior staff agreed to construct a system for staffing. Within several weeks, they had worked out a system to triage patients to other facilities and increased their use of travel nurses. The leadership team then began to work out a new budget for the hospital, anticipating that this would be a long process.

INTRODUCTION

Leadership is essential within health systems; but the skill set to excel as a leader can be daunting! In many of the previous chapters the business of leadership has considered the role of managing systems and people and creating the strategies that fit the time, place, challenge, or opportunity. This chapter will focus primarily on the leader's need to create a healthy organization for self and others. This leadership mindset focuses on health and wellbeing for not only the people who are consumers of the organization's services, but also for those who provide the services and that of the leader. It is part of the work in planning for a sustainable and healthy organization. Leaders need to reflect on their own satisfaction, challenge, joy, and the ability to care for themselves as well as the health of the organization. Attention will be focused on leader wellbeing personally and within the context of organization. The leader's vision of themselves as a healthy person and leader, their ability to do a "checkup" on their successes and challenges, whether their work is bringing them joy, and how resilient they are when things get tough is a critical part of a healthy self. In addition, being a healthy leader includes applying principles of the TRAM model (trust, reliability, accountability, and mindfulness) model. It is important to assess the fit of a leader within an organization. This chapter will begin with a focus on leader well-being and then consider the leader well-being using the TRAM model and an example.

Leader Personal Well-being

A leader many not always succeed in building a high functioning organization. The reasons are many, but leaders must be aware of when their fit with the organization is at odds. Recognizing and responding to a decline of fit between the leader and the organization requires the skill to recognize when a tune-up is in order. It can be painful for a leader to recognize that the elements of an effective and productive team are in jeopardy and that the once thriving leader or organization needs help. It may be time for the leader to seek other opportunities or it may be time to evaluate the opportunity to strengthen the requisite knowledge, skills, and attitudes essential for leadership.

Leaders need to be mindful that creating innovative and creative environments can be stressful, highly challenging, sometimes lonely, and often scary. The consequences can lead to burnout and poor performance. Burnout of health professionals is of great concern. Many health systems are looking at ways of having their workforce find meaning and satisfaction in their work. The Institute for Healthcare Improvement has a "joy in work" effort and many health systems are grappling with how to make work more satisfying and reduce the burnout of health professionals which the COVID 19 pandemic has significantly exacerbated. Nurse leaders need to take care of "why" they entered a healthcare discipline. For leaders to help others find joy in their work, they must have joy in their work. This requires emotional self-awareness and self-management to be proactive, innovative and a great leader. It also requires a commitment to knowing the people they work with in a way that demonstrates deep caring and commitment to the individual as well as the collective. Understanding the identities, challenges, and aspirations of everyone is very important.

Constant stress can wear leaders out, both physically and emotionally. Burnout has been described as representing "an erosion in values, dignity, spirit and will—an erosion of the human soul" (Maslach and Leiter, 1997, p. 24). Burnout can lead to faulty decision making, ineffective leadership, and decreased productivity. Signs of burnout include feeling emotionally drained and tired in the morning, questioning the meaning of your work and feeling like you are not doing a good job. When these thoughts become prevalent it is time to consider making changes. The culprit leading to burnout is often thought to be overwork, however, this is only one contributing factor. Jimenez (2021) makes a point that the following also contribute to burnout.

Organizational Environment

The culture of an organization as well as the processes governing decision-making and being able to do one's work can vary along a continuum in terms of the level of support provided which is largely determined by the leadership. Lots of things change within organizations and it is not unusual for a leader to find themselves in an organization that no longer reflects their values or style. A mismatch of values of the leader and the organization will create a great deal of stress. Organizations that provide resources, both financial and emotional support, to enable leaders to do the work they need to do helps leaders manage stress. Expectations in health systems include ensuring patient safety, positive performance on quality indicators, management of the dynamics among the various health providers, financing challenges and many more. The stress of knowing people can be harmed by a decision can weigh heavily. The ability to diagnose an impending crisis and deftly manage a way to resolution takes considerable skill. Similar stressors can be found in academic environments and while the risks are different, the stakes can also be high in terms of student outcomes, faculty performance, management of resources, donor relations and many more. The Deming Institute has noted that "A bad system will beat an individual every time" Several key strategies to ameliorate the likelihood of burnout are:

- *Societal and nursing mental models*: Leaders often work long hours. There remains a societal culture that fosters giving over to one's workplace, one's life. This is particularly powerful for nurses. The mental model of nursing is that we stay with our patients until they are stable, or another nurse takes over. We give to others before we take care of ourselves. We work 12 hours a day or longer and as needed with the pandemic, day after day after day. This mental model contributes to nurses being the most trusted profession because we are focused on caring for others. In doing this, we also need to acknowledge that we can only care for others when we have cared for ourselves. When the cup is empty there is nothing to give. This mental model is changing as new generations of nurses emerge which we believe is good.
- *Personality and choices*: Leader's personality such as level of emotional intelligence, experiences, values, beliefs and even genetics can influence response to stress (Johnson, O'Grady, Coetzee, 2021). Therefore, it is critical for leaders to know themselves and to work on the areas that can be enhanced through self-exploration and reflection, mindfulness, coaching, mentoring or other self-awareness and self-improvement modalities. As we better understand neuroscience, we also better understand that we can change behaviors and make choices that help us to take care of ourselves.

The extent of a leader's accountability may feel like an emotional onslaught, some nurse leaders dash from one crisis to the next without taking a breath to center one's self. Taking care of oneself and building resilience is important to managing the diverse and often highly emotional situations in health care because the leader's ability to effectively lead will depend on having the emotional resources associated with resilience. Engaging in mindfulness practices can help leaders experience joy, satisfaction, insight, energy, and success in their work. This means taking the time for mindfulness practices such as meditation, breathing, self-reflection or journaling on a regular basis to manage stressful situations through building their resilience.

In addition, there are practices that can be useful on a day to day, practical level. One practice to manage stressful situations is STOP. Jon Kabot-Zinn a master of mindfulness who developed the Stress Reduction Clinic at the University of Massachusetts Medical School developed a straightforward way to be present in a situation and enhance awareness of internal emotional terrain as well as the external terrain. The STOP steps are:

S: *Stop*. Stop what you are doing and pause momentarily.

T: *Take a breath*. Take a deep breath or several. Deep breathing can anchor you to the present moment.

O: *Observe*. Notice what is happening both outside and inside of yourself. Where has your mind gone? What do you feel? What are you doing?

P: *Proceed*. Continue doing what you were doing or using the information gained during this check-in, change course. (Kabat-Zinn, 2013).

Another practice that can be used to reorient to the present, especially when feeling stressed about a situation is the use of RAIN that has been proposed by Brach (2020). Being present when stressed is difficult if not impossible. RAIN helps to refocus and stands for:

- *Recognize what is happening*: This includes recognizing your thoughts, feelings and behaviors. Saying to yourself what you observe will help identify the stressor that is most important now.
- *Allow the experience to be there, just as it is*: Let the thoughts, feelings and behaviors be as you note them without trying to change them.
- *Investigate with interest and care*: Be curious about why you are feeling the way you are through questions like: What is creating the barrier to being present? What most wants attention? How am I experiencing this in my body? What am I believing? What does this vulnerable place want from me? What does it most need?
- *Nurture with self-compassion*. Recognize that you are uncomfortable and give yourself space to experience it and to then say to yourself that you are alright. Give yourself the gift of self-nurturing to do whatever will move you from a place of suffering or discomfort.

Resilience

There has been significant research on resilience in health care and academic environments. It has been studied for its impact on organizational outcomes including job satisfaction at all levels, team performance, staff turnover, faculty and student outcomes and the leaders "intent to stay." Silsbee, 2018 (p. 155) defines resilience as "the capacity to be resourceful and creative, to make choices, and to take effective action no matter what is going on." He also notes that being resilient requires being aware of your inner state and being present to your current situation. It is often the lack of awareness of our inner state that leads us to feel exhausted, unproductive, and cranky.

Resilience enables the leader to concentrate on the organization's mission, its culture, and its people. Building resilience within self as well as within those who work within the organization can create an environment that retains its leaders and workforce and is strategically managed for the future. Who

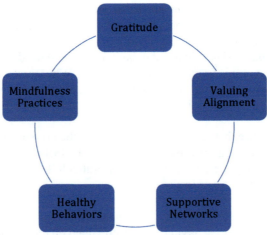

FIGURE 15.1 Building Resilience.

among us would not want to serve as a leader in order to build the infrastructure and environment necessary for managing effectively (culture) an organization that believed in setting a challenge and strategies to succeed (strategic planning) attends to and partners with its people, customers, and key stakeholders (sustainability). Building a resilient organization that collectively strives for success and has strategies in place to manage challenges is a learning organization. This creates an environment that retains its leaders and workforce and strategically plans.

Jimenez (2021) notes that resilience is like a piggy bank. It can be emptied with the constancy of unmanaged stress and needs to be consistently replenished. The ability to build resilience and in turn successfully cope with challenges generally requires a multi-pronged approach as noted in Figure 15.1. The important actions include practicing gratitude and mindfulness, engaging in healthy behaviors including exercise nutrition and sleep, valuing alignment of personal and organizational goals, and having supportive networks of friends and colleagues.

Self-care Strategies

Building a support network of trusted colleagues and friends is important. Having a small circle of very close confidants is important as well as having a larger circle of friends and colleagues who can provide honest input to help problem solve, talk about stress and emotional situations. Practicing gratitude can be very emotionally sustaining. Leaders can do this by reflecting at the beginning of each day three things that they are grateful for. Beginning meetings by thanking all the team members for the work they do and calling out specific examples are also ways of integrating gratefulness practices on a daily basis. In practicing gratitude, it is useful to consider the following (Rosenberg, 2018): What was observed? What need did it meet? How did it make the recipient feel? Saying "great job" is a commonly used phrase by leaders to recognize that someone did something successfully such as managing a difficult, conflictual situation with a patient. A powerful way of expressing gratitude using Rosenberg's model would be to recognize that the nurse was empathetic and clarified what the patient was concerned or fearful about and then took action to address the fear. The interaction of the nurse met the need of the patient to feel cared about and safe.

Continually assessing one's own values for alignment with the organizations will provide information to either realign one's own values, work to realign the values of the organization or decide to leave. Nurse leaders know the importance of engaging in healthy behaviors but are usually better at supporting staff to engage in healthy behaviors than integrating healthy behaviors for themselves, especially when having many tugs on their time. However, adequate sleep, nutrition, exercise, and others are essential to effective leadership by enhancing resilience.

Leaders also need to integrate mindfulness strategies into their leadership that reduces and prevents crises, and builds resilience in oneself and in others. These strategies may include training for self and the team by bringing in mindful coaches or embedding specific mindful practices within team meetings. It should also include the continual evaluation of processes that are making it difficult for people to thrive. For example, a drop in quality scores, an increase in poor patient outcomes, a union action, financial challenges, or high turnover in the nursing staff can create an environment that could impact one's ability to be resilient. Mindfulness practices will help to clarify if the organizational investment in nursing sustains their optimism; if their leadership style fits with the organization's values; and if their own sense of satisfaction with their work aligns with their vision of leadership.

Preparing for and sustaining a leadership role is challenging work. Developing a team that will drive toward a core set of competencies including trust building, high reliability organization principles, social equality, accountability structures and processes and mindfulness is challenging work. It helps to have a structured guide for the development of a team. It can be painful for a leader to recognize that the elements of an effective and productive team are in jeopardy and that the once thriving leader or organization needs help. It may be time for the leader to seek other opportunities or it may be time to evaluate the opportunity to strengthen the requisite knowledge, skills, and attitudes essential for leadership. There are a number of frameworks that can be used as a guide for data driven decision- making, leadership, change management, organizational culture development, diversity, and inclusion as well as the technical tools and resources for data management, quality improvement, innovation and evidence-based practice. Many of these frameworks have been discussed throughout this book. Ideally, the organization will establish, sustain, and advance a system for performance management excellence that will position the organization to be highly productive, competitive, financially solvent and visionary.

LEADER WELL-BEING AND EFFECTIVENESS WITHIN AN ORGANIZATIONAL CONTEXT: THE TRAM MODEL

Leaders are often faced with questions of how good a leader-organization fit is. The fit of a leader with an organization will depend on a number of factors. To help frame such factors, readers may find the "TRAM Model" a useful framework for evaluating fit (Figure 15.2).

TRAM is an acronym for Trust, Reliability, Accountability and Mindfulness. The TRAM Model guides leaders within organizations to create structures and processes that assure that the principles and practices of Trust, Reliability, Accountability and Mindfulness are consistently implemented within the organization. Although this model is theoretical and has not been tested, the belief by the authors of this book is that the application of these evidenced based organizational practices in a coherent and disciplined way will result in organizational performance excellence.

An individual leader may ascribe to these practices to assure leadership effectiveness however it is the contention of the authors that unless an organization's leadership team as a whole commits to these principles and practices, the likelihood of positive impact on organizational performance will be limited. When organizations as a whole make a commitment to implementing the TRAM Model, workforce, consumer and organizational outcomes are likely to improve.

Model Domains

Domains in this model are considered evidence-based practices. The first domain is aimed at building trust at the individual and organizational level among dyads and teams. Building trust is achieved through the application of the behaviors and principles outlined by Stephen MR Covey (2006) in his book, *The Speed of Trust: The One Thing That Changes Everything*. He describes trust as a dynamic between two or more people and is built by the confidence one has in self and others have in an individual. Trust is confidence born of two dimensions: character and competence. Character includes your integrity, motive, and intent with people. Competence includes your capabilities, skills, results, and track record.

The second domain focuses on implementing high reliability principles which requires a commitment by individuals and organizations to implement best practices of high reliability and include robust quality improvement and change management resources. Chassin and Loeb in their classic paper *High-Reliability Health Care: Getting There from Here* (2013) describe these five principles that have become staples of healthcare organizations today promulgated by the Joint Commission and other standard setting organizations. These principles are deference to expertise, reluctance to simplify, sensitivity to operations, commitment to resilience and preoccupation with failure.

The third domain involves implementing processes and structures that result in clear role accountability of individuals and teams and their decision-making rights. McDowell and Mallon (2020) describe these best practices in their monograph: *Getting decision rights right: How effective organizational decision-making can help boost performance*. One organizational tool that is particularly useful in designating specific decision-making roles is the RACI framework, where "RACI" stands for **R**esponsible, **A**ccountable, **C**onsulted, and **I**nformed. The use of this tool by committees, departments and individuals can increase the likelihood of high performing teams who are clear about their roles and responsibilities.

The fourth domain "Mindful Leadership" is an evidence-based strategy to help individuals slow down and find the space to lead using the practices and attitudes of mindfulness. In her book, *Finding the Space to Lead: A Practical Guide to Mindful Leadership* (2015) Janet Marturano describes strategies that leaders can use to move away from a constant state of partial attentiveness and ineffectiveness to one in which more creativity, focus, clarity and compassion are the norm. These practices include meditation; attuning yourself to the feelings and actions of others; exercising daily and finding the space to reflect and be creative.

The Result: Performance Excellence

Organizations and leaders who commit to creating structures and processes of Trust, Reliability, Accountability and Mindfulness and who commit to leading using these practices—that is, assuring the implementation of them throughout an organization, are more likely to advance a high performing organization where the people who work in the organization have meaning and purpose in their work and those served by the organization have their interests and needs met.

Example of the Application of TRAM

The following presents an example of the TRAM model within a complex health system.

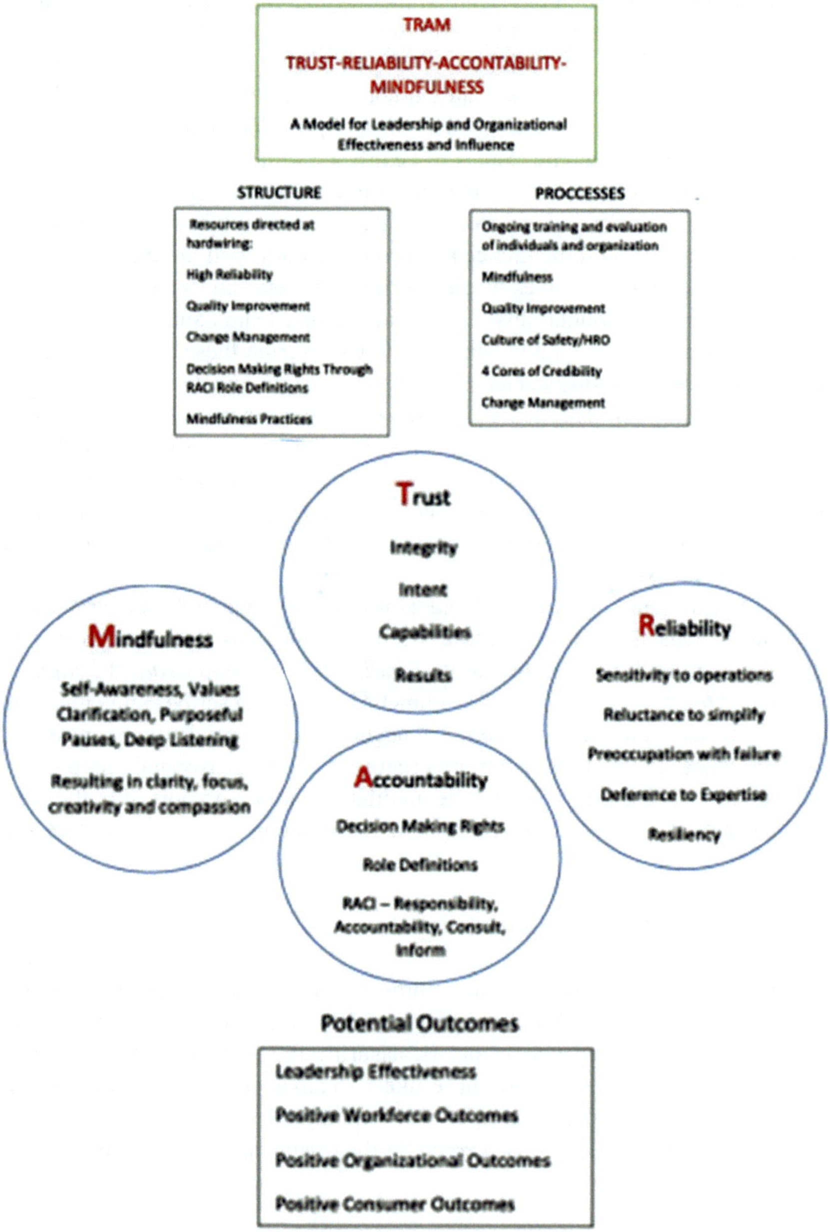

TRAM

TRUST-RELIABILITY-ACCONTABILITY-MINDFULNESS

A Model for Leadership and Organizational Effectiveness and Influence

STRUCTURE

Resources directed at hardwiring:

High Reliability

Quality Improvement

Change Management

Decision Making Rights Through RACI Role Definitions

Mindfulness Practices

PROCCESSES

Ongoing training and evaluation of individuals and organization

Mindfulness

Quality Improvement

Culture of Safety/HRO

4 Cores of Credibility

Change Management

Trust

Integrity

Intent

Capabilities

Results

Mindfulness

Self-Awareness, Values Clarification, Purposeful Pauses, Deep Listening

Resulting in clarity, focus, creativity and compassion

Reliability

Sensitivity to operations

Reluctance to simplify

Preoccupation with failure

Deference to Expertise

Resiliency

Accountability

Decision Making Rights

Role Definitions

RACI – Responsibility, Accountability, Consult, Inform

Potential Outcomes

Leadership Effectiveness

Positive Workforce Outcomes

Positive Organizational Outcomes

Positive Consumer Outcomes

FIGURE 15.2 The TRAM Model.

Jane Stand, FNP-BC, DNP had been working in ambulatory care management and delivery for decades. She was both a provider and manager in a healthcare system in Portland, Oregon with the title of "Chief NP" in a practice since acquiring her DNP degree.

Jane anticipated that many challenges would be forthcoming when accepting the new position, but now, 6 months into the new role, she felt that she underestimated the challenges. She had recently attended a leadership development program and had time to reflect on both her own leadership competencies and fit within the practice and the organization she worked in. These reflections fell into several categories: (1) Her own leadership style and how it mirrored her values (she hoped); (2) Her identity as a nurse leader vs. an organizational leader (was there a difference, she pondered?); (3) Her relationships with her boss, her peers and subordinates; (4) The organizational structure both its' strengths and shortcomings; (5) Challenging relationships with several professional colleagues; (6) The organizational culture involving patient centeredness, patient safety and quality improvement, change and innovation.

Reflection on clinical and leadership practice: At this point in her career, Jane had a good sense of her talents and areas of weaknesses in her leadership style, her relationships with others and her interest in continuing to pursue becoming a more effective person and leader. Her practice with patients and families had always felt like a strong suit for her. She was empathic, caring, expert and inclusive with her patients realizing their unique needs and interests. Her patient satisfaction survey scores were excellent and at times outstanding. She believed this is one reason why she was a person who should lead a practice given her strengths in this arena. However, she often felt overwhelmed and exhausted. She found herself having a hard time focusing on the patient and/or family that she was seeing, rather thinking about what needed to be done next or what administrative tasks she had waiting for her at the end of her day. She did not want to always feel rushed, distracted and overworked. She wondered if there was something she could do to become more centered and less harried.

Another area of struggle and worry for Jane was in her relationships with some colleagues. She had a hard time sharing patients, or co-leading teams. She would rather do things on her own and liked to be in complete control. In this regard, she was not particularly inclusive in her decision making and priority setting. One thing that particularly bothered her, when she had been appointed Lead/Chief NP of the practice five years ago, almost every other advanced practitioner (both NPs and PAs) decided to leave the practice and move to another system. She received feedback from a trusted peer at that time that people did not want to work "under her." They thought she was too controlling.

Consider: **What are some mindfulness strategies Jane could apply to her clinical practice? How can Jane increase the trust that others have in her?**

Jane also had the feeling that people she worked with did not really trust her. She could not put her finger on it, but things that people said made her believe they did not think she would follow through with what she said she would do. She did often change her mind after saying she was going to do something, and she often did not agree with the ideas of others and would just ignore them. She never followed up with people about these things, she did her own thing.

The New Organizational Structure and its Challenges: Jane reported to the Chief Nursing Officer of the hospital and as the nursing director of this practice she was a peer of the Medical Director. The structure called for an MD-RN-Administrator co-leadership structure, but in reality, Jane's "supervising MD" for her advanced practice role was the medical director. In addition, the administrator of this practice held a Vice President, Ambulatory Services title. Jane thought this to be a cumbersome structure in which she never fully felt "equal" to her co-leaders in terms of organizational hierarchy.

The medical director would often make decisions without Jane or the administrator's input. They would often not communicate for weeks at a time and when they did, it was often a rushed encounter. The physicians, NPs, PAs, nurses and support staff who worked in the practice were satisfied, but there was a lot of grumbling about equity in workload, lack of teamwork and respect. Jane sought counsel and direction from the chief nursing officer, but he was often caught up in inpatient flow issues, bed control, staffing crisis and patient safety issues. He also had little experience in the ambulatory setting and was not an advanced practice nurse and although he was smart and he cared about the continuum, it was hard for him to prioritize the issues.

Jane wondered if it was wise for her to be reporting to the CNO given these challenges. She wondered if being a nurse was even helpful to her at this point in her career. Yes, she was an advanced practice nurse with roots in her discipline and highly valued but she couldn't remember the last time she felt like she acted as a nurse or used in everyday practice what she learned in educational preparation. Did she lead like a nurse? Did it matter? Were her views and perspectives different about patient and family centered care than her medical colleagues? She seemed to be at an existential crossroads.

Consider: **Is there a way to increase clarity about Jane's role, her colleagues' roles and relationships, and the individual and shared decision-making authority among members of her leadership team?**

The Organizational Culture: The CEO, COO and CFO of the organization had come to the hospital from another large system and arrived about 8 years ago. Jane thought that they were pretty astute, had a grasp on the realities facing health care delivery and that they had moved the organization in good directions. Jane was bothered however by what she experienced as a lack of interest by them in day-to-day operations. Yes, there were others below them in the hierarchy that were positioned to manage that, but there seemed to be a lack of deference or "holding up" of what providers had to say in terms of patient experience, resource needs and wasteful and unreliable processes. For instance, the provider group asked the administration to consider purchasing a Real Time Locator System so that data-driven operations could improve patient access, flow and provider and staff productivity. This technology would improve reliability in several key quality metrics and is so important to operations. There were many scheduling errors, patients showing up when providers were in the lab or off, lines of patients waiting for phlebotomy service were extensive and errors resulted. Then, when errors occurred, administrative leaders would swoop in with all the solutions for improvement, not engaging front line staff in solutions.

Jane knew there had to be a better way for the organizational leaders to respond to critical elements of the ambulatory operational issues and to engage experts in finding solutions. She considered talking with her co-leadership team about this, but they so infrequently had time to talk with one another, never mind developing a strategy to address these issues.

Consider: How might actions taken by Jane increase her leadership effectiveness and the organizational outcomes?

This case study is a good reminder that leaders may have the best intentions but at times lack an awareness of their own impact on the environment and the people they work with or lead. This is the critical notion of managing oneself, knowing your values, knowing your style and tendencies, and clearly understanding your fit within the organization. The ability to find meaning and balance within the work environment is often a reason an individual stays within an organization. But, moving on when the career goals and organizational fit are no longer working is a choice that leaders should not be afraid to consider.

SUMMARY

This chapter explores a number of the challenges that accompany leadership and some ideas and models about how to manage. The leader, whether new to the role or a seasoned executive, can run up against challenges such as cultural differences, temperament, lack of insight, and response to decision making like Jane experienced. Finding a model such as TRAM that works for a leader who is both new to the role or a seasoned executive can be helpful. This chapter also acknowledges that leadership has many rewards but significant challenges. Seeking out models that work is worth the time and effort.

CRITICAL THINKING QUESTIONS

At the beginning of the chapter academic and clinical vignettes were presented. Please review the vignettes to address the following questions. The questions are specific to the vignettes.

Academic Vignette

1. How could Dr. Blair prepare herself for the new role as Dean of the School of Nursing?
2. What skills will be most essential as she begins the process of working with faculty and staff?
3. The transition from a clinical to an academic environment will require new skills for Dr. Blair. What are some of those skills that she will need?

Clinical Vignette

1. How could the leadership team anticipate funding challenges?
2. How could the team anticipate and manage support for the staff?
3. What opportunities exist to mediate the loss of staff?

REFERENCES

Brach, T. (2021). RAIN: Recognize, allow, investigate, nurture. https://www.tarabrach.com/rain/

Covey, S. (2006). *The Speed of Trust. The One Thing That Changes Everything.* New York: Free Press

Chassin, M.R. & Loeb, J.M. (2013). High-Reliability Health Care: Getting There from Here. *The Milbank Quarterly*, Vol. 91, No. 3, 2013 (pp. 459–490) ©2013 The Authors. The Milbank Quarterly published by Wiley Periodicals Inc. on behalf of Milbank Memorial Fund.

Jimenez, J.M. (2021). *The Burnout Fix: Overcome Overwhelm, Beat Busy, and Sustain Success in the New World of Work.* McGraw-Hill Education.

Johnson, J., O'Grady, E., & Coetzee, M. (2021). *Intentional therapeutic relationship:*

Advancing care in healthcare. DEStech Publishing, Inc.

Kabat-Zinn, J. (2020). Mindfulness STOP skill. https://cogbtherapy.com/mindfulness-meditation-blog/mindfulness-stop-skill#:~:text=Jon%20Kabat%2DZinn%2C%20 a%20prominent,STOP%20skill%2C%20or%20STOP%20Acronym

Maslach, C., & Leiter, M. P. (1997). *The truth about burnout: How organizations cause personal stress and what to do about it*. San Francisco, Calif: Jossey-Bass.

Maturano, J. (2015). *Mindful Leadership*. London: Bloomsbury Press ISBN: 9781620402474

McDowell, T. & Mallon, D. (2020). *Getting decision rights right: How effective organizational decision-making can boost performance.* https://www2.deloitte.com/us/ en/insights/topics/talent/organizational-decision-making.html

Rosenberg, M. (2018). Role of Sincere Gratitude—Session #9—Nonviolent Communication Training—Marshall Rosenberg. Cognitive tech. https://github.com/cognitivetech/Marshall-Rosenberg-NVC/blob/master/NVC-Training-9_Sincere-Gratitude_Marshall-Rosenberg_transcript.md

Silsbee, D. (2018). *Presence-Based Coaching: Cultivating Self-Generative Leaders through Mind, Body, and Heart*. Jossey-Bass.

CHAPTER 16

Our Past and Future: Reflections

INTRODUCTION

Our authorship team took great pleasure in writing this book about leadership. Many of our own experiences as leaders influenced the content we chose to write about and the examples of leadership and case studies that are highlighted throughout the book. And because we wrote about what we believe is best practice, we wanted the reader to get a sense of who we are and what has influenced our careers and perhaps influenced this book as well. Therefore, each of us has provided a peek under the hood, so to speak, about our pathway to leadership in the beginning of the book. We have each faced the challenges and joys of leadership within health systems and academia, having experienced much of what we have written about including lessons learned, mistakes made, choices considered, and excellence achieved. We have always had a strong sense of purpose and the deep understanding that nursing is more than what most people see or understand. For us, nursing has offered meaningful work, a vehicle for social change, a sense of professional community, and life-long friendships across the generations. Few career opportunities provide the intimate privileges afforded nurses, whether caring for individuals, families, or communities in times of need or supporting students, through the transformations that education can bring. For us, there are no second thoughts about the paths we have chosen.

We wrote this book to share what we value about nursing, the intense challenges it presents, and the significant commitment it requires. Nursing is an adventure whose landscape is ever changing. Nursing rewards in incredible ways, teaches many lessons about life, joy, heartache, and the human condition. Nursing knowledge and the application of that knowledge to practice is science-based. Yet, ask a nurse what they value most about nursing and you may hear a story about the wonders of living, the respect for dying, and the more artful aspects of care well-delivered. Like many others, we have also come to the painful realization that Whiteness dominates our workforce and many of our traditions, and that structural racism has affected our own pathways, and those of our peers, students, and those we serve. The nursing profession and the healthcare organizations in which we serve require intentional actions to remedy the inequities that exist today; these inequities must be eliminated. As leaders, these are the commitments we make as we move forward.

Looking back, we see more clearly the ways in which we managed or failed to manage the challenges we faced. As we close our book, we offer some reflections on our paths, and particularly some of the positive influences and the mistakes we have made. We hope these reflections offer hope to others wanting to lead.

REFLECTIONS: CATHERINE GILLISS

After I accepted my first deanship, I sought the advice of a number of leaders on things they wished they had known. One conversation stood out. My friend, a college president, grabbed the small napkin under his cola drink and took out his pen. He made some x's, o's, and lines, all to illustrate his point that the most common mistake made by new leaders: going too fast. His napkin drawing was intended to show me that the leader needed to stay ahead of everyone else, but not so far ahead that the connection to the followers was lost. Despite his advice, I made the mistake (and a number of others) and learned the meaning of the phrase: You cannot lead when no one follows. The leader's approach to engagement and pace of change do matter.

Leaders who are selected from outside an organization enter with fresh eyes and often see barriers, opportunities/strengths, and weaknesses that those who have lived within the organization no longer see. It is tempting to want to change things before taking the time to understand them. A true story (but not my own): A new dean began the first official day of her appointment with a strategic planning workshop. She had no relationship with the school or its faculty and staff, but her plans signaled that she intended to implement change. In fact, it is rumored that she actually said, "There is a new sheriff in town." The example, extreme in nature, is a reminder of both the need to engage the community and its members and pace change after a careful assessment of the situation and review of driving and restraining forces. In other words, the leader should understand the forces working for and against change.

I saw many opportunities for change in my first leadership position and, in fact, I understood from the university president to whom I reported directly that I had been hired to implement long needed changes. That might have all been true, but I did not yet understand what the faculty thought about change (globally) or some of the specific changes I believed were needed. The faculty and staff took great pride in their history, a history filled with firsts that I thought did not accurately describe the current organization. Further, they took pride in activities that were not highly prized by the university or the associated health system. By neglecting to respond to the dominant values, the faculty missed the chance to "show up" in the future of this university; they remained proudly ensconced in their history.

As I set about to make the changes that I understood had been requested by the president, I did not adequately engage the faculty. I failed to fully appreciate their pride and the need to build the future on the accomplishments of the past, connecting to the future with respect for history and for their revered leaders. I did not engage the faculty in advisory task forces. We did not launch a community strategic planning process that invited participation of all faculty and staff. The signs of resistance I noted, I interpreted as personal and not a sign that the organization was resisting. As a result, I never stopped to think about change management, from an organizational point of view. I saw members of the faculty as "good guys" and "bad guys." I experienced the resistance as personal: Some were with me, and some were against me.

Only after a very critical review of my stewardship did I enlist some organizational experts who helped me understand the need to move away from seeing individuals as problems, and toward seeing individual behavior as a reflection of the forces (restraining and driving) within the organization, the so-called canary in the coal mine. In other words, when troubling or unexpected issues emerge, the leader is presented with the opportunity to pause and examine the messages. Individuals and small groups carry important information to the leader, but the leader must be able to hear the message. By engaging, listening, and putting pieces together, the leader has a better chance staying close to the organization and leading through change. When the faculty becomes the problem, the leader has lost the opportunity to effectively lead change.

For me, having begun my nursing career in psychiatry and loving the social and behavioral sciences, this insight reignited my passions about applied social sciences and the possibilities that leadership could be a richly rewarding professional focus.

REFLECTIONS: BOBBIE BERKOWITZ

I distinctly remember sitting in my high school classroom in the spring of 1968. It was the end of the day, and I was talking with one of my close friends who told me he had enlisted in the military and would leave for Vietnam soon after our graduation. He did not return as he was killed in action. He was not the only young man in our small rural school to die in the conflict. The Vietnam War defined many of my views about the military, our society, our country, politics, and my role in the profession I had chosen. I was not alone in this experience, nor was I alone in protesting the war. I gained many skills and insights during my participation as an activist, and as most of my friends experienced, we felt that our beliefs were righteous. At the same time, I was studying to become a nurse and there was limited tolerance for students to take time off to join a protest march. I was conflicted about my priorities and yet I knew that the profession I had chosen was exactly right for me.

After graduation I worked in a large health system caring for cancer patients. I wanted to be a public health nurse and although these positions were hard to find, after a year in cancer care I found a position in a rural county in northern Washington State. Practice as a public health nurse in a rural community with significant poverty and the challenges for families living on the edge was probably more than I had bargained for. What I did not know at the time was that this experience in that rural community and the challenges working with families in crisis would define my entire career. My passion for nursing and for those I served gave me the resilience and a pathway to a long career in leadership, policy, and academic roles.

One cannot overestimate the value of mentors early in one's career. I had two in my first public health role; the health officer and the nursing director gave me every opportunity to grow. They encouraged me to pursue a master's degree, and when I graduated and returned to the health department I was promoted to my retiring mentor's position as nursing director. I was supported when I pursued my PhD knowing that I would no doubt seek a new role where I could continue to grow. After eight years in this incredibly supportive environment, I was recruited to be the chief nursing officer for a large urban health department. That position launched so many opportunities: deputy secretary for the Washington State Department of Health; a move to the University of Washington School of Public Health as the program officer for a ten year long grant from the Robert Wood Johnson Foundation that was designed to build public health infrastructure across states and communities; chair of the Department of Psychosocial and Community Health at the University of Washington School of Nursing; and finally to the position of dean of the Columbia University School of Nursing. I have had a wonderful career, from a young activist to a university dean. I sometimes wonder how it happened and how leadership became fundamental to my passion for justice, equity, service, and impact. I think it has a lot to do with strategy and resilience.

I believe that the pursuit of leadership involves a great deal of strategic thinking and knowing when to take the right opportunity. I believe that we build strategic thinking from our interest in problems to be solved that sometimes seem out of our reach. So, we develop a way to harness what we know and feel and create a clear way forward. We learn about the challenge of change, we seek guidance, we build alliances, and we regularly question the motives that drive us to make sure we stay true to the best in us. We must constantly be tuned into opportunities to act but also to be tuned into what may not be the right opportunity for a particular challenge.

Leadership is steeped in understanding the motivations of individuals and groups and the ability to make sense of the dynamics of a team. Leadership is also about the ability to listen and confirm how individuals and teams are processing and reacting to their own individual challenges. It can be difficult at times to intervene with a troubled employee, particularly when the issues include bullying, discrimination, and lack of the knowledge and compassion to continue in the position. As a leader, I have experienced these challenging conversations and it never gets easier; but the resolve to assure a safe and respectful environment is what leadership is about.

After many years of both successes and failures in leadership, I think the most important lesson I have learned is to trust my thought process and problem-solving skills, trust key partners, constantly check my reality, utilize my team, and learn how to take criticism and gracefully accept the advice of mentors. It is very difficult to succeed on one's own.

REFLECTIONS: JEAN JOHNSON

It is incredibly rewarding to see a vision come to fruition and know that barriers to achieving that vision can be overcome. For me, that vision was to build a school of nursing at George Washington University, an institution that has been my primary base for most of my professional career. While I loved and found very meaningful the leadership opportunities during my career at GW first as a nurse practitioner on the geriatrics team, then as program director for the GW nurse practitioner program, followed by appointment as senior associate dean for health sciences, building a school that would be a major contributor to nursing education was a dream.

The very first milestone on my path to making the school of nursing a reality was to believe this was possible. I had to believe that it was possible in order to get others to believe the possibility. This belief was based on my faith in the capacity of the faculty to create change and address the nursing shortage that was threatening the health system. Nursing degree programs were spawned from a Department of Nursing Education housed in the Health Sciences Programs that was part of the School of Medicine and Health Sciences. As senior associate dean of Health Sciences, I was in a position to support the development of nursing degree programs by leveraging the Health Sciences courses, faculty, and funds. Once we decided a school of nursing was a goal, we moved quickly and offered a fully approved and accredited master's program in 2006, Doctor of Nursing Practice Program in 2008, and an accelerated Bachelor's program in 2010. During the process of building the degree programs we gained the support of several stakeholders including the administrative leadership of the medical center and the university. In fact, some of the university Board of Trustee members thought we already had a school because we had created the degree programs.

School status was important in order to have a voice at the highest levels of the university and to recruit the best and brightest faculty and be influential within nursing education. To create the school, we had to be clear about the vision, which was to provide excellence in nursing education, create new knowledge to continuously improve care and contribute to the health of our community and nation. This vision resonated with stakeholders and provided the overall context for more specific information.

Our vision had to be accompanied by a strategic plan that incorporated a credible financial plan of how this was going to happen. The main source of income for GW is tuition dollars and the school of nursing had to be able to stand on its own financially, covering both direct and indirect costs. Having started the degree programs gave us the tuition base to support a free-standing school of nursing. In addition, we were able to negotiate $1 million of seed funding from the medical center as the school of nursing was going to be a school within the medical center umbrella that included the School of Medicine and Health Sciences and the School of Public Health.

The strategic plan included getting the approvals for the school within a very ambitious timeline of eight months. During this time frame, we needed a series of approvals, first from the Health Sciences faculty and then the faculty of the School of Medicine and Health Sciences, then the University Faculty Senate, and finally the Board of Trustees. Each stakeholder group had its own review and approval process that included having to have committee level review before going to the full group. We mapped out an approval timeline and went about writing reports and proposals for each set of approvals and setting up meetings. There was unanimous approval and active support from the Health Sciences and School of Medicine and Health Sciences faculty. However, not everyone was enthusiastic about the prospect of a school of nursing.

The stakeholder group that presented a real threat to moving the school forward was the University Faculty Senate. Members of the Senate were concerned about having a new school that would continue to be part of the GW Medical Center because ten years prior the School of Public Health was approved with the promises that they would meet the requirements of being a school. However, the school did not meet the requirements and Faculty Senate members carried their resentment about public health forward to the school of nursing proposal. The Senate approached the School of Nursing by establishing a special School of Nursing Oversight Committee to review the progress of the school and make a final recommendation to the full Faculty Senate on whether to approve the school or not. Senate approval was critical because the issue would not go to the Board of Trustees without the approval of the Faculty Senate. Understanding the history and concerns was very important to figuring out how to get out of the Public Health shadow.

Our initial strategy was to get the members of the School of Nursing Oversight Committee to understand that we were well on the way to meeting the requirements and understood their concern. No matter what information we gave them, they were hesitant to support the school. It became clear that the mantra coming from the members was, "I have heard those promises before" and that there was a need for a different strategy. The new strategy was to change the composition of the committee in order to include a voice that supported the school of nursing. There were several well-respected faculty members with whom I had a long-standing relationship and who were willing to volunteer to serve on the committee. The committee did not feel they could refuse the requests of these faculty to participate so the strategy of changing the conversation among committee members was accomplished. A day before a full Faculty Senate meeting, a crucial committee meeting took place that would determine if the members would support the approval of the school. This determination would influence the decision of the full Faculty Senate.

We had worked to present information that would address the committee's concerns, but at the end of that meeting, it was not clear whether the new members could sway the decision. In what turned out to be a very emotionally charged meeting, the committee voted to support the School of Nursing. Just to make sure that the Faculty Senate would approve the school, the nursing faculty recruited nurses from all over the city to be present at that meeting. On the day of the meeting, the room was packed with nurses and the chair of the School of Nursing Oversight Committee noted that he was extremely pleased to recommend support of the school since there were so many nurses in the room. Faculty Senate support for the school was unanimous and that meeting has become legend in terms of the power of nurses influencing decisions. The Board of Trustees went on to also unanimously vote to approve the school. After celebrating the accomplishment, we then focused on the work of building the structure, policies, and procedures of the school. But that is another leadership story.

Lessons learned in the work of leading the effort to create a school can be summed up as: believe change is possible, be bold, include everyone, do your homework in understanding people's positions on issues and why they hold those positions, create a plan and be willing to re-think it, do not take anything for granted, and it is about relationships and trust. The key element to stress is the importance of relationships. Relationships are the cornerstone of leading change.

REFLECTIONS: PAULA MILONE-NUZZO

I became a nurse in 1973 and by 1986, I began having academic leadership opportunities. While I had not initially planned a career in administration, in retrospect, I made myself open to the opportunities and took advantage of them as they arose. I stepped into temporary positions when people unexpectedly resigned and sought opportunities that would give me the chance to grow as a leader. In the course of a career, there are going to be opportunities that you create for yourself and those that happen very unexpectedly. For example, creating an opportunity for yourself might be when you know that there will be an open position and you get the necessary knowledge and skill needed to be the top candidate. An unexpected opportunity might be when someone goes on a leave of absence or resigns, and you are asked to fill the leadership position on a temporary basis. Being open and ready to take advantage of those opportunities can be the difference between moving up in a career or being stagnant. Each of these opportunities provide experiences that you can take to the next opportunity that comes your way.

In 2003, I was asked to be the Director of the Penn State School of Nursing. The School of Nursing was a constituent unit of a very successful College of Health and Human Development (HHD) that has a robust research portfolio and exceptional academic programs. The School of Nursing had a strong history of providing high quality nursing education to students across the Commonwealth but was not a research- intensive environment. When I was hired, the Dean of HHD said he wanted me to create a research environment similar to the other departments in HHD. While it was one of the largest schools of nursing in the country at the time (well over 2000 students), it was not well known in the nursing community and quite frankly, not well known within Penn State. It was clear that there was an opportunity to build on this incredible academic base to advance the School of Nursing. During the 14 years I lead the nursing programs, we built a strong research infrastructure with great research productivity, continued to develop exceptional academic programs growing to over 2800 students, advanced our reputation both in the university and in the national nursing community, and separated from HHD to become a College of Nursing with an independent dean. It was an incredible leadership experience.

I learned so much in my role as leader at Penn State. I had a foundation in how to lead from my years as associate dean at Yale School of Nursing, but having primary responsibility for a large school that needed and wanted change had its challenges. As I reflect on my role at that time, I was confronted with the task of working with an incredible faculty and staff to create a vision for the College of Nursing's future and design a plan to implement that future. It was an interesting combination of retaining the 30,000-foot view and vision while having to work on the ground to facilitate the initiatives. Neither one of those strategic approaches alone would have allowed us to accomplish what we had accomplished in those years.

I also learned a great deal about myself as a leader during my tenure at Penn State. I learned that I love working with faculty as both a leader and a colleague. Being part of scholarly discussions with faculty who are asking important questions, contributing to the science of nursing and to the profession was invigorating. It was important for me to make time in my schedule to participate in these kinds of meetings, not as the leader but as one of a group of scholars. I also learned how important hearing the student voice was in making good organizational decisions. As a leader, it is very easy to get so far away from the critical constituents in an academic program, the faculty, and the students, that you miss perspectives that should be integral in the decision-making process. Spending time with students allowed me to hear their voice and helped me to execute my role more effectively.

After 14 years as leader of the nursing programs at Penn State, first Director, and then Inaugural Dean, I had an opportunity to engage in the next leadership challenge of my career, becoming the President of the MGH Institute of Health Professions (IHP) in 2017. The IHP is a graduate school for individuals interested in becoming a health care professional in nursing or the rehabilitation sciences and was founded on the principles of interprofessional education and practice. So, after forty years in nursing and nursing education, I was in the role of leading an interprofessional community of scholars. It was in this role that I faced some of the most difficult challenges and some of the most rewarding experiences of my career.

The role of college president, even at a small, single focused college such as the IHP is complex and demanding, even on the really good days. Being the president of an interprofessional college meant that I had to make sure, from the start, I thought more broadly than just as a nurse. Each program at the IHP deserved a leader that treated them as the most important entity in the organization. Having that broad view meant that I had to begin by deepening my knowledge of and appreciation for each discipline at the IHP. Understanding their profession and their curriculum was essential to being able to have meaningful discussions with the leaders in the rehabilitation sciences. My conversation with the IHP nursing leaders felt natural and easy, and I wanted the same feeling with all the IHP department leaders. Being an organizationally minded leader was essential to being successful in this role.

The other challenges came from reflecting on what I enjoyed most about my years at Penn State and understanding how to have some of those opportunities in this new role. At the IHP, the President serves as the CEO of the organization, in strong liaison with our corporate partners, the Massachusetts General Hospital, and Mass General Brigham. There is a provost who is the vice president for academics and a vice president for administration and chief financial officer. In addition, each school has a dean and program directors under them. In this structure, it is clear that the president is pretty far removed from both faculty and students. And in order to keep the lines of authority clear, I had to be careful not to drop too deeply into the academic structure, a place where I felt most comfortable, which was the responsibility of the provost. Learning those boundaries was important to appropriately executing my role. Also, learning how to have the opportunity to engage in the kinds of activities with faculty and students that I find most fulfilling was equally as important. I began having lunches with student government leaders to hear their thoughts about their experiences at the IHP. I attended events where students and faculty were sharing their research or scholarship, and I had individual meetings with researchers so I could understand their research enough to be able to explain it to a potential donor. I asked to meet with the Faculty Senate at their regularly scheduled meetings to provide a brief report and stand for questions. And when I was asked, I rarely said no to an opportunity to participate in an IHP event. These experiences have allowed me to have those fulfilling experiences that keep me excited and energized in my role.

As I reflected on my work as a college president, I realized how important it has been for me to rely on my core values as well as the values of the organization that I am leading. As a situation gets more chaotic, being able to rise above the chaos and sort through the noise to see the essence of the situation is the mark of a true leader. Being able to actively listen, show authentic compassion and navigate the problem-solving process using values such as truthfulness, transparency and integrity as a guide are essential. I know I will look back on these years of leadership and wish I did some things differently and other things better but knowing that I led with purpose and integrity is important for how I envision my legacy.

REFLECTIONS: PAT REID PONTE

Organizations are not democracies, but they are replete with power politics. I returned from a two week vacation many years ago and met with my boss. She told me that she was concerned about a conflict in my leadership team. I knew exactly what the conflict was, but I was surprised by the fact that she knew about it. Upon further questioning by me, I discovered that my boss had agreed to meet with one of the members of my leadership team. This person, who reported directly to me, confided to my boss that there was a major conflict about an organizational restructuring plan that was being mapped out by me and my team. He told my boss that he was very distressed by the way he was being treated by other members of my leadership team and by me and he wanted my boss to know this. He told my boss that he did not agree with the restructuring plan. My boss reassured my subordinate that she would address the issue with me on return from my vacation, which she did.

I learned a few lessons from this experience. If a member of your leadership team seeks out and speaks with your boss about a concern regarding you and your decisions or leadership, without your involvement and knowledge, this is a major red flag. This is called insubordination. If this happens and your boss entertains this engagement, this is another major red flag. Neither should happen, and it does not happen in healthy organizations.

That said, leaders at all levels in organizations are subject to making mistakes in judgment based on their own abilities. If it happens once and you appropriately address it will likely not happen again. If it happens more than once and you do not address it, you must face the consequences.

In the above scenario, in the first instance of your subordinates seeking out and confiding in your supervisor, the following actions might be helpful:

- Let your supervisor know that you are disappointed in her decision to speak with your subordinate and let her know that if it happens again without your knowledge, you would need to take serious steps. You could say, "If it happens again, I will resign," but you may not want to at this point.
- Schedule a time for the three of you to meet to discuss the concerns of the subordinate and at that time, let the subordinate know that if he decides to do this again, he will be asked to resign. Do this in the presence of your supervisor.

If you decide not to take this action after a situation like this happening once, it would be important to do it the second time, because there likely will be a second time.

Covey (2006) describes how trust is built and maintained between individuals and in groups. Four cores of credibility are at play in developing and maintaining and/or recovering trust. The *first core* of credibility is integrity, which is defined as acting in accordance with your values and beliefs. The *second core* is intent, which has to do with one's motives, agendas and resulting behavior. Trust grows when motives are straightforward and based on mutual benefit. These first two cores comprise one's character. The *third core* is capabilities, which are the abilities one has that inspires confidence: talents, attitudes, skills, knowledge, and style. The *fourth core* is results, which refers to one's track record and performance in getting things done. These second two cores comprise one's competence.

In the situation above, the actions of both my boss and my subordinate resulted in me not trusting their intentions. Reciprocally, neither my boss or my subordinate likely trusted my intentions.

Although I did not fully resolve this situation in an effective way, my team and I accomplished much good work in the organization. It however came with a price. It was a very stressful and difficult time for me and my team.

Another important point for consideration. Organizations are not designed to behave like democracies. There is no room for a two-power political system. There is one leader, and that leader requires followers to be honest with them. However, loyalty can co-exist with disagreements, respectful debate and effective conflict resolutions as the norm.

The most effective leaders create relationships with individuals and groups that encourage dialogue and debate, effective conflict management, trust, transparency, honesty, and humility. Unfortunately, organizations with such effective leaders at the top are relatively rare.

This book provides knowledge, skills, attitude, and abilities that help leaders lead effectively with trust and humility as a centerpiece. And although decisions and priorities sometimes do fall to the top leader of an organization, the most successful and effective organizations keep decision-making and priority setting with the experts who are most knowledgeable and who need to operationalize them to meet the organization's mission.

SUMMARY

Our personal stories began this book, and they end it. We have shared our experiences of the challenges, adventures, and the rewards of our leadership work in academic and service delivery organizations, as well as our work in professional associations, policy formulation and analysis, knowledge development, government, and politics. We have taken on roles with and without nursing titles, knowing that nursing and leadership expertise combined is recognized as a valuable asset that is not discipline specific.

We acknowledge that there are significant challenges within our society including structural racism, inadequate health care for many, social determinants of health, lack of a living wage for all, and more; all of these factors reduce the the opportunity for people to be healthy and thrive. Nurses are taking on these challenges through effective, collaborative, and decisive organizational leadership. We hope that the evidence and experience described in this book will serve as a foundation and an inspiration for nurse leaders everywhere as they take on these enormous challenges for the health and well-being of all people.

COMMITMENTS FOR THE ORGANIZATIONALLY MINDED LEADER

As we close this book, we want to leave the reader with a few brief thoughts that might represent the true north of our approach to leadership. These are not comprehensive, but represent some high-level ideas to keep in mind as you take up the work of leading with an organizational perspective:

- You are each person's leader. Be there for each one: fair, just, and humble.
- Listen to learn before speaking or concluding.
- Stay focused on the organization, understanding that the individual behaviors you see are sometimes related to the organizational dynamics.

- Attend to the organization, its culture, and its ability to support the individuals who live and work within it, so that these same individuals will be able to carry on the work of the organization.

REFERENCE

Covey, S. (2006). *The Speed of Trust*. New York, New York: Simon & Schuster.

Index

Biographies

Bobbie Berkowitz

Dr. Berkowitz began her career as a public health nurse in rural Washington State. She served as Chief of Nursing for the Seattle-King County Department of Health and Deputy Secretary for the Washington State Department of Health prior to academic positions with the University of Washington and Columbia University. Her significant contributions include public health systems development, population health, health policy and health equity. She served on the Washington Health Care Commission to respond to the need for a comprehensive approach to a health system that was stressed with increasing costs and a growing uninsured population. She joined the Washington State Department of Health in 1993 as Deputy Secretary.

In 1996, Dr. Berkowitz led an initiative designed to focus nationally to modernize states' public health statutes and improve quality, enhance utilization of information technology, create performance management systems, and nurture public health leadership. Dr. Berkowitz served as the Primary Investigator and Program Director for this grant through 2006. During this time, she joined the faculty of the UW School of Nursing as Chair for the Department of Psychosocial and Community Health.

She became Dean of the Columbia University School of Nursing and Sr. Vice President of the Columbia University Irving Medical Center 2010. During this time she served as President of the American Academy of Nursing and an active member of the National Academy of Medicine (NAM). She retired from Columbia in 2018 and returned to her home in Seattle. She currently serves on the Board of Trustees for the Swedish Health System in Washington State, the National Advisory Board for the University of California at Davis

353

Health System, the Board of Trustees of the Nurse-Family Partnership, and Board of Advisors for the University of Washington School of Nursing.

CATHERINE L. GILLISS

Catherine L. Gilliss serves as the Dean and Margretta M. Styles Professor of Nursing and Associate Vice Chancellor at the University of California San Francisco. Her career in nursing has focused on nursing education and, over the last 30 years, the work of leading in academic environments. In addition to her leadership role at UCSF, she held the position of dean at Yale University's School of Nursing and as dean and vice-chancellor at Duke University's School of Nursing. Prepared as a psychiatric-mental health CNS and an adult nurse practitioner, she was an early proponent of the integration of behavioral health into primary care services. She focused on the family and chronic illness during her doctoral and post-doctoral studies and published one of the seminal texts on the topic: Toward a Science of Family Nursing. Her interest in human behavior in the context of social systems drove her toward leadership roles and the underlying scholarship. In 2020, she founded the Leadership Institute at UCSF with her UCSF Health peers.

JEAN JOHNSON

Dr. Johnson is the founding dean of the George Washington University School of Nursing (GWSON), professor emerita and an executive coach. She is a Fellow in the American Academy of Nursing and was awarded the Lifetime Achievement Award by the National Organization of Nurse Practitioner Faculty. As a longtime geriatric nurse practitioner she focused her research and policy work on patient safety and quality improvement in long-term care and nursing education. She was a faculty member of the Quality and Safety Education for Nurses and worked to disseminate the competencies nationwide. She has been a leader in establishing educational and practice standards for advanced practice registered nurses as the co-chair of the National Task Force on Evaluation Criteria for Nurse Practitioner Programs and chair of the task force to establish a regulatory model for advance practice nursing. As national program director for a Robert Wood Johnson Foundation project to develop the primary care capacity in underserved areas. She has served as president of the National Organization of Nurse Practitioner Faculties and president of the American College of Nurse Practitioners and served on the Institute of Medicine (IOM) Committee on the Future of Primary Care. She has continued work at University of Cape Town South Africa (SA) following the completion of a Fulbright award.

PAULA MILONE-NUZZO

Paula Milone-Nuzzo, PhD, RN, FHHC, FAAN, began her role as the MGH Institute of Health Professions sixth president in August 2017. Prior to this current appointment, Dr. Milone-Nuzzo spent the previous 14 years in leadership roles at the College of Nursing at The Pennsylvania State University, serving as Inaugural Dean and Professor since 2008. She is a widely published and nationally recognized nursing leader. Prior to Penn State, Dr. Milone-Nuzzo was Professor and Associate Dean for Academic Affairs at Yale School of Nursing.

Workforce development and health care careers have been the focus of her scholarly activities. Shortly after her arrival at Penn State in 2003, then-Governor of Pennsylvania Ed Rendell appointed her to the Pennsylvania Center for Health Careers, where she served on the Leadership Council for six years. In 2015, she was named chair of the advisory board for the Pennsylvania Action Coalition of the Future of Nursing: Campaign for Action—an organization whose goal is transforming the nursing profession to better meet the nation's health needs. Dr Milone-Nuzzo currently serves on the Massachusetts Healthcare Collaborative, a group of health care leaders charged by Governor Baker to address the healthcare workforce needs in Massachusetts.

Among her many awards are the Distinguished Colleague Award from the Pennsylvania Higher Education Nursing Schools Association, the Service Award from the Pennsylvania Center for Health Careers, the Beverly Koerner Outstanding Alumni Award for Education in Nursing from the University of Connecticut, the Nightingale Award for Excellence in Nursing, and the Leader of Leader Award from the National Student Nurses Association. She is a Fellow of the National Association for Home Care and Hospice, and a Fellow of the American Academy of Nursing, for which she served as Treasurer and board member.

Dr. Milone-Nuzzo received her Bachelor of Science in Nursing from Boston College, Master of Science in Nursing in Community Health Nursing and Education from the University of Connecticut, and PhD in Higher Education Administration from the University of Connecticut. She also completed an invitational post-doctoral seminar in Gerontological Research at the Hartford Institute at the Rory Meyers College of Nursing at New York University.

PATRICIA REID PONTE

Dr. Reid Ponte is a Clinical Associate Professor at both the Boston College William F. Connell School of Nursing and The Woods College of Advanced Studies, Master of Health Administration Program. She has an appointment as a Professor of Practice at Simmons University, College of Natural, Behavioral and Health Sciences where she teaches in the DNP Nurse Executive Leadership Program and at the University of Washington School of Nursing in the Clinical Informatics Patient Centered Technology Program

She is a member of the board of trustee at Lahey Hospital and Medical Center in Burlington, MA and the Beth Israel Lahey Health System Quality, Patient Experience and Assessment Committee.

Before her appointments as a faculty member at Boston College in 2018, Dr. Reid Ponte served as Chief Nursing Officer and Senior Vice President of Patient Care Services at the Dana-Farber Cancer Institute and the Executive Director of Oncology Nursing and Clinical Services at Brigham and Women's Hospital in Boston, Massachusetts for 17 years. During that time she served as a project co-pi of an NCI U54 and U56 grant establishing an accelerated BSN to PhD Program and a Post-Doctoral Fellowship Program in Oncology and Health Disparities with the University of MA, Boston.

She also held clinical and leadership positions at the Brigham and Women's Hospital, Massachusetts General Hospital and the Tufts-New England Medical Center where she began her nursing career in 1976.

She received a research intensive Doctor of Nursing Science degree in 1989, and a Masters of Nursing Science degree in 1979 both from Boston University and a Bachelor of Science in Nursing from the University of Massachusetts, Amherst. She was a 2001 Robert Wood Johnson Nurse Executive Fellow and is an active member of the American Academy of Nursing. She served as a member and Chair of the American Nurses Credentialing Center (ANCC) Commission on Magnet Recognition between 2006 and 2014 and as a member and then President of the ANCC Board until 2019. Her scholarly work focuses on health care quality, patient and family centered care, and health system leadership.

FOREWORD CONTRIBUTORS BIOGRAPHIES

MARILYN P. CHOW, PhD, RN, FAAN

Dr. Marilyn Chow is a recognized expert in leadership, innovation regulation of nursing practice, workforce policy and primary care. Her career has focused on promoting the role of nurses in primary care, advanced practice, and hospital-based care. Although she has held academic appointments, including at the University of California San Francisco where she was one of the first nurses prepared as a pediatric nurse practitioner, she is considered among the most accomplished nurse leaders in health care delivery.

For 16 years, she served as Vice President of National Patient Care Services and Innovation for Kaiser Permanente, during which time she also directed the Robert Wood Johnson Executive Nurse Fellows Program. Dr. Chow served on a number of national boards, including The Joint Commission At-Large Nursing Representative to the Board of Commissioners, the Joint Commission

Resources Board, and chaired the Joint Commission Nursing Advisory Council. She holds an appointment as a non-salaried professor at the UCSF, where she advises on the eponymous Chow Imagine Fund, which supports innovative leadership solutions for the care environment.

A fellow of the American Academy of Nursing, Dr. Chow as named an American Academy of Nursing Living Legend in 2018.

ANGELA BARRON MCBRIDE, PhD, RN, FAAN

Dr. Angela McBride's career has influenced thought on the roles of women in society, as humans, as mothers, as workers and as leaders. Prepared to practice in psychiatric mental-health nursing and with a doctoral degree in psychology, her career helped shape thinking about the experiences of women in ways earlier described as "not like men"—when men were assumed to be normative. Her early writings explored Motherhood (The Growth and Development of Mothers) and a later writing focused on Leadership (The Growth and Development of Nurse Leaders). Her career contributions, including scholarship, teaching, academic and organizational leadership have spanned sixty years and stretched boundaries of thought and integrated sectors to create opportunities. She is a boundary spanner.

Dr. McBride spent most of her career at the Indiana University School of Nursing (IUSON), where she served as dean (1991–2003) and now holds the title Dean Emerita. She was the first associate dean for research at IUSON and later a member of the National Advisory Council for both the National Institute of Mental Health and NIH Office of Women's Health Research. She was the first nurse appointed to the Indiana University Health Board (2004–2016), providing the opportunity to bring nursing to the board table and to better connect nursing education and nursing service delivery. She served as president of the Sigma Theta Tau International and the American Academy of Nursing. She was a member of the national advisory council of the National Academy of Medicine's (formerly the Institute of Medicine)/Robert Wood Johnson Health Policy Fellowship Program and the advisory council of the Robert Wood Johnson Foundation's Executive Nurse Fellows Program.

Dr. McBride was named an American Academy of Nursing Living Legend in 2006.